Essentials of
Medical Terminology

Third Edition

To my loving parents,
Bill and Renee Ozorio,

and to my brothers,
Michael, Stephen, and Timothy

Essentials of Medical Terminology

Third Edition

Juanita J. Davies

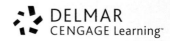
DELMAR
CENGAGE Learning™   Australia Canada Mexico Singapore Spain United Kingdom United States

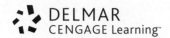

Essentials of Medical Terminology
Juanita J. Davies

Vice President, Health Care
Business Unit:
William Brottmiller

Director of Learning Solutions:
Matthew Kane

Acquisitions Editor:
Matthew Seeley

Editorial Assistant:
Megan Tarquinio

Product Manager:
Debra Myette-Flis

Marketing Director:
Jennifer McAvey

Marketing Manager:
Michele McTighe

Marketing Coordinator:
Chelsey Iaquinta

Technology Product Manager:
Carolyn Fox

Production Director:
Carolyn Miller

Content Project Manager:
Thomas Heffernan

> For product information and technology assistance, contact us at
> **Cengage Learning Customer & Sales Support, 1-800-354-9706**
>
> For permission to use material from this text or product,
> submit all requests online at **cengage.com/permissions**
> Further permissions questions can be emailed to
> **permissionrequest@cengage.com**

ExamView® and ExamView Pro® are registered trademarks of FSCreations, Inc. Windows is a registered trademark of the Microsoft Corporation used herein under license. Macintosh and Power Macintosh are registered trademarks of Apple Computer, Inc. Used herein under license.

Library of Congress Control Number: 2007011938

ISBN-13: 978-1-4018-9019-3

ISBN-10: 1-4018-9019-9

Delmar Cengage Learning
5 Maxwell Drive
Clifton Park, NY 12065-2919
USA

Cengage Learning products are represented in Canada by Nelson Education, Ltd.

For your lifelong learning solutions, visit **delmar.cengage.com**

Visit our corporate website at **www.cengage.com**

Notice to the Reader
Publisher does not warrant or guarantee any of the products described herein or perform any independent analysis in connection with any of the product information contained herein. Publisher does not assume, and expressly disclaims, any obligation to obtain and include information other than that provided to it by the manufacturer. The reader is expressly warned to consider and adopt all safety precautions that might be indicated by the activities described herein and to avoid all potential hazards. By following the instructions contained herein, the reader willingly assumes all risks in connection with such instructions. The publisher makes no representations or warranties of any kind, including but not limited to, the warranties of fitness for particular purpose or merchantability, nor are any such representations implied with respect to the material set forth herein, and the publisher takes no responsibility with respect to such material. The publisher shall not be liable for any special, consequential, or exemplary damages resulting, in whole or part, from the readers' use of, or reliance upon, this material.

Printed in China by China Translation & Printing Services Limited
4 5 6 7 8 12 11 10 09

Contents

Preface   x
How to Use this Book   xiii
How to Use *Essentials of Medical Terminology*, Third Edition StudyWARE™   xvi

PART I   **BASIC MEDICAL TERMINOLOGY   1**

CHAPTER 1   LEARNING MEDICAL TERMS   3
1.1   Pronunciation Guide   4
1.2   The Parts of Medical Terms   5
1.3   How to Analyze Medical Terms   6
1.4   Terms with No Prefix   6
1.5   Terms with No Root   7
1.6   Terms with Two Roots   7
1.7   The Combining Vowel   7
1.8   The Combining Form   9
1.9   Plurals   10
1.10   Putting It All Together   13

CHAPTER 2   ROOTS OF EACH BODY SYSTEM   15
2.1   Anatomy and Physiology   16
2.2   Levels of Organization   16
2.3   Organ Systems   16
2.4   Common Anatomical Roots   18
2.5   Putting It All Together   30

CHAPTER 3   SUFFIXES   33
3.1   Additional Word Parts   34
3.2   Suffixes Used to Indicate Pathologic Conditions   35
3.3   Suffixes Used to Indicate Diagnostic Procedures   40
3.4   Suffixes Used to Indicate Surgical Procedures   43
3.5   General Suffixes   45
3.6   Adjectival Suffixes   46
3.7   Putting It All Together   47

CHAPTER 4   PREFIXES   52
4.1   Additional Word Parts   53
4.2   Prefixes Referring to Direction and Position   54
4.3   Negative Prefixes   63

4.4   Prefixes Referring to Numbers   64
4.5   Miscellaneous Prefixes   65
4.6   Summary of Prefixes That Have the Same Meaning   67
4.7   Summary of Prefixes That Have the Opposite Meaning   67
4.8   Putting It All Together   68

PART II   BODY SYSTEMS   71

CHAPTER 5   BODY ORGANIZATION   73
5.1   Cavities and the Arrangement of Body Parts   74
5.2   Directional Terminology   75
5.3   Planes of the Body   81
5.4   Additional Word Parts   82
5.5   Term Analysis and Definition   83
5.6   Abbreviations   85
5.7   Putting It All Together   85

CHAPTER 6   THE INTEGUMENTARY SYSTEM AND RELATED STRUCTURES   87
6.1   Anatomy and Physiology of the Skin   88
6.2   Related Organs   90
6.3   Additional Word Parts   92
6.4   Term Analysis and Definition   93
6.5   Cosmetic Surgery   101
6.6   Common Injuries and Diseases   104
6.7   Abbreviations   105
6.8   Putting It All Together   105
6.9   Review of Vocabulary   110
6.10 Medical Terms in Context   113

CHAPTER 7   THE SKELETAL SYSTEM   115
7.1   Anatomy and Physiology of Bone   116
7.2   Description of the Skeleton   117
7.3   Joints   126
7.4   Additional Word Parts   128
7.5   Term Analysis and Definition   128
7.6   Common Diseases of the Skeletal System   144
7.7   Abbreviations   146
7.8   Putting It All Together   147
7.9   Review of Vocabulary   151
7.10 Medical Terms in Context   155

CHAPTER 8   THE MUSCULAR SYSTEM   158
8.1   Skeletal Attachments   160
8.2   Major Skeletal Muscles   161
8.3   Additional Word Parts   163
8.4   Term Analysis and Definition   163
8.5   Common Diseases   169
8.6   Abbreviations   170
8.7   Putting It All Together   170

8.8   Review of Vocabulary   173

8.9   Medical Terms in Context   176

CHAPTER 9   THE NERVOUS SYSTEM   177

9.1   Divisions of the Nervous System   178

9.2   Functions of the Nervous System   178

9.3   Nerve Cells   180

9.4   Synapses   181

9.5   The Central Nervous System   182

9.6   The Peripheral Nervous System   187

9.7   Additional Word Parts   189

9.8   Term Analysis and Definition   189

9.9   Common Diseases   199

9.10   Abbreviations   200

9.11   Putting It All Together   201

9.12   Review of Vocabulary   204

9.13   Medical Terms in Context   207

CHAPTER 10   THE EYES AND EARS   209

10.1   Eye   210

10.2   Additional Word Parts   215

10.3   Term Analysis and Definition Pertaining to the Eye   216

10.4   Common Diseases of the Eye   226

10.5   Abbreviations Pertaining to the Eye   228

10.6   Ear   229

10.7   Term Analysis and Definition Pertaining to the Ear   232

10.8   Common Diseases of the Ear   236

10.9   Abbreviations Pertaining to the Ear   237

10.10   Putting It All Together   237

10.11   Review of Vocabulary Pertaining to the Eye   243

10.12   Review of Vocabulary Pertaining to the Ear   246

10.13   Medical Terms in Context   248

CHAPTER 11   THE ENDOCRINE SYSTEM   251

11.1   Central Endocrine Glands   254

11.2   Peripheral Endocrine Glands   256

11.3   Additional Word Parts   260

11.4   Term Analysis and Definition   261

11.5   Common Diseases   267

11.6   Abbreviations   268

11.7   Putting It All Together   269

11.8   Review of Vocabulary   272

11.9   Medical Terms in Context   274

CHAPTER 12   THE CARDIOVASCULAR SYSTEM   277

12.1   Structure of the Heart   278

12.2   Conduction System   282

12.3   Blood Pressure   284

12.4   Heart Sounds   284

12.5   Blood Vessels   284
12.6   Circulation   287
12.7   Additional Word Parts   289
12.8   Term Analysis and Definition   289
12.9   Common Diseases   298
12.10 Abbreviations   299
12.11 Putting It All Together   301
12.12 Review of Vocabulary   304
12.13 Medical Terms in Context   306

CHAPTER 13   BLOOD, IMMUNE, AND LYMPHATIC SYSTEMS   309
13.1   Blood   310
13.2   Additional Word Parts   313
13.3   Term Analysis and Definition Pertaining to Blood   314
13.4   Common Diseases of Blood   318
13.5   Abbreviations Pertaining to Blood   319
13.6   Immune System   319
13.7   Lymphatic System   320
13.8   Term Analysis and Definition Pertaining to the Immune and Lymphatic Systems   325
13.9   Common Diseases of the Lymphatic and Immune Systems   327
13.10 Abbreviations Pertaining to the Immune and Lymphatic Systems   328
13.11 Putting It All Together   328
13.12 Review of Vocabulary Pertaining to Blood   332
13.13 Review of Anatomical Terms Pertaining to the Immune and Lymphatic Systems   334
13.14 Medical Terms in Context   335

CHAPTER 14   THE RESPIRATORY SYSTEM   337
14.1   Nose, Nasal Cavities, and Paranasal Sinuses   339
14.2   Pharynx, Larynx, and Trachea   340
14.3   Bronchi and Lungs   342
14.4   Additional Word Parts   345
14.5   Term Analysis and Definition   345
14.6   Common Diseases   356
14.7   Abbreviations   358
14.8   Putting It All Together   359
14.9   Review of Vocabulary   363
14.10 Medical Terms in Context   366

CHAPTER 15   THE DIGESTIVE SYSTEM   368
15.1   Oral Cavity   370
15.2   Pharynx   371
15.3   Esophagus   372
15.4   Stomach   372
15.5   Small Intestine   373
15.6   Large Intestine   375
15.7   Accessory Organs   376
15.8   Peritoneum   378
15.9   Additional Word Parts   379
15.10 Term Analysis and Definition   380
15.11 Common Diseases   392
15.12 Abbreviations   393

15.13 Putting It All Together   395
15.14 Review of Vocabulary   401
15.15 Medical Terms in Context   404

CHAPTER 16   THE URINARY AND MALE REPRODUCTIVE SYSTEMS   406
16.1   Urinary System   407
16.2   Additional Word Parts   413
16.3   Term Analysis and Definition Pertaining to the Urinary System   413
16.4   Common Diseases of the Urinary System   423
16.5   Abbreviations Pertaining to the Urinary System   425
16.6   Male Reproductive System   427
16.7   Term Analysis and Definition Pertaining to the Male Reproductive System   429
16.8   Common Diseases of the Male Reproductive System   434
16.9   Abbreviations Pertaining to the Male Reproductive System   435
16.10 Putting It All Together   436
16.11 Review of Vocabulary Pertaining to the Urinary System   442
16.12 Review of Vocabulary Pertaining to the Male Reproductive System   444
16.13 Medical Terms in Context   446

CHAPTER 17   THE FEMALE REPRODUCTIVE SYSTEM AND OBSTETRICS   448
17.1   Structures of the Female Reproductive System   449
17.2   Menstrual Cycle   453
17.3   Menopause   454
17.4   Additional Word Parts   454
17.5   Term Analysis and Definition Pertaining to the Female Reproductive System   455
17.6   Common Diseases of the Female Reproductive System   465
17.7   Abbreviations Pertaining to the Female Reproductive System   467
17.8   Obstetrics   468
17.9   Term Analysis and Definition Pertaining to Obstetrics   471
17.10 Obstetrical Conditions   474
17.11 Abbreviations Pertaining to Obstetrics   475
17.12 Putting It All Together   476
17.13 Review of Vocabulary Pertaining to the Female Reproductive System   481
17.14 Review of Obstetrical Vocabulary   484
17.18 Medical Terms in Context   485

APPENDIX A   WORD PART TO DEFINITION   488

APPENDIX B   DEFINITION TO WORD ELEMENT   495

INDEX 503

Preface

Who This Book Is for

Essentials of Medical Terminology, Third Edition is designed specifically for learners taking a one-semester medical terminology course. Every word of the text has been written with the goal of making it possible for a wide range of learners to acquire a basic medical terminology vocabulary in 15 to 16 weeks. The exercises and Instructor's Manual are practical, straight forward, and extensive enough that most instructors will not need to supplement them. The Instructor's Manual makes it possible for the text to be used in a variety of learning modes and environments. Answers to the exercises are provided in the Instructor's Manual on the Electronic Classroom Manager.

Strategy for Learning

Learners should master Chapter 1 before moving on to other chapters. It describes a simple method of analyzing medical terms that has proved effective for my own students over the years. Chapters 2, 3, and 4 introduce standard roots, suffixes, and prefixes. These chapters should also be learned before other chapters. The remaining chapters teach the terms associated with each body system in a variety of sequences to suit your needs. They contain just enough anatomy and physiology to make the chapters interesting and the terms easily understood, but not so much that the learners get bogged down.

Part of completing a chapter is doing the exercises in the text as well as on the CD-ROM. Learners should also take personal responsibility for studying the terminology tables and self-testing for mastery. Because the tables are the heart of the text, they are designed to make learning and remembering the terms as easy as possible. Terms are chunked in association with common word elements. Tables are placed where it makes the most sense from a learning perspective. Explanatory notes are used when extra information will enhance the learning experience.

Essentials of Medical Terminology, Third Edition is a useful and effective learning tool. Several features are incorporated into each chapter to help you master the content. Review the "How to Use this Book" section on page xiii for a detailed description and benefit of each feature.

New to This Edition

SPECIAL FEATURES
- Common diseases to each body system.
- A new section titled Medical Terms in Context has been added to help the learner understand the word as it is used in a medical report.
- New illustrations have been added to facilitate learning.
- Information boxes titled *Effects of Aging* are included to highlight conditions common to the aging population.
- New terms have been added throughout the text.
- Appendix A translates the medical word part to English.
- Appendix B translates English to its medical word part.

CHANGES TO THE CHAPTERS

Chapter 5, Body Organization—Planes of the body have been added.

Chapter 6, The Integumentary System and Related Structures—A new section on cosmetic surgery has been added. Common diseases: burns, skin cancer.

Chapter 7, The Skeletal System—Common diseases: bone cancers and fractures.

Chapter 8, The Muscular System—Common diseases: carpal tunnel syndrome, muscle strain, and muscular dystrophy.

Chapter 9, The Nervous System—Common diseases: brain tumor, multiple sclerosis, Parkinson's disease, and seizure disorder.

Chapter 10, The Eyes and Ears—Common diseases: cataracts, errors of refraction, glaucoma, macular degeneration, deafness, and Meniere's disease.

Chapter 11, The Endocrine System—Common disease: diabetes mellitus.

Chapter 12, The Cardiovascular System—Common diseases: aneurysm, cardiac arrest, cerebral vascular accident (stroke), and myocardial infarction.

Chapter 13, The Blood, Immune, and Lymphatic Systems—Learning is enhanced by the expansion of information on stem cells. Common diseases: leukemia and AIDS.

Chapter 14, The Respiratory System—Common diseases: asthma, emphysema, lung cancer, and pneumonia.

Chapter 15, The Digestive System—Common diseases: Crohn's disease and ulcers.

Chapter 16, The Urinary and Male Reproductive Systems—Common diseases: renal failure, voiding disorders, urinary retention, and benign prostatic hypertrophy.

Chapter 17, The Female Reproductive System and Obstetrics—breast cancer, sexually transmitted diseases, placenta previa, pre-eclampsia, and uterine inertia.

Comprehensive Teaching and Learning Resources

ESSENTIALS OF MEDICAL TERMINOLOGY, THIRD EDITION STUDYWARE™

The StudyWARE™ CD-ROM offers an exciting way to gain additional practice in working with medical terms. The quizzes and activities help you remember even the most difficult terms. See "How to Use *Essentials of Medical Terminology*, Third Edition StudyWARE™" on page xvi for details.

THE ELECTRONIC CLASSROOM MANAGER

The Electronic Classroom Manager is a robust, computerized tool for your instructional needs. A must-have for all instructors, this comprehensive, convenient CD-ROM contains:

- **The Instructor's Manual** is designed to help you with lesson preparation and performance assessment. It includes:
  - Developing a Medical Terminology Course—comprises two sample syllabi (15-week and 10-week course), as well as grading policy ideas and test and quiz suggestions
  - Chapter tests for each of the 17 chapters in the text
  - Midterm exam
  - Final exam
  - Word-part quizzes for each of the body system chapters
  - Answers to review exercises in the text

- **Exam View®Computerized Testbank** contains over 500 questions. You can use these questions and you can add your own questions to create review materials or tests.
- **PowerPoint® Presentations** are designed to aid you in planning your class presentations. If a learner misses a class, a printout of the slides for a lecture makes a helpful review page.

Electronic Classroom Manager, ISBN 1-4018-9020-2

About the Author

Juanita Davies has taught anatomy and medical terminology since 1973. She has also written extensively on the subject of medical terminology. Her early work includes *A Programmed Learning Approach to Medical Terminology* and a computerized testbank containing 15,000 questions that learners have been using since 1985. Her first book with Delmar, *Modern Medical Language*, is a combination of anatomy and medical terminology. Her third book, *A Quick Reference to Medical Terminology*, is a handy quick reference to common medical terms and their meanings. Her fourth book, *Illustrated Guide to Medical Terminology*, is a comprehensive book with extensive illustrations and easy-to-understand writing.

Acknowledgments

Special thanks to Debra Myette-Flis, Senior Product Manager, whose experience and knowledgeable advice greatly improved the quality of this text. Thank you also to the production and editorial staff for their suggestions and support in completing this project.

And to my husband, Jim, thank you for taking time out of your busy schedule to proofread the final manuscript. Your assistance was invaluable.

Reviewers

Special appreciation goes to the following reviewers for their insights, comments, suggestions, and attention to detail, which were very important in guiding the development of this textbook.

Patricia J. Bishop, RN, MSN
Nursing Faculty
Ursuline College, Breen School of Nursing
Pepper Pike, Ohio

Sharon S. Chambers, MEd
Associate Professor
Fulton-Montgomery Community College
Johnstown, New York

Betsy Fuller, PT, EdD
Dean of Health Sciences
Becker College
Worcester, Massachusetts

Janet E. Warner, MSN, RN
Assistant Professor
Southern Utah University Nursing Program
Cedar City, Utah

How to Use this Book

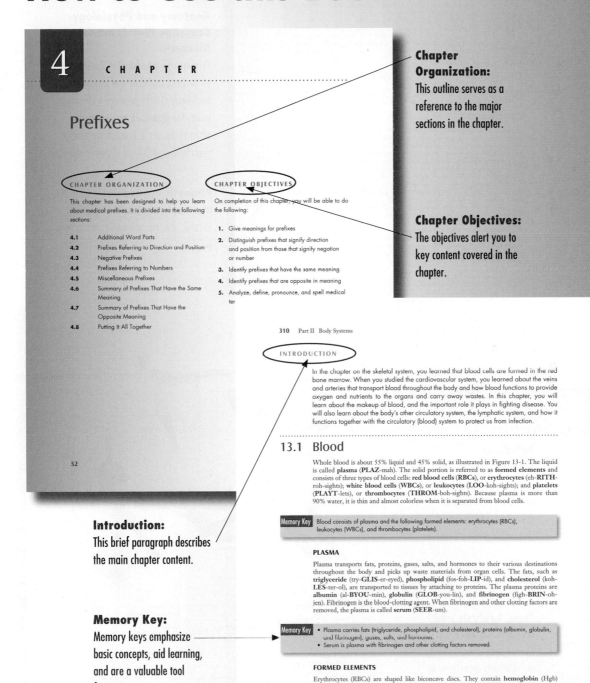

Chapter Organization:
This outline serves as a reference to the major sections in the chapter.

Chapter Objectives:
The objectives alert you to key content covered in the chapter.

Introduction:
This brief paragraph describes the main chapter content.

Memory Key:
Memory keys emphasize basic concepts, aid learning, and are a valuable tool for review.

---

4 CHAPTER

Prefixes

CHAPTER ORGANIZATION

This chapter has been designed to help you learn about medical prefixes. It is divided into the following sections:

4.1   Additional Word Parts
4.2   Prefixes Referring to Direction and Position
4.3   Negative Prefixes
4.4   Prefixes Referring to Numbers
4.5   Miscellaneous Prefixes
4.6   Summary of Prefixes That Have the Same Meaning
4.7   Summary of Prefixes That Have the Opposite Meaning
4.8   Putting It All Together

CHAPTER OBJECTIVES

On completion of this chapter, you will be able to do the following:

1.   Give meanings for prefixes
2.   Distinguish prefixes that signify direction and position from those that signify negation or number
3.   Identify prefixes that have the same meaning
4.   Identify prefixes that are opposite in meaning
5.   Analyze, define, pronounce, and spell medical ter

52

INTRODUCTION

In the chapter on the skeletal system, you learned that blood cells are formed in the red bone marrow. When you studied the cardiovascular system, you learned about the veins and arteries that transport blood throughout the body and how blood functions to provide oxygen and nutrients to the organs and carry away wastes. In this chapter, you will learn about the makeup of blood, and the important role it plays in fighting disease. You will also learn about the body's other circulatory system, the lymphatic system, and how it functions together with the circulatory (blood) system to protect us from infection.

13.1   Blood

Whole blood is about 55% liquid and 45% solid, as illustrated in Figure 13-1. The liquid is called **plasma** (**PLAZ**-mah). The solid portion is referred to as **formed elements** and consists of three types of blood cells: **red blood cells** (**RBCs**), or **erythrocytes** (eh-**RITH**-roh-sights); **white blood cells** (**WBCs**), or **leukocytes** (**LOO**-koh-sights); and **platelets** (**PLAYT**-lets), or **thrombocytes** (**THROM**-boh-sights). Because plasma is more than 90% water, it is thin and almost colorless when it is separated from blood cells.

> **Memory Key** Blood consists of plasma and the following formed elements: erythrocytes (RBCs), leukocytes (WBCs), and thrombocytes (platelets).

PLASMA

Plasma transports fats, proteins, gases, salts, and hormones to their various destinations throughout the body and picks up waste materials from organ cells. The fats, such as **triglyceride** (try-**GLIS**-er-eyed), **phospholipid** (fos-foh-**LIP**-id), and **cholesterol** (koh-**LES**-ter-ol), are transported to tissues by attaching to proteins. The plasma proteins are **albumin** (al-**BYOU**-min), **globulin** (**GLOB**-you-lin), and **fibrinogen** (figh-**BRIN**-oh-jen). Fibrinogen is the blood-clotting agent. When fibrinogen and other clotting factors are removed, the plasma is called **serum** (**SEER**-um).

> **Memory Key** • Plasma carries fats (triglyceride, phospholipid, and cholesterol), proteins (albumin, globulin, and fibrinogen), gases, salts, and hormones.
> • Serum is plasma with fibrinogen and other clotting factors removed.

FORMED ELEMENTS

Erythrocytes (RBCs) are shaped like biconcave discs. They contain **hemoglobin** (Hgb) (**hee**-moh-**GLOH**-bin), a protein that contains iron and has the ability to bind with oxygen and carbon dioxide. This ability enables the blood to transport oxygen to the organ cells and carbon dioxide away from them. Erythropoiesis, the maturation process for red blood cells, involves several stages. In the second-to-last stage, the cell is called a **reticulocyte** (reh-**TICK**-you-loh-sight). After the reticulocyte becomes an erythrocyte, it leaves the red

Effects of Aging:
This feature highlights common conditions among the aging population.

Effects of Aging

In Chapter 8, you learned that the decreased levels of testosterone, estrogen, and the growth hormone that occur with aging can cause muscle atrophy. These are not the only hormones that decrease. In fact, all hormones produced by the endocrine system decrease in production levels and activity as we age. However, because the body can produce far higher levels of hormones than we typically need, the loss of capacity is usually symptomless, or results in mild incapacity. For instance, the ability of the pancreas to produce insulin decreases, particularly in those over 65. In its mildest form, the result is higher than normal blood sugar levels for a longer period after a meal. However, this can lead to the development of diabetes in more severe cases.

11.5 Common Diseases

DIABETES MELLITUS

Diabetes mellitus (**dye**-ah-**BEE**-teez **MEL**-ih-tus) (**DM**) is a disease in which the body is unable to use sugar to produce energy. One cause is insufficient insulin secreted from the pancreas. Another cause is the production of ineffective insulin. When either of these occur, sugar is unable to move from the blood into body cells where it is normally used to produce energy. The result is abnormally high levels of blood glucose, known as hyperglycemia. It is a major symptom of diabetes. The normal blood glucose level is 70 to 100 mg/dL. Patients with blood glucose levels greater that 126 mg/dL are considered to be diabetic.

When the body doesn't have enough glucose, it breaks down fats and proteins for its energy. Over a long period of time, this results in a buildup of toxic wastes called **ketones** (**KEE**-tohnz). The condition is called **ketoacidosis** (**kee**-toh-**ass**-ih-**DOH**-sis). The excess sugars and ketones in the blood cause many diabetic complications such as blindness, arteriosclerosis, heart attacks, and gangrene of the lower extremities (loss of blood supply to the lower extremities causes decay of tissues).

There are two major types of diabetes.

Type 1 is an abrupt end to insulin production, often before the age of 25. This is thought to be due to an autoimmune reaction (the body's own antibodies destroy the pancreatic cells). Other factors such as genetics, viruses, and the environment might trigger the autoimmune reactions.

Type 2 is a reduction in insulin production, and often occurs after the age of 40. The pancreas continues to produce insulin, but one or two factors compromise that production: The pancreas produces reduced amounts of insulin; or body tissue fails to accept insulin into its cells for energy. Genetic factors and obesity play a role in the majority of cases. Obesity requires that the pancreas work harder to produ... cells wear out, and insulin production decreases.

Treatment for type 1 diabetes includes diet, ... betes is controlled by diet, exercise, and drugs th... on its own. Some type 2 diabetics will also need i...

Anatomy and Physiology Coverage Plus Common Diseases:
Terminology introduced in the context of the basic anatomy and physiology of each body system provides a reference point. The **diseases** you will most often encounter in practice are clearly described in each body system chapter.

Phonetic Pronunciation:
Important terms are followed by easy-to-read, phonetic pronunciations to help you learn how to say terms correctly.

---

168 Part II Body Systems

FIGURE 8-3
Types of muscle action

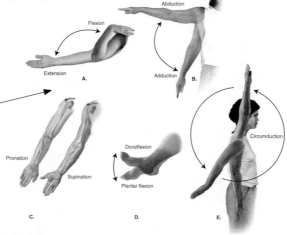

Full-Color Illustrations:
Full-color illustrations act as visual enhancements to help you learn medical terminology.

Term Analysis and Definition Section:
Keeps it simple by clustering or "chunking" new terms to make retention easier.

	-kinesia	movement; motion
Term	**Term Analysis**	**Definition**
bradykinesia (**brad**-ee-kih-**NEE**-zee-ah) (**brad**-ee-kih-**NEE**-shuh)	brady- = slow	slow movement
dyskinesia (**dis**-kih-**NEE**-zee-ah)	dys- = bad; difficult; painful; poor	impairment of muscle movement
hyperkinesia (**high**-per-kye-**NEE**-zee-ah)	hyper- = excessive; above normal	excessive movement

12.11 Putting It All Together

Putting It All Together:
Extensive exercises include short-answer, matching, building medical words, spelling, identification, and defining exercises.

Exercise 12-1   SHORT ANSWER

1. List the structures through which blood passes as it circulates through the body. Start with the right atrium and end with the superior and inferior venae cavae.

2. Differentiate between the pericardium, myocardium, endocardium, and epicardium. Which structure is the same as the visceral pericardium?

3. What is the function of the conduction system? List five structures of the conduction system. Which structure is known as the pacemaker? Why?

4. Define:
   a. systolic pressure
   b. diastolic pressure
   c. sphygmomanometer
   d. P wave
5. How are arteries and veins named?

Exercise 12-2   OPPOSITES

Give the opposite of the following terms.
1. vasodilation
2. hypertension
3. bradycardia
4. diastole

TABLE 17-6

REVIEW OF DIAGNOSTIC TERMS PERTAINING TO OBSTETRICS

1. amniocentesis	2. pelvimetry	3. ultrasonography

Review of Vocabulary:
A comprehensive review at the end of each chapter includes terms categorized into the following groups: anatomy and physiology; pathology; diagnosis; and clinical and surgical procedures. This summary helps reinforce terms learned throughout the chapter.

17.15 Medical Terms in Context

After you read the following Discharge Summary, answer the questions that follow it. Use your text, medical dictionary, or other references if necessary.

Medical Terms in Context:
This end-of-chapter feature encourages understanding of terms as they are used in medical reports.

DISCHARGE SUMMARY

ADMISSION DIAGNOSIS: GRADE 1 ENDOMETRIAL CARCINOMA OF THE UTERUS.

CLINICAL HISTORY: This 48-year-old gravida 2, para 1 was brought in for a total abdominal hysterectomy and bilateral salpingo-oophorectomy. Investigations done in the office, including endometrial biopsy for vaginal bleeding, revealed grade 1 endometrial carcinoma.

The patient had a left mastectomy eight years ago for breast cancer. Because of recurrence, she was placed on Tamoxifen.

INVESTIGATIONS: Hemoglobin was 13.4, platelets 186, white count 5.4. Her postoperative hemoglobin was 11.45.

TREATMENT AND PROGRESS: The patient was taken to the operating room. A vertical midline incision was made; a total abdominal hysterectomy and bilateral salpingo oophorectomy were performed without complications. Total blood loss was approximately 210 ml.

Postoperatively, she did well and remained afebrile throughout. Peritoneal washing revealed benign cytology. Final pathology revealed bilateral adnexa showing salpingitis with no malignancy. The uterus showed a grade 1 adenocarcinoma. The endometrium also showed focal hyperplasia with leiomyomas.

The patient was discharged home on Tylenol #3. She will be followed up in the office in four weeks' time.

MOST RESPONSIBLE DIAGNOSIS: GRADE 1 ADENOCARCINOMA OF THE UTERUS

How to Use Essentials of Medical Terminology, Third Edition StudyWARE™

The StudyWARE™ software helps you learn terms and concepts in *Essentials of Medical Terminology*, Third Edition. As you study each chapter in the text, be sure to explore the activities in the corresponding chapter in the software. Use StudyWARE™ as your private tutor to help you learn the material in your *Essentials of Medical Terminology*, Third Edition textbook.

Getting started is easy. Install the software by inserting the CD-ROM into your computer's CD-ROM drive and following the on-screen instructions. When you open the software, enter your first and last name so the software can store your quiz results. Next, choose a chapter from the menu to take a quiz or explore one of the activities.

Menus:
You can access the menus from wherever you are in the program. The menus include Quizzes, Activities, and Scores.

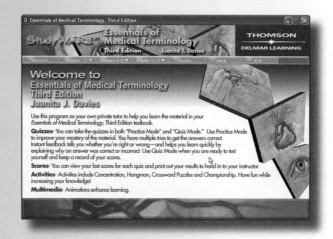

Animations:
Animations help you visualize concepts.

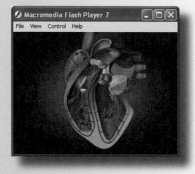

Quizzes:

Quizzes include multiple-choice and fill-in-the-blank questions. You can take the quizzes both in Practice Mode and in Quiz Mode. Use Practice Mode to improve your mastery of the material. You have multiple tries to get the answer correct. Instant feedback tells you whether you're right or wrong—and helps you learn quickly by explaining why an answer was correct or incorrect. Use Quiz Mode when you are ready to test yourself and keep a record of your scores. In Quiz Mode, you have one try to get each answer right, but you can take each quiz as many times as you want.

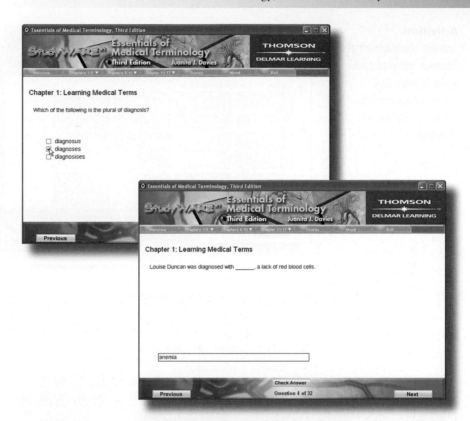

Scores:

You can view your final scores for each quiz and print your results to hand in to your instructor.

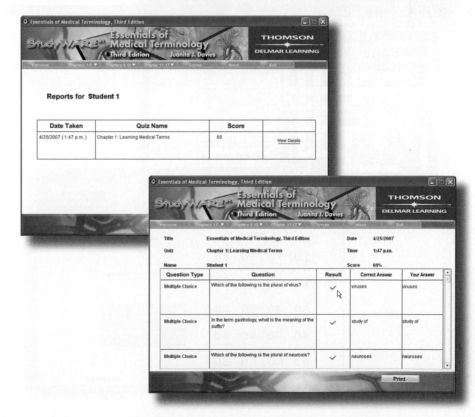

Activities:

Activities include concentration, hangman, crossword puzzles, and a *Jeopardy!*-style championship game. Have fun while increasing your knowledge!

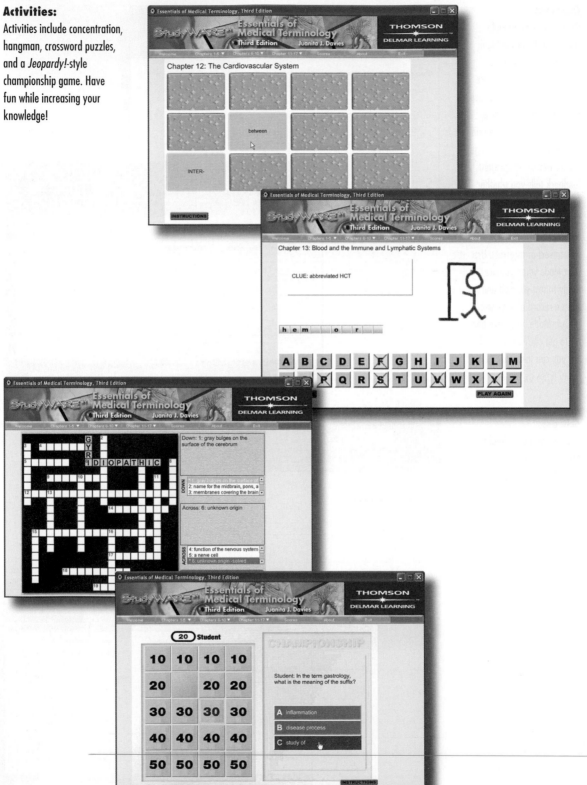

Basic Medical Terminology

1 LEARNING MEDICAL TERMS

2 ROOTS OF EACH BODY SYSTEM

3 SUFFIXES

4 PREFIXES

Learning Medical Terms

CHAPTER ORGANIZATION

This chapter will help you become familiar with basic medical terms. It is divided into the following sections:

1.1   Pronunciation Guide

1.2   The Parts of Medical Terms

1.3   How to Analyze Medical Terms

1.4   Terms with No Prefix

1.5   Terms with No Root

1.6   Terms with Two Roots

1.7   The Combining Vowel

1.8   The Combining Form

1.9   Plurals

1.10 Putting It All Together

CHAPTER OBJECTIVES

On completion of this chapter, you will be able to do the following:

1. Pronounce medical terms

2. Define parts that make up medical terms

3. Analyze component parts of medical terms

4. Identify words with no prefixes or roots

5. Understand when a combining vowel is used or not used

6. Distinguish between a combining vowel and a combining form

7. Pluralize medical terms

INTRODUCTION

Medical terminology is used to describe such things as parts of the body, locations in the body, bodily functions, diseases, surgical and clinical procedures, measurements, medical instruments, and many others. Each medical term describes in a single word something that would otherwise require several words to express. For example, the term *appendicitis* is a short form of saying "inflammation of the appendix."

Medical terminology is most easily learned by using an organized approach called **term analysis**, which is what this chapter is about. When you have mastered term analysis, you will be ready to learn the meanings of the most common parts of medical terms, which are the subjects of Chapters 2, 3, and 4. All of the remaining chapters deal with medical terminology used in relation to the various systems of the human body.

At various places in the book, you will find short summaries of information called **memory keys**. Their purpose is to make study and review easier. They are also a useful way for you to check your understanding of key concepts as you read through the text. There are also lots of exercises at the end of each chapter, which allow you to test yourself to ensure that you have learned the essentials.

At the end of Chapters 6 through 17, there is a review of the terms pertinent to the body system being studied. The medical terms have been grouped into specialties; that is, all the anatomical terms are grouped together, all the pathologic terms are grouped together, and all the diagnostic and surgical terms are grouped together. As a review, you can define the term in the space provided.

1.1   Pronunciation Guide

Correct spelling is very important in medicine. Often, the best spellers have accurate pronunciation, but the proper pronunciation of a medical term is not always obvious. To help you, in their first appearance in this book, all difficult terms are typed in bold print and are followed by a common pronunciation. Each term is spelled phoenetically, using combinations of letters that are commonly known to have a particular sound. Many terms have more than one accepted pronunciation, so do not be surprised if from time to time your instructor prefers a pronunciation different from the one given in this book. In these cases, simply strike out the pronunciation given here, and replace it with the version your instructor prefers.

The system of pronunciation used in this book is simple. The most strongly emphasized syllable is written in bold type with capital letters (e.g., **BOLD**). Any syllable with secondary emphasis is written in bold but without capitals (e.g., **bold**).

Table 1-1 outlines the major features of the pronunciation system.

TABLE 1-1

Sound	Pronunciation	Example
a in b**a**t	ah	acute (ah-**KYOOT**)
a in l**a**ne	ay	pain (**PAYN**)
e in b**e**t	eh	hematemesis (**hee**-mah-**TEM**-eh-sis)
e in b**ee**t	ee	ileitis (**ill**-ee-**EYE**-tis)
i in b**i**t	ih	adipose (**AD**-ih-pohs)
i in b**i**te	eye or igh	rhinitis (rye-**NIGH**-tis) ileitis (**ill**-ee-**EYE**-tis)
o in l**o**t	o	prognosis (prog-**NOH**-sis)
o in t**o**te	oh	myeloma (**my**-eh-**LOH**-mah)
u in b**u**t	u	abduction (ab-**DUCK**-shun)
u in c**u**te	yoo	acute (ah-**KYOOT**)
tion in lo**tion**	shun	abduction (ab-**DUCK**-shun)

1.2   The Parts of Medical Terms

Medical terms are made up of the following word elements: **prefixes**, **roots**, and **suffixes**. Not all terms have all three parts, but let's start by looking at an example that does.

> peri**arthr**itis (**per**-ee-ar-**THRIGH**-tis)
>
> peri-   prefix
> **arthr**   root
> -itis   suffix

The first part is the prefix. Whenever a prefix stands alone in this book, it is followed by a hyphen (for example, the prefix in the above example, if standing alone, would be written as peri-). You will learn all the common prefixes in Chapter 4. The root in the example (**arthr**) is in the middle, in bold type. In this book, all roots are in bold type, so that you can easily identify them. You will get an introduction to the common roots in Chapter 2. The last part of our example is the suffix. Whenever a suffix stands alone in this book, it is preceded by a hyphen (e.g., -itis). Suffixes are dealt with in Chapter 3. When you learn the common prefixes, roots, and suffixes, you will be able to understand the meaning of terms you have not seen before by simply analyzing the term using the method described in the next section.

Memory Key   The parts of medical terms are prefixes, roots, and suffixes.

1.3   How to Analyze Medical Terms

When you analyze a term, always start with the suffix. Look again at the example in section 1.2. The suffix is -itis, which means "inflammation." Now look at the prefix, peri-. It means "around." By combining these two, you know that the term refers to "inflammation around something." Now look at the middle of the term. It is the root "**arthr**," meaning joint. Putting it all together, we learn that peri**arthr**itis means inflammation around a joint. It is important that you fully understand the proper procedure for analyzing terms.

Memory Key To analyze a term, always start with the suffix. Then go to the beginning of the word; it will be either a prefix or a root. If there is an additional part in that term, it will be a root.

1.4   Terms with No Prefix

Some terms have no prefix. An example is

arthritis (ar-**THRIGH**-tis)

-itis   suffix meaning "inflammation"
arthr   root meaning "joint"

The meaning of the complete medical term, reading from the suffix to the beginning of the word, is "inflammation of a joint."

Table 1-2 gives additional examples of terms with no prefix.

TABLE 1-2

EXAMPLES OF TERMS WITH NO PREFIX

Term	Definition
gastritis (gas-**TRY**-tis)	inflammation of the stomach
hepatitis (**hep**-ah-**TYE**-tis)	inflammation of the liver
carditis (kar-**DYE**-tis)	inflammation of the heart
adenitis (**ad**-eh-**NIGH**-tis)	inflammation of a gland
cardiology (**kar**-dee-**OL**-oh-jee)	study of the heart
gastrology (gas-**TROL**-oh-jee)	study of the stomach
hepatology (**hep**-ah-**TOL**-oh-jee)	study of the liver

Memory Key Some terms have a suffix and a root, with no prefix.

1.5 Terms with No Root

Some terms consist of a prefix and suffix, with no root at all. An example is

neoplasm (**NEE**-oh-plazm)

neo-   prefix meaning "new"
-plasm   suffix meaning "growth"

The meaning of the complete term is "new growth."

1.6 Terms with Two Roots

Some terms have two roots followed by a suffix. Examples are

osteoar**thr**itis (**oss**-tee-oh-ar-**THRIGH**-tis)

-itis   suffix meaning "inflammation"
-**oste**/o   root meaning "bone"
arthr   root meaning "joint"

The meaning of the complete term is inflammation of the bone and joint.

gastro**enter**itis (**gas**-troh-en-ter-**EYE**-tis)

-itis   suffix meaning "inflammation"
gastr/o   root meaning "stomach"
enter/o   root meaning "intestine"

The meaning of the complete term is "inflammation of the stomach and intestine."

When two roots are combined, there will be an additional vowel placed between them to make pronunciation easier. This is called a **combining vowel**, which is discussed in the next section.

> **Memory Key**   When a term has two roots, they are joined with a combining vowel and are followed by a suffix.

1.7 The Combining Vowel

A combining vowel is a vowel, usually *o*, that combines two roots or a root and a suffix. Using the example *osteoarthritis*, you can see that the vowel *o* joins the two roots *oste* and *arthr*. The *o* in this case is a combining vowel. Its only purpose is to aid pronunciation. Similarly, in *gastroenteritis*, the combining vowel *o* joins the two roots *gastr* and *entr*. Gastroenteritis means inflammation of the stomach and intestines.

In the preceding examples, a combining vowel is used between two roots, as in osteoarthritis and gastroenteritis. But when a root is followed by a suffix, a combining vowel is used *only when the suffix begins with a consonant*. In Table 1-2, the term *cardiology* uses the combining vowel *o* between the root and suffix because the suffix -logy begins with a consonant.

> **cardi**ology (**kar**-dee-**OL**-oh-jee)
>
> -logy   suffix meaning "the study of"
> **cardi**   root meaning "heart"
> /o   combining vowel

In the example *gastritis*, there is no combining vowel between the word root **gastr** and the suffix -itis because the suffix starts with a vowel.

> **gastr**itis (gas-**TRY**-tis)
>
> -itis   suffix meaning "inflammation"
> **gastr**   root meaning "stomach"

Although *o* is by far the most common combining vowel, occasionally *e* or *i* is used. An example using *e* is **chol**elith (**KOH**-lee-lith), meaning "gallstones," and an example using *i* is **dent**iform (**DEN**-tih-form), meaning "shaped like a tooth."

> **chol**elith (**KOH**-lee-lith)
>
> -lith   suffix meaning "stone"
> **chol**   root meaning "gall"
> /e   combining vowel
>
> **dent**iform (**DEN**-tih-form)
>
> -form   suffix meaning "shape"
> **dent**   root meaning "tooth"
> /i   combining vowel

Note that in the examples *cholelith* and *dentiform*, the combining vowel is used because the suffix starts with a consonant. Rare exceptions to this rule are the terms *biliary* (**BILL**-ee-air-ee), which means "pertaining to the bile ducts," and *angiitis* (**an**-jee-**EYE**-tis), which refers to inflammation of a blood vessel. Angiitis is also frequently written angitis (an-**JEYE**-tis).

Table 1-3 provides examples of when a combining vowel is used and not used.

TABLE 1-3

PROPER USE OF A COMBINING VOWEL

Term	Explanation
gastritis (gas-**TRY**-tis)	no combining vowel is used because the suffix -itis starts with a vowel
gastrology (gas-**TROL**-oh-jee)	the combining vowel is used because the suffix -logy starts with a consonant

continued on page 9

Table 1-3 *continued from page 8*

Term	Explanation
cephalgia (seh-**FAL**-jee-ah)	no combining vowel is used because the suffix -algia starts with a vowel
hepatopathy (**hep**-ah-**TOP**-ah-thee)	the combining vowel is used because the suffix -pathy starts with a consonant

Memory Key   A combining vowel is used between two roots. Between a root and a suffix, the combining vowel is used when the suffix begins with a consonant.

1.8   The Combining Form

You have already learned what a combining vowel is. The **combining form** is the name given to a root that is followed by a combining vowel. For example, the root **arthr**, written in its combining form, is

arthr/o

Notice that in many of the preceding examples, the root is separated from the combining vowel by a slash (/). This indicates that the *o* may or may not be used in a medical word. Other examples of combining forms are provided in Table 1-4. Note that the combining form is often easier to pronounce than the root alone.

Memory Key   The combining form is the root plus the combining vowel.

TABLE 1-4

ADDITIONAL EXAMPLES OF COMBINING FORMS

Combining Form	Root	Meaning
gastr/o	**gastr**	stomach
hepat/o	**hepat**	liver
aden/o	**aden**	gland
cardi/o	**cardi**	heart

. . . .

1.9 Plurals

Plurals are formed in various ways, depending on which letters are at the end of a term. To form the plural of singular terms ending in *is*, change the *i* to an *e*, as shown in the following examples:

Singular	Plural
diagnosis (**dye**-ag-**NOH**-sis)	diagnoses (**dye**-ag-**NOH**-seez)
pelvis (**PEL**-vis)	**pelv**es (**PEL**-veez)
neurosis (new-**ROH**-sis)	**neuro**ses (new-**ROH**-seez)

To form the plural of many singular words ending in *us*, change the *us* to an *i*, as shown in the following examples:

Singular	Plural
bronchus (**BRONG**-kus)	**bronch**i (**BRONG**-kye)
bacillus (bah-**SILL**-us)	**bacill**i (bah-**SILL**-eye)
calculus (**KAL**-kyoo-lus)	**calcul**i (**KAL**-kyoo-lye)
embolus (**EM**-boh-lus)	**embol**i (**EM**-boh-lye)

There are a few exceptions. For example, the plural of *virus* (**VYE**-rus) is *viruses* (**VYE**-rus-ez), and the plural of *sinus* (**SIGH**-nus) is *sinuses* (**SIGH**-nus-ez).

The plural of singular words ending in *a* is formed by adding an *e* to the word, as shown in the following examples. Modifiers in Latin must agree with the noun. For example, the plural of *vena cava* is *venae cavae*.

Singular	Plural
sclera (**SKLEHR**-ah)	sclerae (**SKLEHR**-ee)
scapula (**SKAP**-yoo-lah)	scapulae (**SKAP**-yoo-lee)
vena cava (**VEE**-nah **CAV**-ah)	venae cavae (**VEE**-nee **CAV**-ee)

Singular terms ending in *um* are pluralized by changing the *um* to an *a*, as shown in the following examples:

Singular	Plural
acetabulum (**ass**-eh-**TAB**-yoo-lum)	acetabula (**ass**-eh-**TAB**-yoo-lah)
capitulum (ka-**PIT**-yoo-lum)	capitula (ka-**PIT**-yoo-lah)
septum (**SEP**-tum)	septa (**SEP**-tah)
diverticulum (**dye**-ver-**TICK**-yoo-lum)	diverticula (**dye**-ver-**TICK**-yoo-lah)

To form the plural of singular words ending in *ix* or *ex*, change the ending to *ices*, as shown in the following examples:

Singular	Plural
cal**ix** (**KAY**-licks)	cal**ices** (**KAY**-lih-seez)
cerv**ix** (**SER**-vicks)	cerv**ices** (**SER**-vih-seez)
ind**ex** (**IN**-decks)	ind**ices** (**IN**-dih-seez)
var**ix** (**VAR**-icks)	var**ices** (**VAR**-ih-seez)

Singular words ending in *oma* are made plural by the addition of a *ta* or *s*, as shown in the following examples:

Singular	Plural
adenoma (**ad**-eh-**NOH**-mah)	**aden**omata or **aden**omas (**ad**-eh-no-**MA**-tah) (**ad**-eh-**NOH**-mahz)
carcinoma (**kar**-sih-**NOH**-mah)	**carcin**omata or **carcin**omas (**kar**-sin-oh-**MA**-tah) (**kar**-sin-**OH**-mahz)
fibroma (figh-**BROH**-mah)	**fibr**omata or **fibr**omas (figh-broh-**MA**-tah) (figh-**BROH**-mahz)

To form the plural of singular words ending in *nx*, change the *x* to *g* and add *es*, as shown in the following examples:

Singular	Plural
laryn**x** (**LAR**-inks)	laryn**ges** (**LAR**-in-jeez)
phalan**x** (**FAH**-lanks)	phalan**ges** (fah-**LAN**-jeez)

To form the plural of singular words ending in *on*, change the *on* to an *a* or simply add an *s*, as shown in the following example:

Singular	Plural
ganglion (**GANG**-glee-on)	**gangli**a or **gangli**ons (**GANG**-glee-ah) (**GANG**-glee-onz)

To form the plural of singular words ending in *ax*, change the *ax* to *aces*, as shown in the following example:

Singular	Plural
thorax (**THOH**-racks)	**thor**aces (**THOH**-rah-sees)

Memory Key	Remember the following rules:		
	is→es	um→a	nx→nges
	us→i	ix or ex→ices	on→a, or simply add an *s*
	a→ae	oma→omata; omas	ax→aces

1.10 Putting It All Together

Exercise 1-1   FILL IN THE BLANKS

1. The three parts of a medical term are the _prefix_ , _root_ , and _suffix_ .

2. The component part usually found at the end of a medical word is the _suffix_ .

3. When you analyze a medical term, you start with the _suffix_ , and then define the _prefix_ .

4. The root in periarthritis is _arthr_ .

5. The difference between the combining form and combining vowel is _the form includes the root and the vowel_ .

Exercise 1-2   TRUE OR FALSE

1. The term *carditis* has no prefix.   (T)   F

2. An example of a word with no root is *gastrology*.   T   (F)

3. In the term *hepatopathy*, the combining vowel is used because the suffix starts with a consonant.   (T)   F

4. A combining vowel is not used between two roots.   T   (F)

5. The prefix peri- means "around."   (T)   F

Exercise 1-3   SINGULARS AND PLURALS

Give the plural for the following singular forms.

Singular	Plural
1. thorax	*thoraces*
2. neurosis	*neuroses*
3. ganglion	*ganglions ganglia*
4. virus	*viruses*
5. phalanx	*phalanges*
6. fibroma	*fibromata*
7. varix	*varices*
8. diverticulum	*diverticula*
9. scapula	*scapulae*
10. embolus	*emboli*

Give the singular for the following plural forms.

Plural	Singular
1. larynges	*larynx*
2. carcinomas	*carcinoma*
3. calices	*calix*
4. acetabula	*acetabulum*
5. sclerae	*sclera*
6. bronchi	*bronchus*
7. diagnoses	*diagnosis*
8. sinuses	*sinus*
9. septa	*septum*
10. indices	*index*

Roots of Each Body System

CHAPTER ORGANIZATION

This chapter will help you learn basic anatomical roots. It is divided into the following sections:

2.1	Anatomy and Physiology
2.2	Levels of Organization
2.3	Organ Systems
2.4	Common Anatomical Roots
2.5	Putting It All Together

CHAPTER OBJECTIVES

On completion of this chapter, you will be able to do the following:

1. Define anatomy and physiology
2. Describe the levels of organization into which the body is arranged
3. Name the body systems
4. Define and spell common anatomical roots

INTRODUCTION

This chapter starts by introducing you to some basic concepts related to the study of the human body. It will prepare you for learning the roots you need to know for this and the following chapters on suffixes and prefixes.

The roots in this chapter are grouped according to body systems. You will find it much easier to remember each root if you associate it with a mental picture of the organs to which it refers. The roots you encounter in this chapter will give you a foundation, a base for building medical terms found in Chapters 3 and 4. Additional roots pertinent to each body system can be found in Chapters 6 through 17. Note that the roots in the tables of this chapter are expressed in their combining forms, as described in Chapter 1.

2.1   Anatomy and Physiology

Two terms you will encounter often in this text are **anatomy** and **physiology**. Anatomy is the study of the parts of the body. The names and locations of the muscles of the body exemplify anatomy. Physiology is the study of how the body parts work. Gas exchange at the alveolar-capillary membrane is an example of physiology.

Memory Key	Anatomy is the study of structure. Physiology is the study of function.

2.2   Levels of Organization

All life consists of microscopic living structures called **cells**, which perform various functions in the body. Regardless of their function, all cells are similar in structure. They have an outer membrane and various internal structures that absorb nutrients, create protein, fight bacteria, excrete wastes, and store various products created within the cell. In other words, the cell is a structural and functional unit despite its size. Cells make up the cellular level, which is the first level of organization of the body. The next level is called **tissue**. Cells combine to make tissues such as muscle and bone. Tissues combine to make up **organs**, such as the heart and liver. Related organs make up **organ systems**, such as the cardiovascular and skeletal systems. All of the organ systems go together to form the human body. To summarize, the levels of organization are cells, tissues, organs, organ systems, and the entire body (the organism). Figure 2-1 illustrates these levels of organization. Later in this chapter, all of the individual organ systems are illustrated.

Memory Key	The levels of organization of the body, from smallest to largest, are cells, tissues, organs, systems, and organism.

2.3   Organ Systems

Twelve organ systems (often called body systems) make up the human body. They are: integumentary, skeletal, muscular, digestive, nervous, endocrine, eyes and ears, cardiovascular, lymphatic and immune, respiratory, urinary, and reproductive systems. These systems work together to perform all the necessary functions of life. Figures 2-2 through 2-13 illustrate all of these systems. Included with each figure is a list of the common anatomical roots of each system.

FIGURE 2-1
Levels of organization

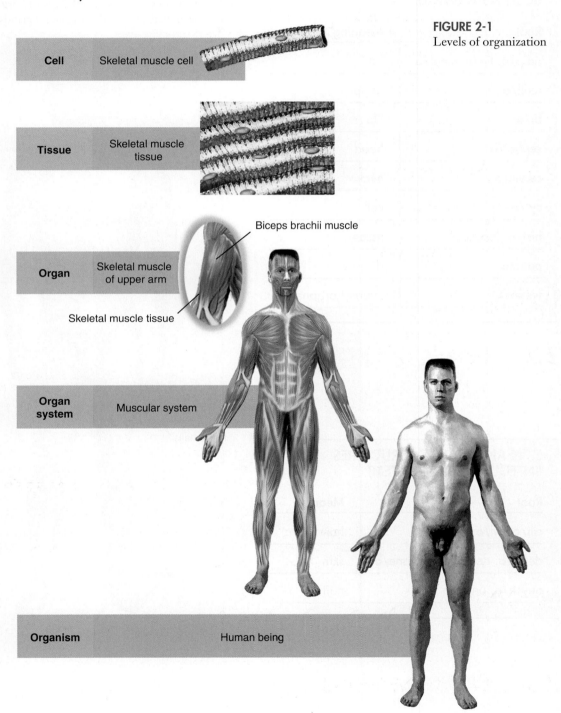

Cell Skeletal muscle cell

Tissue Skeletal muscle tissue

Biceps brachii muscle

Organ Skeletal muscle of upper arm

Skeletal muscle tissue

Organ system Muscular system

Organism Human being

2.4   Common Anatomical Roots

BODY AS A WHOLE

Root	Meaning
adip/o; lip/o; steat/o	fat
axill/o	armpit
bi/o	life
cephal/o	head
cervic/o	neck
cyt/o	cell
hist/o; histi/o	tissue
path/o	disease
viscer/o	internal organs

SKIN AND RELATED STRUCTURES (INTEGUMENTARY SYSTEM)

Root	Meaning
cili/o; pil/o	hair
derm/o; dermat/o; cutane/o	skin
onych/o; ungu/o	nail

FIGURE 2-2
Integumentary system: skin and accessory organs such as hair, nails, sweat glands, and oil glands

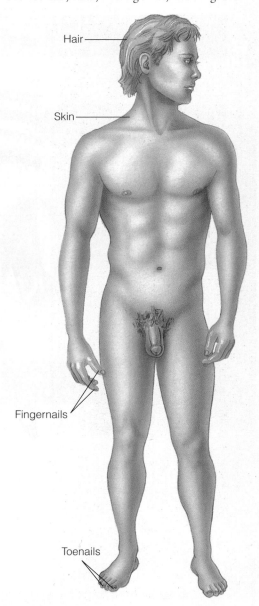

Hair

Skin

Fingernails

Toenails

SKELETAL SYSTEM

Root	Meaning
arthr/o	joint
chondr/o	cartilage
crani/o	skull
cost/o	rib
myel/o	bone marrow (also means spinal cord)
oste/o	bone
pelv/o; **pelvi/i**	pelvis
spin/o	spine; spinal (vertebral) column; backbone
vertebr/o; **spondyl/o**	vertebra

FIGURE 2-3
Skeletal system: bones, cartilage, and joints

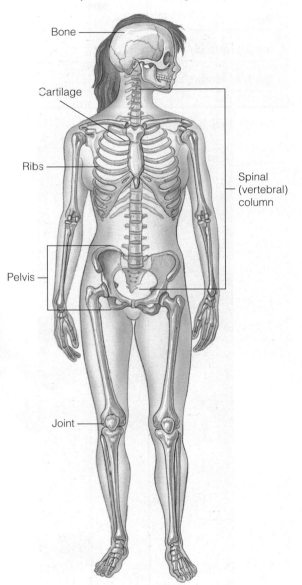

MUSCULAR SYSTEM	
Root	**Meaning**
my/o; muscul/o	muscle
tend/o; tendin/o	tendon

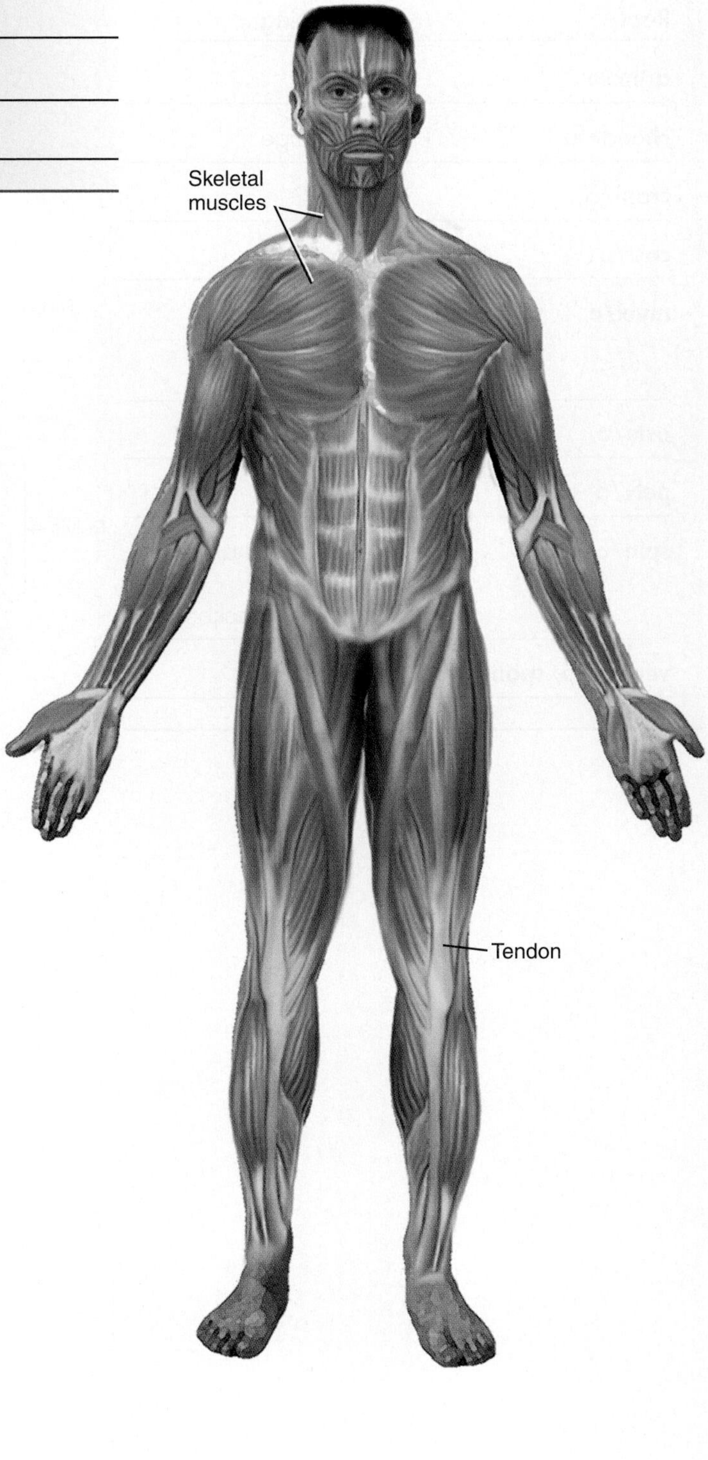

FIGURE 2-4
Muscular system: muscles and tendons

Skeletal
muscles

Tendon

NERVOUS SYSTEM; EYES, EARS

Root	Meaning
blephar/o	eyelid
cerebr/o; encephal/o	brain
myel/o	spinal cord (also means bone marrow)
neur/o	nerve
ophthalm/o; ocul/o	eye
ot/o	ear

FIGURE 2-5
Nervous system and organs of special sense: brain, spinal cord, nerves, eyes, and ears

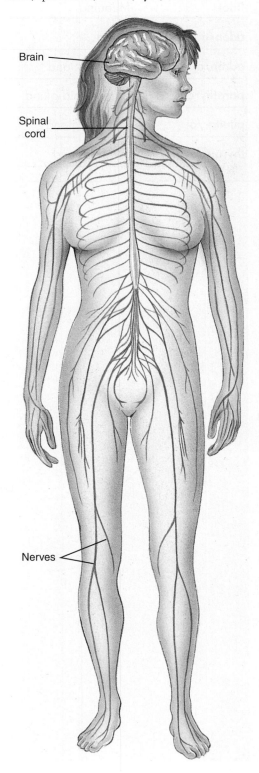

Brain

Spinal cord

Nerves

ENDOCRINE SYSTEM

Root	Meaning
aden/o	gland
adren/o	adrenal gland
parathyroid/o	parathyroid gland
pituitar/o	pituitary gland
thyroid/o	thyroid gland

FIGURE 2-6
Endocrine system: pituitary, thyroid, parathyroid, adrenal, and pineal glands; thymus, portions of the hypothalamus and the pancreas; ovaries, and testes.

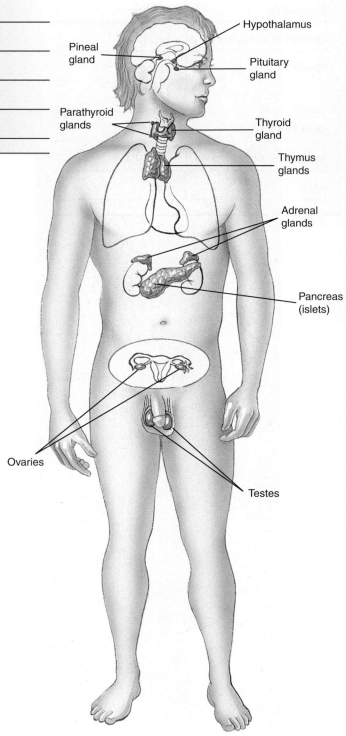

CIRCULATORY SYSTEM

Root	Meaning
angi/o; vascul/o; vas/o	vessel
arteri/o	artery
cardi/o	heart
hem/o; hemat/o	blood
ven/o; phleb/o	vein

FIGURE 2-7
Circulatory system: heart, arteries, veins, capillaries, and blood

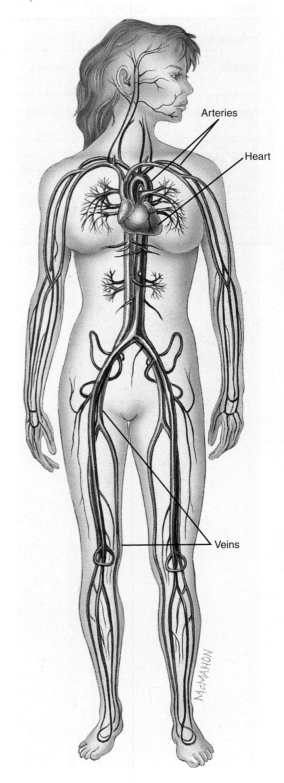

Arteries

Heart

Veins

McMAHON

LYMPHATIC AND IMMUNE SYSTEMS

Root	Meaning
adenoid/o	adenoids
lymph/o	lymph (clear, watery fluid)
lymphaden/o	lymph glands; lymph nodes
lymphangi/o	lymph vessels
splen/o	spleen
tonsill/o	tonsils

FIGURE 2-8
Lymphatic and immune systems: thymus, bone marrow, spleen, tonsils, lymph nodes, lymph capillaries, lymph vessels, lymphocytes, and lymph

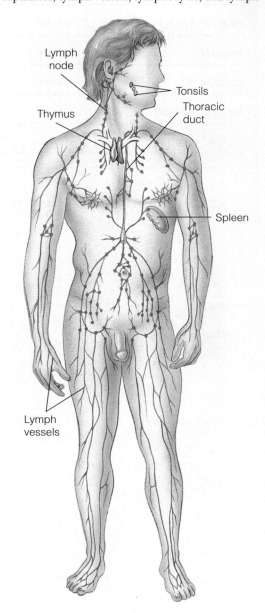

RESPIRATORY SYSTEM

Root	Meaning
alveol/o	air sac; alveolus
bronch/o; bronchi/o	bronchus
bronchiol/o	small bronchial tubes
laryng/o	voice box; larynx
nas/o; rhin/o	nose
pharyng/o	throat; pharynx
phren/o	diaphragm
pneum/o; pneumon/o; pulmon/o	lungs
thorac/o	chest
trache/o	windpipe; trachea

FIGURE 2-9
Respiratory system: lungs, nasal cavity, pharynx, larynx, trachea, bronchi, and bronchioles

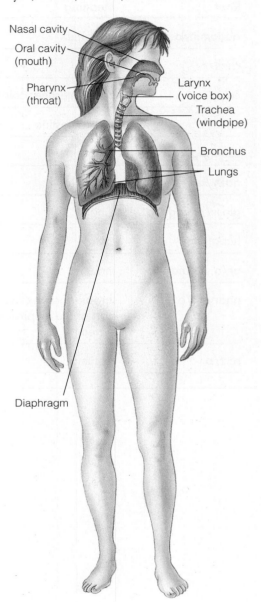

DIGESTIVE SYSTEM

Root	Meaning
abdomin/o	abdomen
cheil/o	lips
col/o	large intestine; colon
enter/o	small intestine
esophag/o	esophagus
gastr/o	stomach
gloss/o; lingu/o	tongue
hepat/o	liver
or/o; stomat/o	mouth
pharyng/o	throat; pharynx (also part of the respiratory system)
rect/o	rectum

FIGURE 2-10
Digestive system: mouth, pharynx, esophagus, stomach, small intestine, large intestine, salivary glands, pancreas, gallbladder, and liver

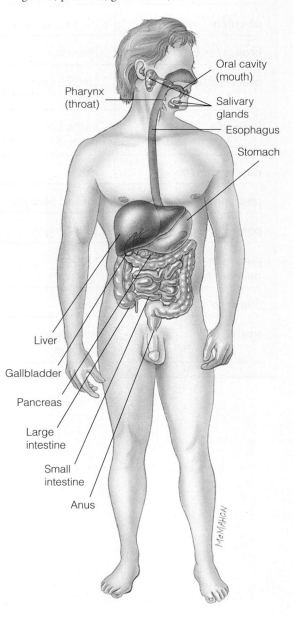

URINARY SYSTEM

Root	Meaning
cyst/o	bladder
ren/o; nephr/o	kidneys
ureter/o	ureters
urethr/o	urethra

FIGURE 2-11
Urinary system: kidneys, ureters, urinary bladder, and urethra

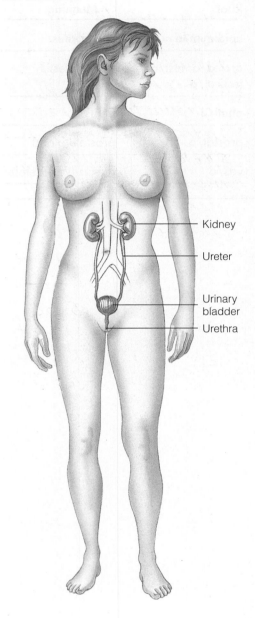

MALE REPRODUCTIVE SYSTEM

Root	Meaning
epididym/o	epididymis
orchid/o; **test/o**; **testicul/o**	testicle; testis
phall/o	penis
prostat/o	prostate gland
vas/o	ductus (vas) deferens

FIGURE 2-12
Male reproductive system: testes, epididymides, ductus deferens, ejaculatory ducts, penis, seminal vesicles, and prostate gland

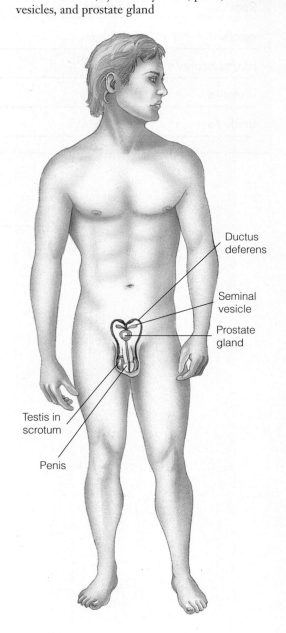

Ductus deferens

Seminal vesicle

Prostate gland

Testis in scrotum

Penis

FEMALE REPRODUCTIVE SYSTEM

Root	Meaning
colp/o; **vagin/o**	vagina
gynec/o	female
mast/o; **mamm/o**	breast
oophor/o; **ovari/o**	ovary
salping/o	fallopian tubes; uterine tubes
uter/o; **hyster/o**; **metr/o**	uterus
vulv/o	vulva; external genitalia

FIGURE 2-13
Female reproductive system: ovaries, uterine tubes, uterus, vagina, vulva (external genitalia), and mammary glands

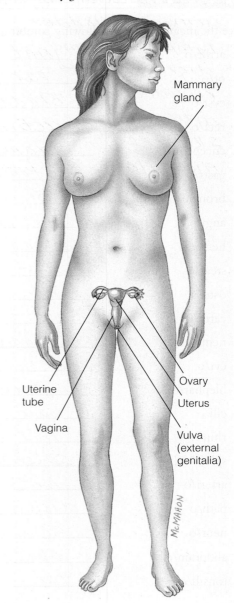

2.5 Putting It All Together

Exercise 2-1 DEFINITIONS

Give the meaning of the following combining forms.

1. arthr/o _____ joint _____
2. ot/o _____ ear _____
3. cyst/o _____ bladder _____
4. rect/o _____ rectum _____
5. encephal/o _____ brain _____
6. gastr/o _____ stomach _____
7. bronchi/o; bronch/o _____ bronchial tube _____
8. angi/o _____ vessel _____
9. hemat/o _____ blood _____
10. steat/o _____ fat _____
11. oste/o _____ bone _____
12. cardi/o _____ heart _____
13. nephr/o _____ kidney _____
14. cyt/o _____ cell _____
15. blephar/o _____ eyelid _____
16. cili/o _____ hair _____
17. rhin/o _____ nose _____
18. splen/o _____ spleen _____
19. arteri/o _____ artery _____
20. path/o _____ disease _____
21. neur/o _____ nerve _____
22. abdomin/o _____ abdominal _____
23. tonsill/o _____ tonsills _____
24. myel/o _____ bone marrow / spinal cord _____
25. bi/o _____ life _____
26. trache/o _____ trachea _____
27. ophthalm/o _____ eye _____
28. hepat/o _____ liver _____

29. viscer/o   _organs_

30. cephal/o   _head_

Exercise 2-2   ROOTS

Give the root for each of the following words.

1. armpit   _axill_
2. head   _cephal_
3. nail   _ungu / onych_
4. cartilage   _chondro_
5. skull   _crani_
6. tendon   _tendin_
7. eye   _ophthalm_
8. small intestine   _enter_
9. colon   _col_
10. tongue   _gloss / lingu_
11. ductus deferens   _vas_
12. thyroid gland   _thyroid_
13. vein   _phleb_
14. lung   _pneumo_
15. chest   _thorac_
16. lymph vessels   _lymphangi_
17. external genitalia   _vulv_
18. testicle   _testi_
19. epididymis   _epi_
20. ovary   _ovari_

Exercise 2-3   SHORT ANSWER

1. Define anatomy and physiology. _anatomy - study of body parts._
physiology - how body parts work.

2. Name 12 body systems and at least two organs in each. _____

respiratory - lungs

cardiovascular - heart

urinary - bladder, kidneys

lymph / immune - spleen, tonsils

digestive - stomach, colon

reproductive - uterus, penis

integumentary - skin

skeletal - all muscles. ⤴

muscular - all bones ⤵

nervous - brain, spinal cord

endocrine - pancreas, ovaries

Suffixes

CHAPTER ORGANIZATION

This chapter will help you learn about medical suffixes. It is divided into the following sections:

3.1   Additional Word Parts

3.2   Suffixes Used to Indicate Pathologic Conditions

3.3   Suffixes Used to Indicate Diagnostic Procedures

3.4   Suffixes Used to Indicate Surgical Procedures

3.5   General Suffixes

3.6   Adjectival Suffixes

3.7   Putting It All Together

CHAPTER OBJECTIVES

On completion of this chapter, you will be able to do the following:

1. Spell and give the meaning for suffixes

2. Distinguish suffixes that signify pathologic conditions from those that signify diagnostic and surgical procedures

3. Identify suffixes used to convert medical nouns to adjectives

4. Analyze, define, pronounce, and spell medical terms in this chapter

INTRODUCTION

You learned in Chapter 1 that suffixes are the first word parts to examine when analyzing a term. The most common suffixes are grouped into four sections in this chapter. In each section, you will find the suffix definition first, followed by examples of terms using the suffix. Each example is accompanied by a pronunciation guide, term analysis, and a definition. Make sure you know the pronunciation first. Then work to remember the meaning.

You may find that in this and other chapters, memory aids are useful. Many learners realize that remembering suffix, prefix, and root meanings is aided by associating them with a particular visualization or other sensory association. For example, the first suffix, -algia, means "pain." It may be best remembered by recalling a particular pain you have experienced and associating it with the suffix. Similarly, you might remember the second suffix, -cele, by imagining a huge hernia coming out of your intestine when you say the suffix to yourself. The more outrageous the imagined association, the more likely you are to remember.

3.1   Additional Word Parts

The following roots and prefix will also be used in this chapter to build medical terms.

Root	Meaning
acr/o	top; extremities
carcin/o	cancer
don/o	donates
fluor/o	luminous
glyc/o	sugar
pharmac/o	drug
physi/o	nature
practition/o	practice
sect/o	cut

Prefix	Meaning
micro-	small

3.2   Suffixes Used to Indicate Pathologic Conditions

Pathology means the study of disease processes. The following suffixes describe disease, symptoms, or abnormalities.

	-algia	pain
Term	**Term Analysis**	**Definition**
cephalgia (sef-**AL**-jee-ah)	**cephal/o** = head	headache
arthralgia (ar-**THRAL**-jee-ah)	**arthr/o** = joint	joint pain
otalgia (oh-**TAL**-jee-ah)	**ot/o** = ear	earache
	-cele	**hernia (protrusion or displacement of an organ through a structure that normally contains it)**
cystocele (**SIS**-toh-seel)	**cyst/o** = bladder	hernia of the urinary bladder; protrusion of the bladder onto the vaginal walls (see Figure 3-1)

FIGURE 3-1
Cystocele

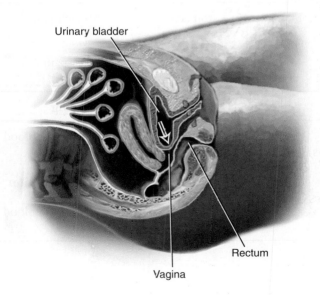

Urinary bladder

Rectum

Vagina

FIGURE 3-2
Rectocele

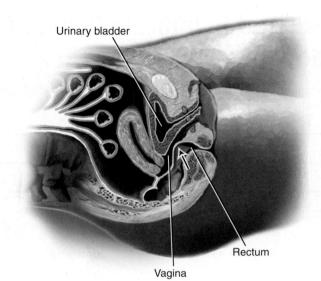

Urinary bladder

Rectum

Vagina

Term	Term Analysis	Definition
rectocele (**RECK**-toh-seel)	**rect/o** = rectum	hernia of the rectum; protrusion of the rectum onto the vaginal wall (see Figure 3-2)
encephalocele (en-**SEF**-ah-loh-**seel**)	**encephal/o** = brain	hernia of the brain
	-dynia	**pain**
gastrodynia (**gas**-troh-**DIN**-ee-ah)	**gastr/o** = stomach	stomach pain
mastodynia (**mas**-toh-**DIN**-ee-ah)	**mast/o** = breast	breast pain
	-emesis	**vomiting**
hematemesis (**hee**-mah-**TEM**-eh-sis)	**hemat/o** = blood	vomiting of blood
	-emia	**blood condition**
glycemia (glye-**SEE**-mee-ah)	**glyc/o** = sugar	sugar in the blood

	-ia	state of; condition
Term	**Term Analysis**	**Definition**
pneumonia (new-**MOH**-nee-ah)	**pneumon/o** = lung	condition of the lung (most commonly known as an inflammation of the lung)
	-itis	**inflammation (the redness, swelling, heat, and pain that occur when the body protects itself from injury)**
enteritis (**en**-ter-**EYE**-tis)	**enter/o** = small intestine	inflamed small intestine
stomatitis (**sto**-mah-**TYE**-tis)	**stomat/o** = mouth	inflamed mouth
spondylitis (**spon**-dih-**LYE**-tis)	**spondyl/o** = vertebra	inflamed vertebra

Memory Key   Inflammation has two *ms*; inflamed has only one *m*.

	-lysis	destruction; separation; breakdown
hemolysis (hee-**MOL**-ih-sis)	**hem/o** = blood	breakdown of blood

Memory Key   To remember the meaning of -lysis, think of the word *analysis*, meaning to "break down or separate into parts."

	-malacia	softening
cerebromalacia (**ser**-eh-broh-mah-**LAY**-shee-ah)	**cerebr/o** = brain	softening of the brain
chondromalacia (**kon**-droh-mah-**LAY**-shee-ah)	**chondr/o** = cartilage	softening of cartilage

Term	Term Analysis	Definition
	-megaly	**enlargement**
visceromegaly (**VIS**-er-oh-**meg**-ah-lee)	**viscer/o** = internal organs	enlargement of the internal organs
	-oma	**tumor; mass**
lipoma (lih-**POH**-mah)	**lip/o** = fat	tumor containing fat
myoma (my-**OH**-mah)	**my/o** = muscle	tumor of muscle
	-osis	**abnormal condition**
nephrosis (neh-**FROH**-sis)	**nephr/o** = kidney	abnormal condition of the kidney
	-pathy	**disease process**
ureteropathy (yoo-**ree**-ter-**OP**-ah-thee)	**ureter/o** = ureter (a tube leading from each kidney)	disease process of the ureter to the bladder for the passage of urine
	-penia	**decrease, deficiency**
cytopenia (**sigh**-toh-**PEE**-nee-ah)	**cyt/o** = cell	deficiency of cells
	-phobia	**irrational fear**
acrophobia (**ack**-roh-**FOH**-bee-ah)	**acr/o** = top, extremities	fear of heights
	-ptosis	**downward displacement; drooping; prolapse; sagging**
blepharoptosis (**blef**-ah-rop-**TOH**-sis)	**blephar/o** = eyelid	drooping eyelid (see Figure 3-3)
nephroptosis (**nef**-rop-**TOH**-sis)	**nephr/o** = kidney	drooping kidney
	-ptysis	**spitting**
hemoptysis (he-**MOP**-tih-sis)	**hem/o** = blood	spitting up blood

FIGURE 3-3
Blepharoptosis

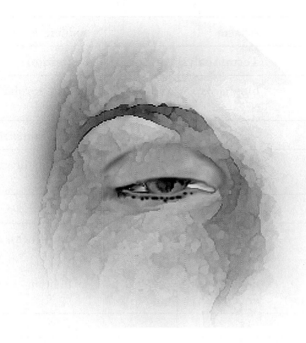

	-rrhage; rrhagia	bursting forth
Term	**Term Analysis**	**Definition**
hemorrhage (**HEM**-or-idj)	**hem/o** = blood	bursting forth of blood; bleeding
gastrorrhagia (gas-troh-**RAY**-jee-ah)	**gastr/o** = stomach	bleeding from the stomach
	-rrhea	flow; discharge
otorrhea (**oh**-toh-**REE**-ah)	**ot/o** = ear	discharge from the ear
	-rrhexis	rupture
splenorrhexis (**splee**-nor-**ECKS**-sis)	**splen/o** = spleen	ruptured spleen
	-sclerosis	hardening
arteriosclerosis (ar-**teer**-ee-oh-skleh-**ROH**-sis)	**arteri/o** = artery	hardening of the arteries

Term	-spasm	sudden, involuntary contraction
Term	**Term Analysis**	**Definition**
blepharospasm (**BLEF**-ah-roh-spazm)	**blephar/o** = eyelid	sudden, involuntary contraction of the eyelid
	-stenosis	**narrowing; stricture**
phlebostenosis (**fleb**-oh-steh-**NOH**-sis)	**phleb/o** = vein	narrowing of a vein
	-y	**process**
neuropathy (new-**ROP**-ah-thee)	**neur/o** = nerve **path/o** = disease	disease process of the nerve
microencephaly (**my**-kroh-en-**SEF**-ah-lee)	micro- = small **encephal/o** = brain	small brain

3.3 Suffixes Used to Indicate Diagnostic Procedures

Diagnosis of pathologic conditions involves using many different standard procedures, depending on the symptoms displayed by the patient. Common suffixes associated with diagnostic procedures are listed next.

Term	-gram	record; writing
Term	**Term Analysis**	**Definition**
lymphangiogram (lim-**FAN**-jee-oh-**gram**)	**lymphangi/o** = lymph vessel	record of the lymph vessel (by the use of x-rays)
	-graph	**instrument used to record**
cardiograph (**KAR**-dee-**oh**-graf)	**cardi/o** = heart	instrument used to record heart activity

	-graphy	process of recording; producing images
Term	**Term Analysis**	**Definition**
computed **tomo**graphy (CT scan) (toh-**MOG**-rah-fee)	**tom/o** = to cut	x-ray beam rotates around the patient detailing the structure at various depths. The information is computer analyzed and converted to a picture of the body part. Common body parts studied in this fashion include the abdomen, kidneys, brain, and chest. *NOTE:* Another type of scan is the nuclear medicine scan. X-rays are not used as they are in CT scans. An image of a body organ is taken after a radioactive substance known as a tracer has been introduced into the body. The tracer travels through the bloodstream to the body organ being studied, and gives off small amounts of radiation that are detected by a special camera called a gamma camera, which produces an image called a scan. Nuclear medicine scans are commonly of bone, brain, liver, lung, thyroid, and heart.
mammography (mam-**OG**-rah-fee)	**mamm/o** = breast	producing images of the breast (by the use of x-rays) (see Figure 3-4)
myelography (**my**-eh-**LOG**-rah-fee)	**myel/o** = spinal cord	producing images of the spinal cord (by the use of x-rays)
	-meter	instrument used to measure; process of measuring
craniometer (**kray**-nee-**OM**-eh-ter)	**crani/o** = skull	instrument used to measure the skull
	-metry	to measure; measurement
pelvimetry (pel-**VIM**-eh-tree)	**pelv/i** = pelvis	measurement of the pelvis. *NOTE:* A pelvimetry is performed to confirm the size of the maternal pelvis in situations in which the pelvis is thought to be too small for the delivery of the baby.

FIGURE 3-4
Mammography

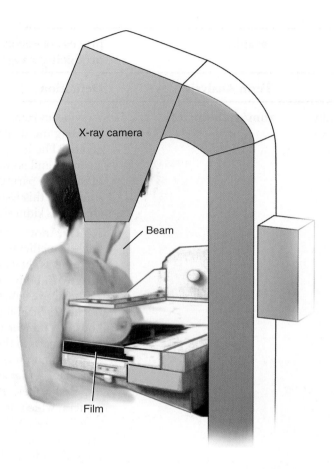

	-opsy	to view
Term	**Term Analysis**	**Definition**
biopsy (**BYE**-op-see)	**bi/o** = life	a procedure involving the removal of a piece of living tissue, which is then microscopically examined for any abnormalities
	-scope	**instrument used to visually examine (a body cavity or organ)**
bronchoscope (**BRONG**-koh-skohp)	**bronch/o** = bronchus	instrument used to visually examine the interior of the bronchus (for examples of endoscopes, see Figure 4-1)

	-scopy	process of visually examining (a body cavity or organ)
Term	**Term Analysis**	**Definition**
bronchoscopy (brong-**KOS**-koh-pee)	**bronch/o** = bronchus	process of visually examining the bronchus
fluoroscopy (floo-**ROS**-keh-pee)	**fluor/o** = luminous	x-ray of moving structures, such as the movement of substances through the digestive tract *NOTE:* In this term, *-scopy* does not mean the process of visually examining a body cavity or organ. A fluoroscopy produces an image of a structure on a fluorescent screen rather than on a single x-ray film. This procedure has the advantage of allowing observation of structures as they move.

3.4   Suffixes Used to Indicate Surgical Procedures

If the diagnosis indicates that surgery is required, then the appropriate surgical procedures will be recommended. Common suffixes associated with surgical procedures are listed next.

	-centesis	surgical puncture to remove fluid
Term	**Term Analysis**	**Definition**
abdominocentesis (ab-**dom**-ih-noh-sen-**TEE**-SIS)	**abdomin/o** = abdomen	surgical puncture to remove fluid from the abdomen
thoracocentesis (**thoh**-rah-koh-sen-**TEE**-sis)	**thorac/o** = chest	surgical puncture of the chest wall to remove excess fluid from around the lungs
	-desis	surgical binding; surgical fusion
arthrodesis (ar-throh-**DEE**-sis)	**arthr/o** = joint	surgical fusion of a joint

	-ectomy	excision; surgical removal
Term	**Term Analysis**	**Definition**
oophorectomy (oh-**of**-oh-**RECK**-toh-mee)	**oophor/o** = ovary	excision of the ovary
tonsillectomy (ton-sih-**LECK**-toh-me)	**tonsill/o** = tonsils	excision of the tonsils
	-pexy	**surgical fixation**
nephropexy (**NEF**-roh-**peck**-see)	**nephr/o** = kidney	surgical fixation of the kidney
	-plasty	**surgical reconstruction; surgical repair**
orchidoplasty (**OR**-kid-oh-**plas**-tee)	**orchid/o** = testicle	surgical reconstruction of the testicle
	-rrhaphy	**suture; sew**
colporrhaphy (kol-**POR**-ah-fee)	**colp/o** = vagina	suturing of the vagina
	-stasis	**stoppage; stopping; controlling**
hemostasis (**he**-moh-**STAY**-sis)	**hem/o** = blood	stoppage of blood
	-stomy	**new opening; artificial opening**
tracheostomy (**tray**-kee-**OS**-toh-mee)	**trache/o** = trachea; windpipe	new opening into the trachea
	-tome	**instrument used to cut**
myotome (**MY**-oh-tohm)	**my/o** = muscle	instrument used to cut muscle
	-tomy	**process of cutting; incision**
tenotomy (teh-**NOT**-oh-mee)	**ten/o** = tendon	process of cutting a tendon

3.5 General Suffixes

The following is a list of general suffixes you need to know to understand a great number of medical terms:

	-cyte	**cell**
Term	**Term Analysis**	**Definition**
adipocyte (**AD**-ih-poh-**sight**)	**adip/o** = fat	fat cell
histiocyte; **histo**cyte (**HISS**-tee-oh-**sight**); (**HISS**-toh-**sight**)	**histi/o; hist/o** = tissue	tissue cell
	-er; -ician; -logist; -ist	**specialist; one who specializes; specialist in the study of**
practitioner (prack-**TISH**-un-er)	**practition/o** = practice	one who has obtained the proper requirements to work in a specific field of study
physician (fih-**ZIH**-shun)	**physi/o** = nature	specialist in the study of medicine who has graduated from a recognized school of medicine and is licensed by the appropriate authority to practice
neurologist (new-**ROL**-oh-jist)	**neur/o** = nerve	specialist in the study of the nervous system and its disorders
pharmacist (**FARM**-ah-sist)	**pharmac/o** = drug	specialist licensed to prepare and dispense drugs
	-ion	**process**
section (**SECK**-shun)	**sect/o** = to cut	process of cutting
	-logy	**study of; process of study**
hepatology (hep-ah-**TOL**-oh-jee)	**hepat/o** = liver	study of the liver
physiology (fiz-ee-**OL**-oh-jee)	**physi/o** = nature	study of function (the study of how a structure functions)

Term	Term Analysis	Definition
	-or	**one who; person or thing that does something**
organ **don**or (**DOH**-nor)	**don/o** = donate	one who donates organ tissue to be used in another body
	-plasia	**formation; development**
chondroplasia (**kon**-droh-**PLAY**-zee-ah)	**chondr/o** = cartilage	formation of cartilage
	-poiesis	**production; manufacture; formation**
hematopoiesis (**he**-mah-toh-poi-**EE**-sis)	**hemat/o** = blood	production of blood

3.6   Adjectival Suffixes

Adjectival suffixes describe special qualities or relationships.

Term	Term Analysis	Definition
	-genic	**produced by; producing**
carcinogenic (**kar**-sih-noh-**JEN**-ick)	**carcin/o** = cancer	producing cancer (agent that produces cancer)
	-oid	**resembling**
osteoid (**OS**-tee-oyd)	**oste/o** = bone	resembling bone
	-ole; -ule	**small**
bronchiole (**BRONG**-kee-ohl)	**bronchi/o** = bronchus	small bronchus
venule (**VEN**-yool)	**ven/o** = vein	small vein
	-ac; -al; -ary; -eal; -ic; -ous	**pertaining to**
cardiac (**KAR**-dee-ack)	**cardi/o** = heart	pertaining to the heart

Term	Term Analysis	Definition
renal (**REE**-nal)	**ren/o** = kidney	pertaining to the kidney
mammary (**MAM**-ah-ree)	**mamm/o** = breast	pertaining to the breast
pharyngeal (far-**IN**-jee-al)	**pharyng/o** = throat; pharynx	pertaining to the throat
gastric (**GAS**-trik)	**gastr/o** = stomach	pertaining to the stomach
venous (**VEE**-nus)	**ven/o** = vein	pertaining to a vein

NOTE: Although there are some exceptions, the suffixes meaning "pertaining to" are not generally interchangeable with a given root. For example, one can create the adjectives *renal* and *cardiac*, but not renac, renar, renary, cardiar, cardieal, cardious, or cardiose.

3.7   Putting It All Together

Exercise 3-1   DEFINING SUFFIXES

Define the following suffixes.

Suffixes indicating pathologic conditions:

1. -algia   *pain*
2. -dynia   *pain*
3. -emesis   *vommiting*
4. -osis   *abnormal condition*
5. -cele   *hernia*
6. -malacia   *softening*
7. -oma   *tumor*
8. -penia   *decrease / deficiency*
9. -emia   *blood disorder*
10. -ptosis   *drooping*
11. -rrhage   *bursting forth*
12. -rrhexis   *rupture*
13. -stenosis   *narrowing*

Suffixes indicating diagnostic and surgical procedures:

14. -ectomy _____ to remove. _____
15. -gram _____ record / write. _____
16. -graph _____ instrument for recording _____
17. -opsy _____ to view _____
18. -plasty _____ reconstructive _____
19. -scope _____ instrument used to view _____
20. -tome _____ " " " cut _____

General suffixes:

21. -cyte _____ cell _____
22. -ist _____ person studying _____
23. -ion _____ process _____
24. -logy _____ study of _____
25. -poiesis _____ formation _____

Adjectival suffixes:

26. -genic _____ produced by _____
27. -oid _____ resembling _____
28. -ole _____ small _____
29. -ac; -al; -ary; -eal;
    -ic; -ous _____ pertaining to _____

Exercise 3-2   IDENTIFYING SUFFIXES

Give the suffix for the following:

1. hernia _____

2. instrument used to measure _____

3. blood condition _____

4. inflammation _____

5. destruction _____

6. enlargement _____

7. abnormal condition _____

8. irrational fear _____

9. drooping _____

10. spitting _____

11. flow, discharge _____

12. hardening _____

13. process _____

14. surgical fusion _____

15. process of recording _____

16. to measure _____

17. surgical fixation _____

18. suture _____

19. process of visually examining
    (a body cavity or organ) _____

20. stopping _____

21. instrument used to cut _____

22. cell _____

23. study of _____

24. formation _____

25. resembling _____

Exercise 3-3   IDENTIFYING SUFFIXES MEANING "PERTAINING TO"

Place a check mark beside each suffix that means "pertaining to."

1. -al _____

2. -ous _____

3. -eal _____

4. -oma _____

5. -ary _____

6. -ule _____

7. -ic _____

8. -ole _____

9. -ac _____

10. -oid _____

Exercise 3-4   IDENTIFYING SUFFIXES INDICATING SURGICAL PROCEDURES

Place a check mark beside the suffix indicating a surgical procedure.

1. -sclerosis   _____

2. -ectomy   _____

3. -plasia   _____

4. -stomy   _____

5. -cyte   _____

6. -pexy   _____

7. -rrhaphy   _____

8. -rrhexis   _____

9. -rrhagia   _____

10. -penia   _____

Exercise 3-5   DEFINITIONS

Define the following terms.

1. mastodynia   _____

2. hematemesis   _____

3. enteritis   _____

4. cerebromalacia _____

5. nephrosis   _____

6. blepharoptosis _____

7. otorrhea   _____

8. phlebostenosis _____

9. mammography   _____

10. orchidoplasty _____

11. tenotomy   _____

12. bronchoscopy   _____

13. histiocyte   _____

14. pharmacist   _____

15. chondroplasia _____

Exercise 3-6   USING ADJECTIVAL SUFFIXES

Complete the medical word by using the correct adjectival suffix to indicate "pertaining to."

Example: cardi**ac**. -ac is the adjectival suffix.

1. ren/ _____ *renal*
2. mamm/ _____ *mammary*
3. pharyng/ _____ *pharyngeal*
4. gastr/ _____ *gastric*
5. ven/ _____ *venous*

Exercise 3-7   SPELLING

Place a check mark beside the terms that are spelled incorrectly. Correct the misspelled words.

1. ophorectomy _____
2. inflamation _____ *inflammation*
3. cephalgia _____
4. pelvmetry _____
5. hemolysis _____
6. spleenorrhexis _____
7. physiology _____
8. orchidoplaste _____
9. hemostasis _____
10. practitionor _____ *practitioner*

4 CHAPTER

Prefixes

CHAPTER ORGANIZATION

This chapter has been designed to help you learn about medical prefixes. It is divided into the following sections:

4.1 Additional Word Parts

4.2 Prefixes Referring to Direction and Position

4.3 Negative Prefixes

4.4 Prefixes Referring to Numbers

4.5 Miscellaneous Prefixes

4.6 Summary of Prefixes That Have the Same Meaning

4.7 Summary of Prefixes That Have the Opposite Meaning

4.8 Putting It All Together

CHAPTER OBJECTIVES

On completion of this chapter, you will be able to do the following:

1. Give meanings for prefixes

2. Distinguish prefixes that signify direction and position from those that signify negation or number

3. Identify prefixes that have the same meaning

4. Identify prefixes that are opposite in meaning

5. Analyze, define, pronounce, and spell medical terms in this chapter

Prefixes tell us how, why, where, when, how much, how many, what position, and what direction. This chapter introduces you to the most common prefixes, but starts by listing new roots, suffixes, and their meanings used in this chapter. The remaining sections display the prefix and its meaning first, followed by examples of terms using the prefix. As in Chapter 3, learn pronunciation first, then the meaning.

4.1   Additional Word Parts

The following roots and suffixes will also be used in this chapter to build medical terms.

Root	Meaning
cellul/o	cell
cis/o	to cut
comat/o	deep sleep
digest/o	digestion
duct/o	to draw
later/o	side; lateral
nat/o	birth
sept/o	infection
son/o	sound

Suffix	Meaning
-aise	ease
-ar	pertaining to
-cuspid	projection; cusps
-drome	to run
-form	shape; form

continued on page 54

continued from page 53

Suffix	Meaning
-genous	produced by
-gnosis	knowledge
-mortem	death
-plasm	development; formation
-plegia	paralysis
-version	turning; tilting

4.2   Prefixes Referring to Direction and Position

The following prefixes tell us which direction, where, when, and how much.

	ab-	away from
Term	**Term Analysis**	**Definition**
ab**duct**ion (ab-**DUCK**-shun)	-ion = process **duct/o** = to draw	process of drawing away from (see Figure 8-3B)
	ad-	**toward**
ad**duct**ion (ah-**DUCK**-shun)	-ion = process **duct/o** = to draw	process of drawing toward (see Figure 8-3B)

Memory Key   The prefix ad- means "to draw toward." Remember this example: when you add something, you bring it toward you.

	ante-	before
ante**nat**al (an-tee-**NAY**-tal)	-al = pertaining to **nat/o** = birth	pertaining to before birth, referring to the fetus; prenatal *NOTE:* Fetus is the name given to the unborn infant.

Memory Key The prefix ante- means "before." Both the prefix and its meaning contain the letter *e*, making them easy to remember. Compare with anti- (against) in section 4.3.

	circum-	around
Term	**Term Analysis**	**Definition**
circum**duct**ion (**ser**-kum-**DUCK**-shun)	-ion = process **duct/o** = to draw	process of drawing a part in a circular motion (see Figure 8-3E)
	dia-	**through; complete**
diameter (dye-**AM**-eh-ter)	-meter = measurement	measurement from edge to edge of a circle *NOTE:* In this word, the suffix -meter means measurement not instrument used to measure
diagnosis (**dye**-ag-**NOH**-sis)	-gnosis = knowledge	one disease is differentiated from another disease after complete knowledge of the disease is obtained through a study of the signs and symptoms, and through laboratory, x-ray, and other diagnostic procedures
	ecto-	**outside**
ectogenous (eck-**TOJ**-eh-nus)	-genous = produced by; produced from	produced from the outside; infection that originates from the outside
	endo-	**within**
endoscope (**EN**-doh-skohp)	-scope = instrument used to visually examine a body cavity or organ	instrument used to visually examine a body cavity or organ. *NOTE:* Endoscopes are named after the organ being examined. For example, in Figure 4-1, a gastroscope, laparoscope, and a colonoscope are used to visualize the stomach, abdominal cavity, and colon, respectively.

FIGURE 4-1
Endoscopes: (A) gastroscope;
(B) laparoscope; (C) colonoscope

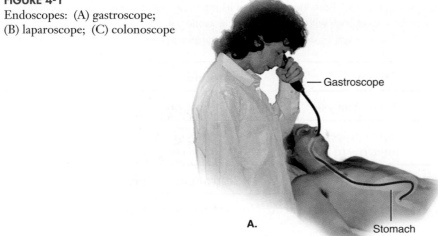

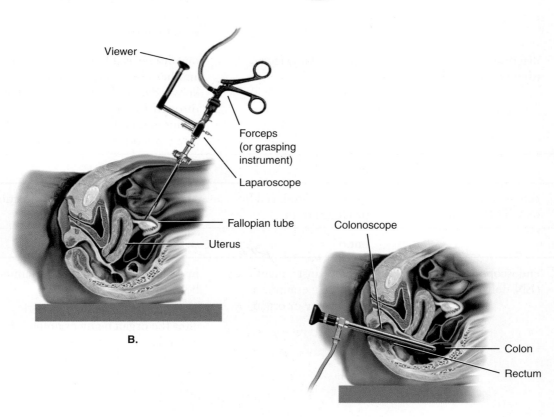

	epi-	upon; on; above
Term	**Term Analysis**	**Definition**
epi**gastr**ic (ep-ih-**GAS**-trick)	-ic = pertaining to **gastr/o** = stomach	pertaining to upon the stomach
	e-; ex-; exo-; extra-	**out; outward; outside**
eversion (ee-**VER**-zhun)	-version = process of turning	process of turning out, as in the turning of the sole of the foot outward (see Figure 4-2)
ex**cis**ion (eck-**SIH**-zhun)	-ion = process **cis/o** = cut	process of cutting out
extra**ocul**ar (**ecks**-trah-**OCK**-you-lar)	-ar = pertaining to **ocul/o** = eye	pertaining to outside the eye

Memory Key   Ex- means "out," as in exit.

FIGURE 4-2
Inversion and eversion

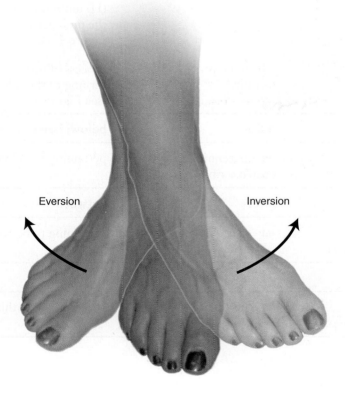

Eversion   Inversion

Term	Term Analysis	Definition
	hyper-	**excessive; above**
hyperplasia (**high**-per-**PLAY**-zha)	-plasia = formation; development	excessive formation; increase in the number of normal cells
	hypo-	**below; under; deficient**
hypo**gastr**ic (high-poh-**GAS**-trick)	-ic = pertaining to **gastr/o** = stomach	pertaining to below the stomach
	in-	**in; into**
in**cis**ion (in-**SIH**-zhun)	-ion = process **cis/o** = to cut	process of cutting into. *NOTE:* Types of incisions include (A) McBurney, over the appendix; (B) Pfannenstiel, a curved lower abdominal incision; (C) subcostal, below the ribs; (D) suprapubic, above the pubic area; (E) transverse, a horizontal incision; (F) midline or epigastric, vertical incision at the midline; (G) paramedian, vertical incision near the midline; and (H) umbilical cord incision, through the umbilicus for scopic surgery (see Figure 4-3).
inversion (in-**VER**-zhun)	-version = process of turning	process of turning in, as in the turning of the sole of the foot inward (see Figure 4-2)
	infra-	**below; beneath**
infra**cost**al (in-frah-**KOS**-tal)	-al = pertaining to **cost/o** = rib	pertaining to below the ribs
	inter-	**between**
inter**cellul**ar (**in**-ter-**SEL**-yoo-lar)	-ar = pertaining to **cellul/o** = cell	pertaining to between the cells
	intra-	**within**
intra**crani**al (**in**-trah-**KRAY**-nee-al)	-al = pertaining to **crani/o** = skull	pertaining to within the skull

FIGURE 4-3
Types of abdominal incisions

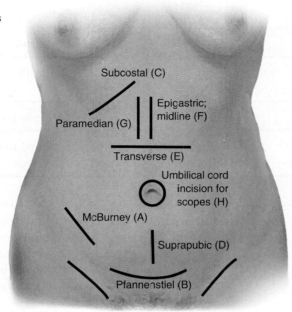

Subcostal (C)

Epigastric;
midline (F)

Paramedian (G)

Transverse (E)

Umbilical cord
incision for
scopes (H)

McBurney (A)

Suprapubic (D)

Pfannenstiel (B)

	meta-	beyond
Term	**Term Analysis**	**Definition**
metaplasia (met-ah-**PLAY**-zha)	-plasia = formation; development	change in formation
metastasis (meh-**TAS**-tah-sis)	-stasis = stopping; controlling	the uncontrolled spread of cancerous cells from one organ to another. *NOTE:* A malignant tumor will undergo metastasis.
	para-	**beside; near**
para**nas**al (par-ah-**NAY**-zal)	-al = pertaining to **nas/o** = nose	pertaining to near the nose
	per-	**through**
per**cutane**ous (**per**-kyou-**TAY**-nee-us)	-ous = pertaining to **cutane/o** = skin	pertaining to through the skin
	peri-	**around**
peri**neur**itis (**per**-ih-nyou-**RYE**-tis)	-itis = inflammation **neur/o** = nerve	inflammation around a nerve

Term	Term Analysis	Definition
	post–	**after**
postmortem (pohst-**MOR**-tehm)	-mortem = death	after death
	pre–	**before; in front of**
prenatal (pre-**NAY**-tal)	-al = pertaining to **nat/o** = birth	pertaining to before birth, referring to the fetus
	pro–	**before**
prodrome (**proh**-drohm)	-drome = to run	symptom or symptoms occurring before the onset of disease. For example, chest pain, tiredness, and shortness of breath are prodromal symptoms of a heart attack.
prognosis (prog-**NOH**-sis)	-gnosis = knowledge	prediction or forecast of the outcome of the disease
	retro–	**back; behind**
retroversion (**ret**-roh-**VER**-zhun)	-version = process of turning	backward turning or tipping of an organ
	sub–	**under; below**
subcutaneous (**sub**-kyoo-**TAY**-nee-us)	-ous = pertaining to **cutane/o** = skin	pertaining to under the skin; for example, subcutaneous fat (see Figure 4-4)
sublingual (sub-**LING**-gwahl)	-al = pertaining to **lingu/o** = tongue	pertaining to under the tongue

FIGURE 4-4
Location of skin and subcutaneous fat

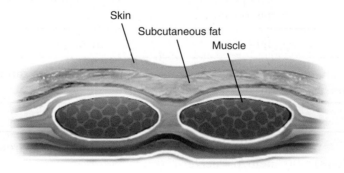

Skin
Subcutaneous fat
Muscle

	supra-	above
Term	**Term Analysis**	**Definition**
suprarenal (**soo**-prah-**REE**-nal)	-al = pertaining to **ren/o** = kidney	pertaining to above the kidney
	trans-	**across**
transection (tran-**SECK**-shun)	-ion = process **sect/o** = cut	process of cutting across (see Figure 4-5)
	ultra-	**beyond**
ultrasonography (**ul**-trah-son-**OG**-) rah-fee)	-graphy = process of recording **son/o** = sound	process of recording an image of internal structures by using high-frequency sound waves; also known as ultrasound (see Figure 4-6)

FIGURE 4-5
Transection

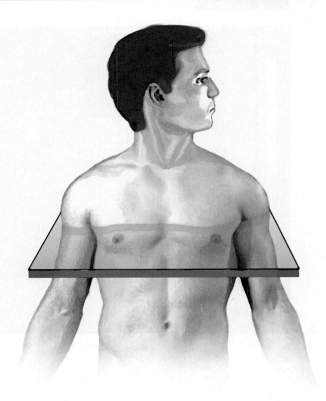

FIGURE 4-6
Ultrasonography:
(A) ultrasonography is often
used to monitor fetal devel-
opment during pregnancy;
(B) fetal ultrasound

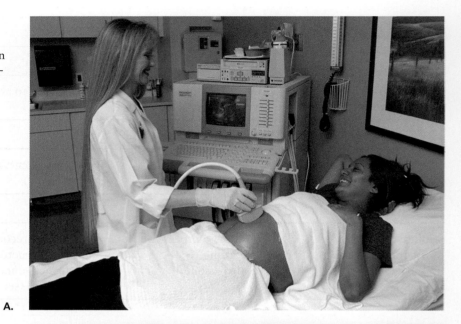

A.

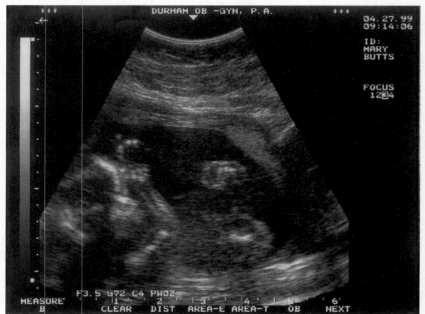

B.

4.3   Negative Prefixes

The following prefixes mean against, not, or lacking.

	anti-	against
Term	**Term Analysis**	**Definition**
antibiotic (**an**-tih-bye-**OT**-ick)	-tic = pertaining to **bi/o** = life	drug used to kill harmful bacteria

> **Memory Key**   The prefix anti- means "against." Both the prefix and its meaning contain the letter *i*, making them easy to remember. Compare with ante- (before) in section 4.2.

	a-; an-	no; not; lack of
aseptic (ay-**SEHP**-tick)	-ic = pertaining to **sept/o** = infection	free from infectious material
anemia (ah-**NEE**-me-ah)	-emia = blood condition	lack of red blood cells (RBCs); lack of hemoglobin (Hgb)

> **Memory Key**   The prefix "a-" is used before roots or suffixes that start with a consonant. The prefix "an-" is used before roots or suffixes that start with a vowel.

	contra-	against; opposite
contralateral (**kon**-trah-**LAH**-ter-al)	-al = pertaining to **later/o** = side	pertaining to the opposite side
	in-	not
indigestible (**in**-dih-**JES**-tih-bl)	-ible = able to be; tending to **digest/o** = digestion	not capable of being digested

4.4 Prefixes Referring to Numbers

The prefixes below tell us how many.

	bi-; di-	**two**
Term	**Term Analysis**	**Definition**
bilateral (bye-**LAT**-er-al)	-al = pertaining to **later/o** = side	pertaining to two sides

Memory Key A bicycle has two wheels.

dissection (dye-**SECK**-shun)	-ion = pertaining to **sect/o** = to cut	to cut into two pieces
	hemi-; semi-	**half**
hemigastrectomy (**hem**-ee-gas-**TRECK**-toh-mee)	-ectomy = excision **gastr/o** = stomach	excision of half the stomach
semicomatose (**sem**-ee-**KOH**-mah-tohs)	semi- = half **comat/o** = deep sleep	state of unconsciousness from which the patient may be aroused
	mono-; uni-	**one**
monocyte (**MON**-oh-sight)	-cyte = cell	blood cell with a single nucleus
unilateral (**you**-nih-**LAT**-er-al)	-al = pertaining to **later/o** = side	pertaining to one side
	multi-; poly-	**many**
multiform (**MUL**-tih-form)	-form = shape; form	having many shapes
polyadenoma (**pol**-ih-ad-eh-**NOH**-mah)	-oma = tumor **aden/o** = gland	tumor of many glands
	quadri-	**four**
quadrilateral (**kwad**-rih-**LAT**-er-al)	-al = pertaining to **later/o** = side	pertaining to four sides

	tri-	three
Term	**Term Analysis**	**Definition**
tricuspid (try-**KUS**-pid)	-cuspid = projection; cusp	three cusps or projections. *NOTE:* The tricuspids or molars are teeth with three projections for grinding and cutting food.

Memory Key   A trio is a group of three.

· ·

4.5   Miscellaneous Prefixes

The following prefixes tell us various qualities.

	ana-	apart; up
Term	**Term Analysis**	**Definition**
anatomy (ah-**NAT**-oh-mee)	-tomy = process of cutting; to cut	the study of the structure of the body. *NOTE:* This term is derived from the fact that, to study structure, one must cut up, or dissect, the body.
	auto-	**self**
autopsy (**AW**-top-see)	-opsy = to view	internal and external examination of the body after death to determine the cause of death; also called necropsy or postmortem examination
	brady-	**slow**
brady**card**ia (**brad**-ee-**KAR**-dee-ah)	-ia = state of; condition **cardi/o** =-heart	pertaining to a slow heartbeat
	dys-	**bad; abnormal; difficult; painful**
dysplasia (dis-**PLAY**-zha)	-plasia = development; formation	abnormal development
	macro-	**large**
macro**cephal**ia (**mack**-roh-seh-**FAY**-lee-ah)	-ia = state of; condition **cephal/o** = head	excessively large head

	mal-	bad
Term	**Term Analysis**	**Definition**
malaise (mah-**LAYZ**)	-aise = ease	a feeling of uneasiness or discomfort; a sign of illness
	micro-	**small**
microscope (**MYE**-kroh-skohp)	-scope = instrument used to visually examine	instrument used to visually examine very small objects
	neo-	**new**
neoplasm (**NEE**-oh-plazm)	-plasm = development; formation	new formation of tissue such as an abnormal growth or tumor
	pan-	**all**
pan**hyster**ectomy (**pan**-hiss-ter-**ECK**-toh-mee)	-ectomy = excision; surgical removal **hyster/o** = uterus	excision of all the uterus
	syn-; sym-	**together; with; joined**
syn**arthr**otic (**sin**-ar-**THRAH**-tick)	-tic = pertaining to **arthr/o** = joint	a type of joint in which the bones are joined
symmetry (**SIM**-eh-tree)	-metry = process of measuring	like parts on opposite sides of the body are similar in form, size, and position

Memory Key syn- becomes sym- before *m*, *b*, and *p*.

	tachy-	fast; rapid
tachy**cardi**a (**tack**-ee-**KAR**-dee-ah)	-ia = condition **cardi/o** = heart	pertaining to fast heartbeat of over 100 beats per minute
	tetra-	**four**
tetraplegia (**tet**-rah-**PLEE**-jee-ah)	**-plegia** = paralysis	paralysis of all four limbs; also known as quadriplegia (**kwad**-rih-**PLEE**-jee-ah)

4.6   Summary of Prefixes That Have the Same Meaning

Some prefixes mean the same thing. For example, epi-, hyper-, and supra- all mean "above." Below is a list of such prefixes:

Meaning	Prefix
above	epi-; hyper-; supra-
against	anti-; contra-
around	circum-; peri-
bad	dys-; mal-
before	ante-; pre-; pro-
below	hypo-; infra-; sub-
half	hemi-; semi-
many	multi-; poly-
one	mono-; uni-;
outside	e-; ex-; extra-; ecto-; exo-
within	endo-; intra-

4.7   Summary of Prefixes That Have the Opposite Meaning

Some prefixes mean exactly the opposite of each other. For example, ab- means "away from" and ad- means "toward." Following is a list of opposite prefixes:

Meaning	Prefix
away from toward	ab- ad-
before after	ante-; pre-; pro- post-

continued on page 68

continued from page 67

Suffix	Meaning
above below	epi-; hyper-; supra- hypo-; infra-; sub-
fast slow	tachy- brady-
excessive deficient	hyper- hypo-
large small	macro- micro-
apart together; with; joined	ana- syn-

4.8   Putting It All Together

Exercise 4-1   DEFINING PREFIXES

Underline, and then define, the prefix in each word.

1. circumduction   _____

2. epigastric   _____

3. hyperplasia   _____

4. infracostal   _____

5. metastasis   _____

6. postmortem   _____

7. retroversion   _____

8. transection   _____

9. contralateral   _____

10. hemigastrectomy   _____

11. tricuspid   _____

12. macrocephalia   _____

13. neoplasm   _____

14. synarthrotic   _____

15. tachycardia   _____

Exercise 4-2 MATCHING

Match the word in Column A with its meaning in Column B.

	Column A		Column B
_____	1. ectogenous	A.	study of structure
_____	2. incision	B.	slow breathing
_____	3. dysplasia	C.	lack of red blood cells
_____	4. bilateral	D.	produced from the outside
_____	5. anatomy	E.	pertaining to between the cells
_____	6. perineuritis	F.	abnormal development
_____	7. anemia	G.	a feeling of uneasiness or discomfort
_____	8. intercellular	H.	pertaining to two sides
_____	9. bradypnea	I.	inflammation around the nerve
_____	10. malaise	J.	process of cutting into

Exercise 4-3 OPPOSITES

Write the prefix that is opposite in meaning to each of the following prefixes.

1. ab- _____

2. ante- _____

3. hyper- _____

4. endo- _____

5. brady- _____

6. micro- _____

7. syn- _____

8. epi- _____

Exercise 4-4 COMPLETION

Complete the word by placing the correct prefix in the blank provided. Definitions are given in the right-hand column.

Example: ***per*** cutaneous   through the skin

1. _____-duction   process of drawing away from

2. _____-natal   before birth, referring to the fetus

3. _____-cision   process of cutting out

4. _____-cision   process of cutting into

5. _____-drome   a symptom occurring before the onset of disease

6. _____-section   process of cutting across

7. _____-digestible   not digestible

8. _____-lateral   pertaining to one side

9. _____-adenoma   tumor of many glands

10. _____-cardia   fast heartbeat

Exercise 4-5 IDENTIFYING PREFIXES WITH THE SAME MEANING

Write the prefixes that mean:

1. bad   _____

2. below   _____

3. above   _____

4. against   _____

5. before   _____

6. around   _____

P A R T II

Body Systems

5 BODY ORGANIZATION

6 THE SKIN (INTEGUMENTARY SYSTEM)

7 THE SKELETAL SYSTEM

8 THE MUSCULAR SYSTEM

9 THE NERVOUS SYSTEM

10 THE EYES AND EARS

11 THE ENDOCRINE SYSTEM

12 THE CARDIOVASCULAR SYSTEM

13 BLOOD AND THE IMMUNE AND LYMPHATIC SYSTEMS

14 THE RESPIRATORY SYSTEM

15 THE DIGESTIVE SYSTEM

16 THE URINARY AND MALE REPRODUCTIVE SYSTEMS

17 THE FEMALE REPRODUCTIVE SYSTEM AND OBSTETRICS

Body Organization

CHAPTER ORGANIZATION

This chapter will help you learn basic anatomy. It is divided into the following sections:

5.1   Cavities and the Arrangement of Body Parts

5.2   Directional Terminology

5.3   Planes of the Body

5.4   Additional Word Parts

5.5   Term Analysis and Definition

5.6   Abbreviations

5.7   Putting It All Together

CHAPTER OBJECTIVES

On completion of this chapter, you will be able to do the following:

1. Name the cavities of the body and their organs
2. Define anatomical position
3. List and define correct terminology used for direction, body planes, and abdominopelvic regions and quadrants
4. Locate the body cavities and abdominopelvic regions and quadrants
5. Analyze, define, pronounce, and spell medical terms in this chapter
6. Define abbreviations common to body organization

INTRODUCTION

This chapter will teach you the common medical terms related to the organization of the body in its various cavities. You will also learn the terms used to describe the positions of the body and the placement of various body parts.

5.1   Cavities and the Arrangement of Body Parts

The body consists of a several cavities, just as a backpack is divided into different sections. The two main body cavities are the **dorsal** (**DOOR**-sal), or back cavity, and the **ventral** (**VEN**-tral), or front cavity. Each is subdivided into smaller additional cavities. The dorsal cavity contains the **cranial** (**KRAY**-nee-al) **cavity** and **spinal** (**SPY**-nal) **cavity**. As the names imply, the cranial cavity contains the brain, and the spinal cavity contains the spinal cord. The spinal cavity is also known as the spinal canal. The ventral cavity contains the **thoracic** (thoh-**RAS**-ick), **abdominal** (ab-**DOM**-ih-nal), and **pelvic** (**PEL**-vick) cavities.

The **diaphragm** (**DYE**-ah-fram), the major respiratory muscle, separates the thoracic cavity from the abdominal cavity. The thoracic cavity contains the heart, lungs, aorta, trachea, and esophagus. The abdominal cavity contains such digestive organs as the stomach, large and small intestines, pancreas, gallbladder, and liver. It also contains the spleen, kidneys, and ureters.

The **pelvic cavity** contains reproductive and urinary organs (excluding the kidneys and ureters). The abdominal and pelvic cavities are frequently referred to as one cavity, called the **abdominopelvic** (ab-**dom**-ih-noh-**PEL**-vick) **cavity**. The body cavities are summarized in Table 5-1 and illustrated in Figure 5-1.

Memory Key • Major cavities are the dorsal and ventral.
  • Subdivisions of the dorsal cavity are the cranial and spinal cavities.
  • Subdivisions of the ventral cavity are the thoracic, abdominal, and pelvic cavities.

TABLE 5-1

SUMMARY OF MAJOR BODY CAVITIES, THEIR SUBDIVISIONS AND ORGANS

SUMMARY OF BODY CAVITIES

MAJOR CAVITIES

Dorsal		Ventral		
Cranial	**Spinal**	**Thoracic**	**Abdominal**	**Pelvic**
↓	↓	↓	↓	↓
contains brain	contains spinal cord	contains heart, lungs, aorta, trachea and esophagus	contains stomach, liver, spleen, kidneys, large and small intestines, pancreas, and gallbladder	contains bladder, urethra, and reproductive organs

FIGURE 5-1
Body cavities

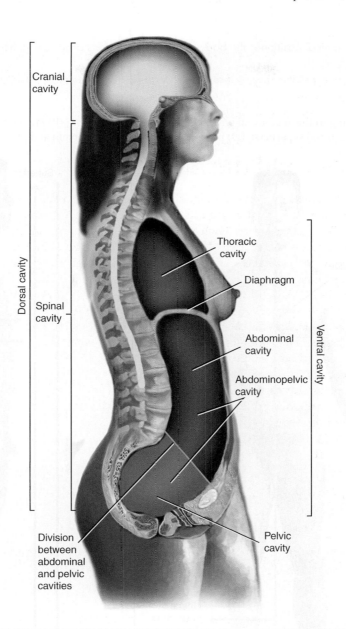

Cranial cavity

Dorsal cavity

Spinal cavity

Thoracic cavity

Diaphragm

Abdominal cavity

Abdominopelvic cavity

Ventral cavity

Division between abdominal and pelvic cavities

Pelvic cavity

5.2   Directional Terminology

ANATOMICAL POSITION

Just as we need directional terms (east, west, etc.) to describe the world in which we live, we need directional terms to describe locations in the body. However, the body can be upright, lying down, and facing different directions. This situation creates a problem in trying to describe location, and it is for this reason that the concept of a standard **anatomical position** was developed (see Figure 5-2A). In the anatomical position, the body is standing erect, arms by the side, with head, palms, and feet facing forward. All directional terms assume that the body is in this position. One must constantly keep the anatomical position in mind when using directional terms.

Memory Key The anatomical position is the body: standing erect, arms at side, with head, palms, and feet facing forward.

FIGURE 5-2
Directional terms relating to the anatomical position: (A) anatomical position; (B) lateral view of the body; (C) directional terms deep and superficial; (D) prone; (E) supine; and (F) dorsum and plantar

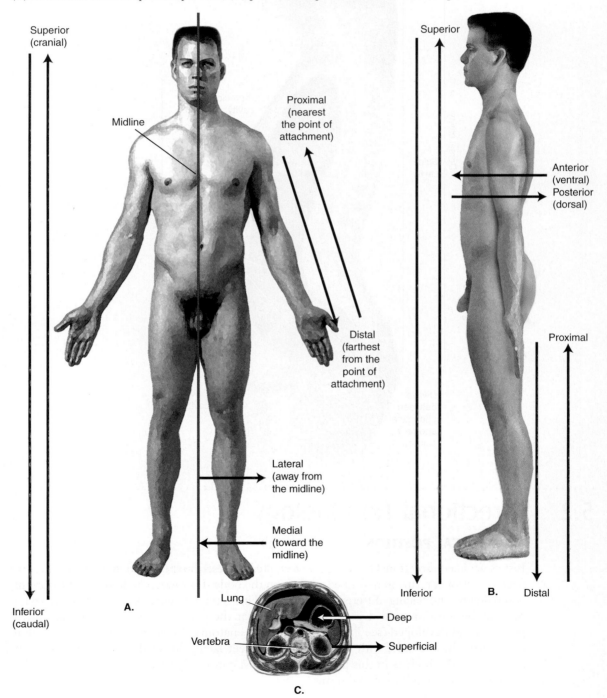

FIGURE 5-2 *continued*

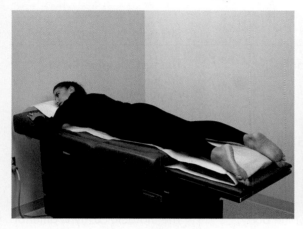

D.

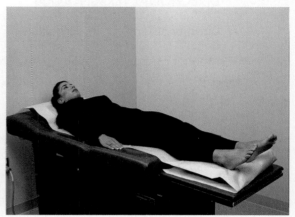

E.

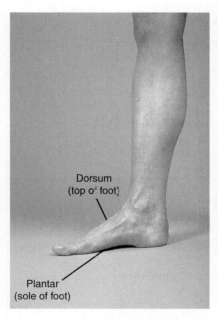

Dorsum
(top of foot)

Plantar
(sole of foot)

F.

DIRECTIONAL TERMS

Directional terms are required for describing the position of body parts, particularly in relation to each other. Table 5-2 lists the directional terms and provides examples of their use. Figure 5-2 illustrates the use of the terms.

TABLE 5-2

DIRECTIONAL TERMINOLOGY

Directional Term	Definition	Example
superior or cranial	above; toward the head	The head is superior to the neck. Cranial nerves originate in the head.
inferior or caudal	below; toward the lower end of the body or tail	The neck is inferior to the head. Caudal anesthesia is injected in the lower spine.
anterior or ventral	front surface of the body; belly side of the body	The thoracic cavity is anterior to the spinal cavity.
posterior or dorsal	back surface of the body	The spinal cavity is posterior to the thoracic cavity.
medial	toward the midline (The midline is an imaginary line drawn down the center of the body from the top of the head to the feet.)	The big toe is medial to the small toe.
lateral	away from the midline	The small toe is lateral to the big toe.
proximal	1. nearest the point of attachment to the trunk. (*NOTE:* This definition is used primarily to describe directions on the arms and legs.) 2. toward the point of origin. (*NOTE:* This definition is used primarily to describe directions pertaining to the digestive tract, with the mouth as the point of origin.)	1. The elbow is proximal to the wrist, and the wrist is proximal to the fingers. 2. The stomach is proximal to the intestines.

continued on page 79

Table 5-2 *continued from page 78*

Directional Term	Definition	Example
distal	farthest from the point of attachment to the trunk; farthest from the point of origin	The knee is distal to the hip, and the ankle is distal to the knee. The intestines are distal to the stomach, and the stomach is distal to the throat.
superficial	near the surface of the body	The skin is superficial to underlying organs.
deep	away from the surface of the body	Muscles are deep to the skin.
supine	lying on the back, face up. (*NOTE:* In relation to the arms, *supine* means the palms are facing toward the front.)	During an operation, the patient may be placed in the supine position.
prone	lying on the abdomen, face down. (*NOTE:* In relation to the arms, *prone* means the palms are facing toward the back.)	During an operation, the patient may be placed in the prone position.
plantar	sole of the foot	Plantar warts are on the sole of the foot.
dorsum	upper portion of the foot	The dorsum of the foot is the top portion.
peripheral	away from the center	Peripheral nerves are the nerves away from the brain and spinal cord. Peripheral blood vessels are in the extremities.

Memory Key   To remember the term *supine*, notice that supine has "up" as part of the word.

ABDOMINOPELVIC REGIONS AND QUADRANTS

The abdominopelvic area of the body has been divided into regions and quadrants for purposes of describing areas of pain and the location of organs within the abdominopelvic cavity. There are nine abdominal regions and four quadrants. Figure 5-3 illustrates the regions. Figure 5-4 illustrates the quadrants.

FIGURE 5-3
Abdominopelvic regions

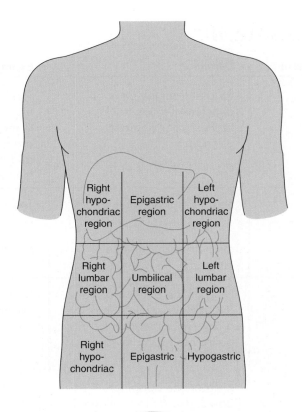

Right hypo-chondriac region	Epigastric region	Left hypo-chondriac region
Right lumbar region	Umbilical region	Left lumbar region
Right hypo-chondriac	Epigastric	Hypogastric

FIGURE 5-4
Abdominopelvic quadrants

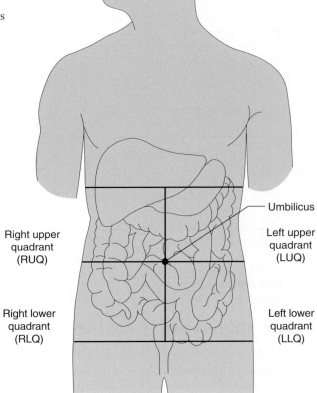

Umbilicus

Right upper quadrant (RUQ)

Left upper quadrant (LUQ)

Right lower quadrant (RLQ)

Left lower quadrant (LLQ)

5.3 Planes of the Body

When internal anatomy is described, we think of the body or organ as being cut or **sectioned** (**SECK**-shunned) in a specific way to make a particular structure clearly visible. Once the body or organ is sectioned, an internal flat surface is exposed. This surface is called a **plane** (**PLAYN**). Because an organ can be cut in different ways, there are different kinds of planes. They are listed in Table 5-3 and illustrated in Figure 5-5.

FIGURE 5-5
Planes of the body

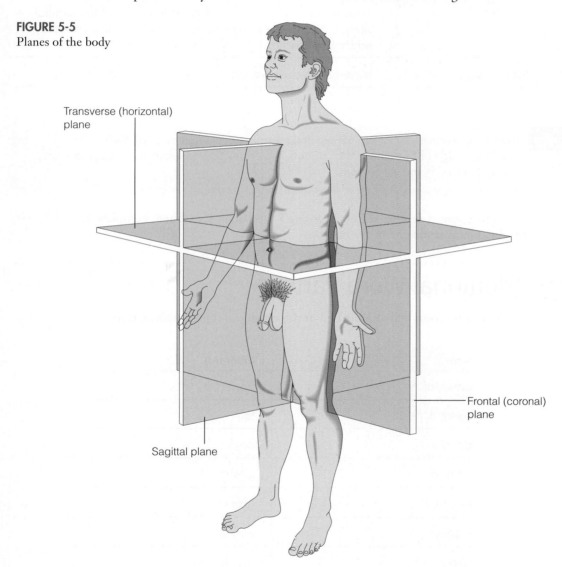

Transverse (horizontal) plane

Frontal (coronal) plane

Sagittal plane

TABLE 5-3

Plane	Definition
frontal; coronal	separates a structure into anterior (front) and posterior (back) portions
Sagittal	separates a structure into right and left sides; if the sagittal section divides the body into equal portions, it is called a **midsagittal** section
transverse; horizontal	separates a structure into superior and inferior portions

Memory Key   To help you remember that sagittal separates a structure into right and left, think of the astrological sign of Sagittarius. With its bow and arrow, Sagittarius can hit a body structure, slicing it into right and left portions.

Before you continue, review Sections 5.1 through 5.3. Then, complete Exercises 5-1 and 5-2 found at the end of the chapter.

5.4   Additional Word Parts

The following roots will also be used in this chapter to build medical terms.

Root	Meaning
anter/o	front
caud/o	tail
dors/o	back
infer/o	inferior
inguin/o	groin
medi/o	middle
phren/o	diaphragm
poster/o	posterior
proxim/o	near

continued on page 83

continued from page 82

Root	Meaning
super/o	superior
ventr/o	front

5.5   Term Analysis and Definition

ROOTS

	gastr/o	stomach
Term	**Term Analysis**	**Definition**
epigastric (ep-ih-**GAS**-trick)	-ic = pertaining to epi- = upon; above	pertaining to upon the stomach (Refers to an abdominal region.)
hypogastric (**high**-poh-**GAS**-trick)	-ic = pertaining to hypo- = below; deficient	pertaining to below the stomach (Refers to an abdominal region.)
	ili/o	**hip**
iliac (**ILL**-ee-ack)	-ac = pertaining to	pertaining to the hip

SUFFIXES

	-al	pertaining to
Term	**Term Analysis**	**Definition**
caudal (**KAW**-dal)	**caud/o** = tail	pertaining to the tail; toward the tail (see Figure 5-2A)
cranial (**KRAY**-nee-al)	**crani/o** = skull	pertaining to the skull (see Figure 5-2A)
dorsal (**DOOR**-sal)	**dors/o** = back	pertaining to the back (see Figure 5-2B) *NOTE:* Think of the dorsal fin of a fish.
inguinal (**ING**-gwih-nal)	**inguin/o** = groin	pertaining to the groin

Term	Term Analysis	Definition
medial (**MEE**-dee-al)	**medi/o** = middle	pertaining to the middle (see Figure 5-2A)
proximal (**PROCK**-sih-mal)	**proxim/o** = near; close	pertaining to that which is near a point of reference (see Figure 5-2A, B)
spinal (**SPYE**-nal)	**spin/o** = spine; spinal column; backbone	pertaining to the spine
ventral (**VEN**-tral)	**ventr/o** = front	pertaining to the front (see Figure 5-2B)
visceral (**VIS**-er-al)	**viscer/o** = internal organ	pertaining to the internal organs
	-ic	**pertaining to**
pelvic (**PEL**-vick)	**pelv/o** = pelvic	pertaining to the pelvis
phrenic (**FREN**-ick)	**phren/o** = diaphragm	pertaining to the diaphragm
thoracic (thoh-**RAS**-ick)	**thorac/o** = chest; thorax	pertaining to the chest
	-ior	**pertaining to**
anterior (an-**TEER**-ee-or)	**anter/o** = front	pertaining to the front of the body or organ (see Figure 5-2B)
inferior (in-**FEER**-ee-or)	**infer/o** = below; downward	pertaining to below or in a downward position; a structure below another structure (see Figure 5-2B)
posterior (pos-**TEER**-ee-or)	**poster/o** = back	pertaining to the back of the body or an organ (see Figure 5-2B)
superior (soo-**PEER**-ee-or)	**super/o** = above; toward the head	pertaining to a structure or organ situated either above another or toward the head (see Figure 5-2B)

5.6   Abbreviations

Abbreviation	Meaning
LLQ	left lower quadrant
LUQ	left upper quadrant
RLQ	right lower quadrant
RUQ	right upper quadrant

5.7   Putting It All Together

Exercise 5-1   TRUE OR FALSE

1. The diaphragm is a muscle.	T	F
2. The liver is located in the pelvic cavity.	T	F
3. The abdominal cavity is inferior to the thoracic cavity.	T	F
4. The big toe is lateral to the small toe.	T	F
5. The wrist is proximal to the elbow.	T	F
6. Prone is lying on the back, face up.	T	F
7. The left iliac region is in the left lower quadrant.	T	F
8. *Supine* refers to the palms facing toward the back.	T	F
9. *Dorsum* may refer to the back portion of a structure.	T	F
10. The right hypochondriac region of the abdomen is in the RUQ.	T	F
11. The coronal plane separates a structure into anterior and posterior portions.	T	F
12. The sagittal plane separates a structure into right and left portions.	T	F

Exercise 5-2   MATCHING

Match each directional term in Column A with its meaning in Column B.

Column A	Column B
_____ 1. superior	A. away from the midline
_____ 2. superficial	B. toward the midline
_____ 3. peripheral	C. near or toward the surface of the body
_____ 4. lateral	D. away from the center

———————   5. proximal   E. farthest away from the point of attachment to the trunk

———————   6. caudal   F. above

———————   7. medial   G. nearest the point of attachment to the trunk

———————   8. distal   H. toward the tail

Exercise 5-3   DEFINITIONS

Underline the root or combining form, and then define the medical word.

1. hypogastric   _____

2. iliac   _____

3. dorsal   _____

4. inguinal   _____

5. visceral   _____

6. cranial   _____

7. phrenic   _____

8. anterior   _____

9. superior   _____

10. thoracic   _____

11. caudal   _____

The Integumentary System and Related Structures

CHAPTER ORGANIZATION

This chapter will help you understand the skin (the integumentary system). It is divided into the following sections:

6.1 Anatomy and Physiology of the Skin

6.2 Related Organs

6.3 Additional Word Parts

6.4 Term Analysis and Definition

6.5 Cosmetic Surgery

6.6 Common Diseases

6.7 Abbreviations

6.8 Putting It All Together

6.9 Review of Vocabulary

6.10 Medical Terms in Context

CHAPTER OBJECTIVES

On completion of this chapter, you will be able to do the following:

1. State the differences among the epidermis, dermis, and subcutaneous tissue as to structure and function

2. Describe how epithelial cells, melanocytes, and keratinocytes are related to the epidermis

3. State the function of fibroblasts, macrophages, mast cells, and plasma cells as they relate to the dermis

4. Describe the structure and function of the hair and nails

5. Name and describe the function of the skin glands

6. Locate the structures of the skin and accessory organs on a diagram

7. Analyze, define, pronounce, and spell medical terms common to the skin

8. Describe common diseases of the skin

9. Define abbreviations common to the skin

INTRODUCTION

This is the first of the body system chapters. For the remainder of the text, you will learn medical terms in the context of the system studied.

The **integumentary** (in-teg-you-**MEN**-tah-ree) system gets its name from the Latin word *integumentum*, meaning "covering." This system is the covering of the body. The skin is by far the major part, but also included are related structures such as hair, glands, and nails.

....

6.1   Anatomy and Physiology of the Skin

Most people do not think of the skin as an organ, but in fact, it is the largest organ of the body. It has two layers. The outer layer is the **epidermis** (ep-ih-**DER**-mis). The inner layer is the **dermis**. Underlying the dermis is the **subcutaneous** (sub-kyoo-**TAY**-nee-us) layer, but it is not regarded as part of the skin. Figure 6-1 illustrates the skin.

> **Memory Key**   The skin consists of the epidermis and the dermis.

EPIDERMIS

As described in Chapter 2, cells make up tissue and tissue makes up organs. The epidermis (an organ), consists primarily of **epithelial** (ep-ih-**THEE**-lee-al) cells. The tissue is known as epithelial tissue, or **epithelium** (ep-ih-**THEE**-lee-um). The epidermis covers the body and lines body cavities and covers organs. Specialized cells called **melanocytes** (meh-**LAN**-oh-sights) are responsible for skin color. These cells produce **melanin** (**MEL**-ah-nin), a pigment. The more melanin produced, the darker the skin. **Keratinocytes** (keh-**RAT**-in-oh-sights), other specialized cells, are important because they produce **keratin** (**KER**-ah-tin), a protein that infiltrates the outermost layer of epithelial cells and makes them tough, waterproof, and resistant to bacteria. The cells that have been filled with keratin are called **keratinized** cells.

There are four layers (strata) of epithelium in the epidermis covering most of the body, but the soles of the feet and palms of the hands have five layers because of the need for extra thickness. This extra layer causes the palms and soles to appear lighter than the rest of the skin, because the melanocytes are found in the deeper layers. At the deepest, or **basal cell**, layer of the epidermis, epithelial cells are constantly being produced, pushing the older cells toward the more superficial layers, where they die and become filled with keratin. This is a continuous process taking about two weeks. The most superficial layer is sometimes called the horny (hornlike) layer, and its medical name is the **stratum corneum** (**STRAY**-tum **KOR**-nee-um). The cells in this layer are continuously being shed.

There are no blood vessels or nerves in the epidermis.

> **Memory Key**   The epidermis consists of epithelial cells, melanocytes, and keratinocytes. The tissue type is epithelium.

FIGURE 6-1
The skin

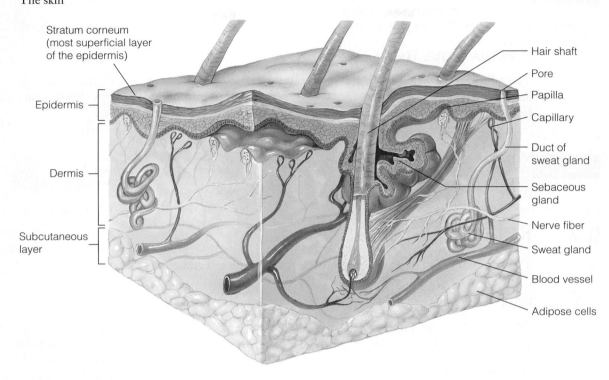

Stratum corneum
(most superficial layer
of the epidermis)

Epidermis

Dermis

Subcutaneous
layer

Hair shaft

Pore

Papilla

Capillary

Duct of
sweat gland

Sebaceous
gland

Nerve fiber

Sweat gland

Blood vessel

Adipose cells

DERMIS

The dermis lies beneath the deepest layer of the epidermis. It is a thick area of **connective tissue** containing hair follicles, blood vessels, nerves, and glands. The dermis contains blood vessels and therefore supplies nutrients for the skin. These blood vessels also help control inner body temperature through a process called thermoregulation. When the body needs to lose heat, the vessels in the dermis dilate (expand), allowing a greater volume of blood to be cooled near the surface. When the body is cold, the same vessels constrict (contract), reducing heat loss. Sensory receptors in the dermis are responsible for our sense of touch. The glands secrete substances necessary for skin maintenance and function (see Glands in section 6.2).

The tissue of the dermis consists of four types of cells, which strengthen and protect the skin: **fibroblasts** (**FIGH**-broh-blasts), **macrophages** (**MACK**-roh-fay-jeez), **mast cells**, and **plasma cells**. Fibroblasts produce collagen (**KAHL**-ah-jen) and elastin. Collagen is the most abundant protein in the body. It is found in bones, tendons, cartilage, and skin. Like a piece of string, collagen can be bent, but it resists breaking and stretching, and therefore makes the skin tough and durable. Elastin is also a protein, but unlike collagen, it allows tissue to stretch and then recoil to its original length. This is evident during pregnancy when the abdominal skin stretches to accommodate the growing fetus. Macrophages engulf bacteria and other potentially harmful foreign substances. Mast cells produce **histamine** (**HISS**-tah-meen), and plasma cells produce **antibodies**. Both histamine and antibodies act against foreign materials.

Memory Key The dermis is connective tissue containing hair follicles, blood vessels, nerves, and glands. It consists of fibroblasts, macrophages, mast cells, and plasma cells.

SUBCUTANEOUS TISSUE

The subcutaneous tissue is a layer of connective tissue that is not part of the skin. It is important because it connects the dermis to the muscles and organs below it. It also contains fatty tissue, which insulates inner structures from temperature extremes.

A summary of the anatomy and physiology of the skin is given in Table 6-1.

Memory Key Subcutaneous tissue connects the dermis to inner structures and provides insulation.

6.2   Related Organs

The hair, nails, and glands are the other organs of the integumentary system.

HAIR

As you can see in Figure 6-2, each hair is a long, slender, tube-shaped structure. It grows from epidermal cells at the base of a tube-like depression called a hair **follicle** (**FALL**-ih-kul). At the lower end of each hair is a bulb. The bottom of the bulb is indented. This indentation is called a hair **papilla** (pah-**PILL**-ah). The papilla contains blood vessels

TABLE 6-1

SUMMARY OF THE ANATOMY AND PHYSIOLOGY OF THE EPIDERMIS AND DERMIS

Epidermis		Dermis	
Cells:	epithelial melanocytes keratinocytes	**Cells:**	fibroblasts macrophages mast cells plasma cells
Tissue:	epithelial tissue	**Tissue:**	connective tissue
Function:	protection	**Function:**	temperature regulation sensation secretion nutrition protection

FIGURE 6-2
Hair and related
structures

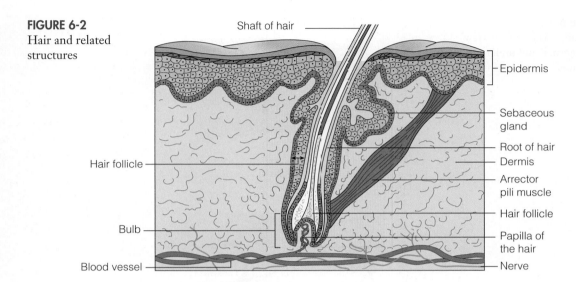

Shaft of hair

Epidermis

Sebaceous
gland

Root of hair

Dermis

Arrector
pili muscle

Hair follicle

Papilla of
the hair

Nerve

Hair follicle

Bulb

Blood vessel

to nourish the hair and promote growth. Hair grows from the root out. As the cells move away from their source of nutrition, they die and become keratinized, forming the shaft of the hair. When a new hair starts to grow, the shaft of hair pushes its way out of the follicle, and then above the surface of the skin. Because melanin production decreases with aging, hair loses its color and turns gray.

Memory Key   Hair is formed in a hair follicle. The shaft of the hair consists of keratinized cells.

NAILS

Nails are epithelial cells that have been keratinized. New cells form at the moon, or **lunula** (**LOO**-noo-lah), pushing the other cells toward the end of the finger or toe along the nailbed underlying the nail. A fingernail is illustrated in Figure 6-3. The cuticle, or **eponychium** (**ep**-oh-**NICK**-ee-um), overlaps onto the nail. It also consists of keratinized epithelial cells, but the keratin is much softer than on the rest of the nail.

Memory Key   The nail and cuticle consist of keratinized epithelial cells.

GLANDS

The skin glands (see Figure 6-1) are very important to the maintenance of skin health and function. **Sebaceous** (seh-**BAY**-shus) **glands** secrete an oil called **sebum** (**SEE**-bum), which keeps the skin soft and waterproof. It also keeps the hair pliable; without sebum, the hair would become brittle and would break.

The **sudoriferous** (**soo**-dor-**IF**-er-us) **glands**, or sweat glands, play a role in thermo-regulation by secreting sweat onto the surface of the skin. Evaporation of the sweat cools the skin.

The **ceruminous** (seh-**ROO**-min-us) **glands** produce **cerumen** (seh-**ROO**-men) in the ear, which is a waxy substance that helps prevent bacterial infection.

FIGURE 6-3
The nail: (A) posterior view; (B) fingernail and underlying structures

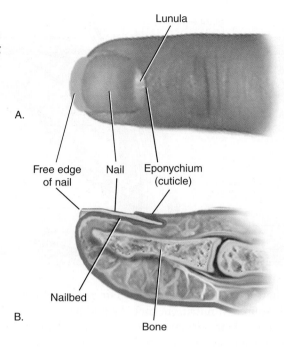

> **Memory Key**   Sebaceous glands secrete sebum to lubricate the skin and hair. Sudoriferous glands secrete sweat to cool the skin. Ceruminous glands secrete cerumen in the ear to prevent infection.

Before you continue, review Sections 6.1 and 6.2. Then, complete Exercises 6-1 and 6-2 found at the end of the chapter.

6.3   Additional Word Parts

The following roots and suffixes will also be used in this chapter to build medical terms.

Root	Meaning
cry/o	cold
leuk/o	white
papill/o	nipple-like
scler/o	hardening
xer/o	dry

Suffix	Meaning
-ism	process
-ium; -um	structure
-sis	state of; condition

6.4   Term Analysis and Definition

ROOTS

	albin/o	white
Term	**Term Analysis**	**Definition**
albinism (**AL**-bih-niz-um)	-ism = process	lack of pigment in the skin, hair, and eyes
	adip/o (see also lip/o and steat/o)	**fat**
adipose (**AD**-ih-pohs)	-ose = pertaining to	pertaining to fat
	bi/o	**life**
skin biopsy (**BYE**-op-see)	-opsy = to view	a piece of living tissue is removed for microscopic examination
	cutane/o (see also derm/o; dermat/o)	**skin**
subcutaneous (**sub**-kyoo-**TAY**-nee-us)	sub- = under -ous = pertaining to	pertaining to under the skin
	cyan/o	**blue**
cyanotic (**sigh**-ah-**NOT**-ick)	-tic = pertaining to	pertaining to a bluish discoloration of skin
	derm/o; dermat/o	**skin**
dermatitis (**der**-mah-**TYE**-tis)	-itis = inflammation	inflammation of the skin (see Figure 6-4)
dermatology (**der**-mah-**TOL**-oh-jee)	-logy = study	study of the skin and its diseases

FIGURE 6-4
Dermatitis caused by
poison oak
*(Courtesy Timothy Berger, MD,
Clinical Professor, University
of California San Francisco,
Department of Dermatology)*

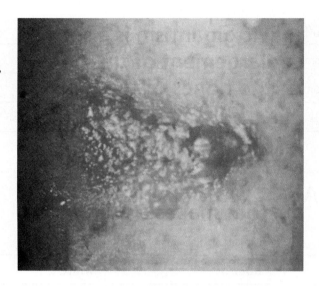

Term	Term Analysis	Definition
dermatologist (**der**-mah-**TOL**-oh-jist)	-logist = one who specializes in the study of	one who specializes in the study of the skin and its diseases
hypodermic (**high**-poh-**DER**-mick)	-ic = pertaining to hypo- = under; below	pertaining to below the skin; subcutaneous. *NOTE:* The prefixes hypo- and sub- cannot be interchanged. Hypo- is used with the root **derm/o**, and sub- is used with the root **cutane/o**.
dermatoplasty (der-**MA**-toh-**plast**-ee)	-plasty = surgical reconstruction	surgical reconstruction of the skin; surgical replacement of injured or diseased skin
	diaphor/e	**profuse sweating**
diaphoresis (**dye**-ah-foh-**REE**-sis)	-sis = state of; condition	state of profuse sweating; hyperhidrosis
	epitheli/o	**covering**
epithelium (**ep**-ih-**THEE**-lee-um)	-um = structure	structure made up of epithelial cells covering the internal and external surfaces of the body
epithelial (**ep**-ih-**THEE**-lee-al)	-al = pertaining to	pertaining to the epithelium

	erythemat/o (see also erythr/o)	red
Term	**Term Analysis**	**Definition**
erythematous (**er**-ih-**THEM**-ah-tus)	-ous = pertaining to	pertaining to a redness of the skin. *NOTE:* Erythematous is an adjective.
	erythr/o	**red**
erythema (**er**-ih-**THEE**-mah)		red discoloration to the skin; erythroderma. *NOTE:* Erythema is a noun.
	hidr/o	**sweat**
anhidrosis (**an**-high-**DROH**-sis)	-osis = abnormal condition a(n)- = no; not; lack of	lack of sweat
hyperhidrosis (**high**-per-high-**DROH**-sis)	-osis = abnormal condition hyper- = excessive; above normal	excessive secretion of sweat; diaphoresis
	kerat/o; keratin/o	**hard; hornlike**
hyperkeratosis (**high**-per-ker-ah-**TOH**-sis)	-osis = abnormal condition hyper- = excessive; above normal	excessive growth of the outer layer of skin (hornlike layer)
keratinocyte (ker-**RAT**-in-oh-sight)	-cyte = cell	cell that produces keratin
	lip/o	**fat**
lipoma (lih-**POH**-mah)	-oma = tumor; mass	tumor or mass containing fat
liposuction (**LIP**-oh-**suck**-shun)	suction = process of aspirating or withdrawing	withdrawal of fat from the subcutaneous tissue. (See Section 6.5, Cosmetic Surgery.)
	melan/o	**black**
melanocyte (mel-**LAN**-oh-sight)	-cyte = cell	cell that produces melanin

	myc/o	**fungus**
Term	**Term Analysis**	**Definition**
dermatomycosis (**der**-mah-toh-my-**KOH**-sis)	-osis = abnormal condition **dermat/o** = skin	fungal infection of the skin
	necr/o	**death**
necrotic tissue (neh-**KROT**-ick)	-tic = pertaining to	pertaining to death of tissues *NOTE:* An example of necrotic tissue is a pressure sore, also known as a bedsore or decubitus ulcer. This is defined as dead skin, usually over a bony prominence, due to a lack of circulation and loss of oxygen to the skin. It may occur when a patient is kept in the same position, without being moved, for an extended length of time (see Figure 6-5).
	onych/o (see also ungu/o)	**nail**
eponychium	-ium = structure epi- = upon; above	structure upon the nail; the cuticle (**ep**-oh-**NICK**-ee-um)
onychomycosis (**on**-ih-koh-my-**KOH**-sis)	-osis = abnormal condition **myc/o** = fungus	fungal infection of the nail
paronychia (**par**-oh-**NICK**-ee-ah)	-ia = condition para- = beside; near	inflammation of the tissue around the nail. *NOTE:* The suffix -itis, meaning "inflammation," is not used in this term (see Figure 6-6).

FIGURE 6-5
Pressure sore or decubitus ulcer
(Permission to reproduce this copyrighted material has been granted by the owner, Hollister Incorporated)

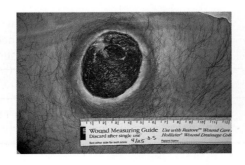

FIGURE 6-6
Paronychia

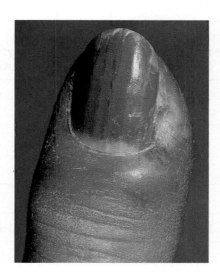

	pil/o	hair
Term	**Term Analysis**	**Definition**
pilosebaceous (**pye**-loh-seh-**BAY**-shus)	-ous = pertaining to **seb/o** = sebum	pertaining to hair follicles and sebaceous glands
	py/o	**pus**
pyogenic (**pye**-oh-**JEN**-ick)	-genic = producing	pus producing. For example, pyogenic bacteria produces pus.
	ras/o	**scrape**
abrasion (ab-**BRAY**-zhun)	-ion = process ab- = away from	scraping away of the superficial layers of injured skin; for example, injury from a floor burn
	rhytid/o	**wrinkle**
rhytidectomy (**RIT**-ih-**DECK**-tah-mee)	-ectomy = surgical excision; removal	removal of wrinkles; facelift
	seb/o	**sebum**
seborrhea (**seb**-oh-**REE**-ah)	-rrhea = flow; discharge	increased discharge of sebum from the sebaceous glands
	steat/o	**fat**
steatoma (**stee**-ah-**TOH**-mah)	-oma = tumor; mass	fatty tumor of the sebaceous glands

	ungu/o	nail
Term	**Term Analysis**	**Definition**
periungual (**per**-ee-**UNG**-gwal)	-al = pertaining to peri- = around	pertaining to around the nail

SUFFIXES

	-dermis; -derma	skin
Term	**Term Analysis**	**Definition**
epidermis (**ep**-ih-**DER**-mis)	epi- = upon; above	above the dermis
erythroderma (eh-**rith**-roh-**DER**-mah)	**erythr/o** = red	redness of the skin; erythema
leukoderma (**loo**-koh-**DER**-mah)	**leuk/o** = white	lack of pigmentation of the skin showing up as white patches; vitiligo
pyoderma (**pye**-oh-**DER**-mah)	**py/o** = pus	any pus-producing disease of the skin
scleroderma (**skleh**-roh-**DER**-mah)	**scler/o** = hardening	abnormal thickening of the dermis, usually starting in the hands and feet
xeroderma (**zer**-oh-**DER**-mah)	**xer/o** = dry	dry skin of a chronic (continuous) nature
	-oma	**tumor; mass**
adenoma (**ad**-eh-**NOH**-mah)	**aden/o** = gland	tumor of a gland
carcinoma (**kar**-sih-**NOh**-mah)	**carcin/o** = cancerous	malignant tumor of epithelial cells. Examples include: **basal cell carcinoma**, a malignant tumor that is the most common and least harmful type of skin cancer usually caused by overexposure to the sun (see Figure 6-7A); and **squamous cell carcinoma**, a malignant tumor that is more harmful and has a faster growing rate and tendency to metastasize (spread) to other body systems (see Figure 6-7B).

FIGURE 6-7

Carcinoma: (A) basal cell; (B) squamous cell *(Courtesy of Robert A. Silverman, MD, Pediatric Dermatology, Georgetown University)*

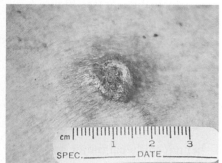

A.

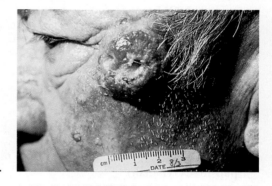

B.

Term	Term Analysis	Definition
hemangioma (heh-**man**-jee-**OH**-mah)	**hem/o** = blood **angi/o** = vessel	a common, benign tumor of blood vessels. Also known as birthmarks or nevi (singular = nevus) (see Figure 6-8).

FIGURE 6-8

Hemangioma

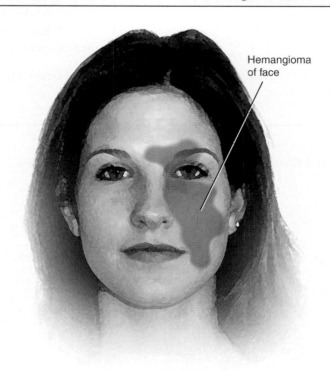

Hemangioma of face

Term	Term Analysis	Definition
melanoma (**mel**-ah-**NOH**-mah)	**melan/o** = black	tumor arising from the melanocytes; usually malignant (see Figure 6-9) *NOTE:* Treatment may include **Mohs'** (**MOHZ**) surgery. The tumor is removed in thin horizontal layers under microscopic examination. Successive layers are removed until microscopic examination reveals no more cancerous cells.
papilloma (**pap**-ih-**LOH**-mah)	**papill/o** = nipple-like	benign epithelial tumor
	-therapy	**treatment**
cryotherapy (**kri**-oh-**THER**-ah-pee)	**cry/o** = cold	destruction of tissue by freezing with liquid nitrogen
laser therapy (**LAY**-zer)	laser = intense beam of light	an intense beam of light is used to remove unwanted tissue. (See Section 6.5, Cosmetic surgery.) *NOTE:* In this example, therapy is used as a word rather than a suffix.
radiotherapy (**ray**-dee-oh-**THER**-ah-pee)	radi/o = x-rays	use of x-rays and radiation to treat cancer

FIGURE 6-9

Melanoma (*Courtesy of Robert A. Silverman, MD, Pediatric Dermatology, Georgetown University*)

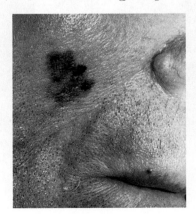

PREFIXES

	derma-	skin
Term	**Term Analysis**	**Definition**
dermabrasion (der-mah-**BRAY**-zhun)	-ion = process ab- = away from **ras/o** = scrape	scraping away of the top layers of skin using sandpaper or wire brushes to remove tattoos or disfigured skin. The skin then regenerates with little scarring (see microdermabrasion in Section 6.5, Cosmetic Surgery).

6.5   Cosmetic Surgery

Cosmetic surgery, also called plastic surgery, consists of a variety of procedures designed to improve appearance. Laser surgery has become the treatment of choice for many conditions. Facial renewal is achieved through several different techniques. Liposuction is commonly utilized to reduce fat deposits. Hair implantation is the most effective treatment for baldness. More extensive procedures involving traditional surgical techniques often require some period of hospitalization.

LASER SURGERY

There are several different types of lasers, but all lasers use an intense beam of light to remove tissue. There is little if any bleeding, surrounding tissue is not harmed, and the versatility of lasers allows them to be used in hard-to-reach, sensitive places.

Lasers are excellent for the removal of the following kinds of skin blemishes:

- Vascular lesions, which are caused by blood vessels that lie too close to the surface of the skin. They include red patches called port-wine stains, spider veins, and raised red marks called strawberry hemangiomas.
- Tattoos
- Pigmented lesions such as moles and age spots
- Unpigmented lesions such as warts and skin tags
- Stretch marks and scars
- Excessive facial or body hair

Lasers are also used in a procedure called laser resurfacing. The outer portion of the stratum corneum (the outer layer of the skin) is removed to achieve wrinkle reduction and the removal of blemishes such as acne scars.

FACIAL RENEWAL

Laser resurfacing is only one method of facial renewal. Chemical peels achieve much the same results using mild acid solutions to remove the part of the stratum corneum. Another procedure that produces similar results is microdermabrasion. This procedure uses a machine to blast the skin with small particles of aluminum oxide or silica.

Wrinkles can also be effectively reduced with injections of a bacteria-containing substance called botox. Botox blocks nerve impulses that activate tiny facial muscles underlying wrinkles. Because these muscles can no longer contract, the wrinkles do not show as much. However, the effects of botox injection last only a few months, and additional injections are required to maintain the effect.

LIPOSUCTION

Liposuction is used to remove fat deposits. A tube attached to a vacuum is placed through a tiny incision in the skin, and the vacuum removes the fat. A procedure called the tumescent technique involves injecting a saline solution and local anesthetic into the fat before the liposuction is done. This reduces postoperative bruising and swelling. If the fat deposits are large, a technique called ultrasound assisted lipoplasty (UAL) might be used. An ultrasound probe is inserted under the skin. It generates ultrasound waves that liquefy the fat, making it easier to remove by suction.

HAIR IMPLANTATION

Some surgeries, accidents, and scalp infections can cause permanent hair loss. However, hormonal changes are the most common cause of nonreversible hair loss in women. A hereditary condition called male pattern baldness is the leading cause for men.

Creams, pills, and lotions can claim only limited success. Thus, several surgical techniques have been developed to fill the great demand for hair replacement. All involve relocating the patient's own hair.

In some patients, a scalp reduction is used. A piece of bald skin is removed so that hair-covered portions can be stitched together. This can be useful to address hair loss from scars due to accidents or surgery. However, it must be used in conjunction with transplantation of the patient's own hair to effectively remedy large bald areas such as those occurring in male pattern baldness.

A variety of techniques are used to transplant the patient's hair—scalp flaps, strip grafts, and plugs. With the scalp flap approach, a relatively large portion of the scalp with dense hair is surgically relocated to a bald area. The scalp flap is sometimes stretched before relocation. Strip grafts involve the surgical relocation of many long narrow portions of hair-covered scalp to bald areas. Plugs are the most common approach. Several small circular areas of hair-covered scalp are relocated. Plugs are relatively successful and do not require general anesthesia. The micro-plug involves hundreds of tiny grafts implanted over multiple sessions. It is popular because it does not leave the clumped look that results from larger plugs.

TREATMENTS REQUIRING HOSPITAL STAY

Abdominoplasty

Known as the tummy tuck, a full abdominoplasty (ab-**DOM**-ih-noh-plas-tee) is a comparatively lengthy procedure (two–five hours) and frequently is done with a general anesthetic. A circular cut is made from hip bone to hip bone, extending down just above the pelvis. A hole is cut around the navel. The skin is separated from the abdominal wall, from the pelvis to the bottom of the rib cage. A large skin flap is lifted. Excess fat is removed and the vertical muscles of the abdomen are pulled closer together and stitched to maintain the new position. Extra skin is then removed from the skin flap and a new hole is cut to fit around the navel. The incisions are then stitched. A tube might be inserted to drain excess fluid. The result is that the abdominal wall is narrowed and firmed, and the skin is tightened.

A partial abdominoplasty involves separating the skin between the pelvis and the navel The skin flap is stretched down and excess skin and fat are removed. The flap is then stitched into place.

Rhytidectomy

A rhytidectomy (**rit**-ih-**DECK**-tah-mee) is a face-lift. It might be performed under twilight (not completely unconscious) or general anesthesia (completely unconscious) and can involve a brief stay as an inpatient, although many are performed on an outpatient basis.

The rhytidectomy is performed on one side of the face at a time. The incision begins inside the hairline in the temple area, and continues in front of the ear and around the ear lobe, then behind the ear into the hairline. The skin is lifted. Excess skin and fat might be removed. Facial muscles and tissues also might be slightly repositioned. The skin is re-draped, and the incision is finely stitched. Results last five to ten years.

Blepharoplasty

A blepharoplasty (**BLEF**-ah-roh-plas-tee) is a surgical procedure to correct drooping upper eyelids and puffy bags below the eyes. It is frequently carried out under a twilight anesthetic, and patients are usually discharged the same day. This procedure is often carried out in conjunction with a rhytidectomy.

An incision is made in the natural skin crease of the upper eyelid. Excess skin, muscle, and fat are removed, and the upper lid is sculpted and finely stitched.

For the lower eyelid, excess fat can usually be removed from the inside of the lid, thus avoiding an incision. After the fat is removed, skin wrinkling is increased and might be treated with laser exfoliation to stimulate the growth of new collagen and shrink the skin. If the lower lid is excessively baggy and saggy, an incision might be made to remove fat and excess skin. The lid is then finely stitched. Results last for years, and might be permanent.

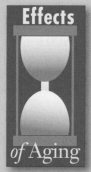

Effects of Aging on the Integumentary System

As people age, the body's collagen starts to break down. Because cellular division also slows with aging, collagen production in the fibroblasts slows. The result is that lost collagen is not fully replaced, and thus the skin becomes loose and wrinkles start to appear in what was once smooth, tight skin.

The number of keratinocytes and melanocytes also decreases, thus, the skin gradually loses its tough outer, keratinized surface. It becomes thinner and more transparent.

The sebaceous glands decrease their production of oils, resulting in dry, itchy skin.

Irregular production of melanin by melanocytes gives rise to brown-colored freckles called age spots or liver spots.

The result of all of these processes is that aged skin is marked with wrinkles and age spots, and becomes dry and thin. Coupled with damage due to smoking and sun exposure, the overall result is decreased skin vitality.

Hair is also affected by the aging process. Hair follicles are less active, and the hair becomes thinner. Some follicles cease hair production altogether, resulting in permanent hair loss.

....

6.6   Common Injuries and Diseases

BURNS

Destruction of the skin by heat, chemicals, electricity, or radiation is called a **burn**. Burns can be classified as first degree, second degree, third degree, or fourth degree, depending on the extent of damage to the epidermis, dermis and deep tissue.

> **First-degree burn** (superficial burn) involves the epidermis. There is erythema but no blisters. An example is a sunburn.
> **Second-degree burn** (partial-thickness burn) involve the epidermis and upper portion of the dermis. The skin is erythematous. There may or may not be blisters.
> **Third-degree burn** (full-thickness burn) involves the epidermis and all of the dermis. The skin is black and charred. The subcutaneous tissue may be damaged.
> **Fourth-degree burn** involves the epidermis, dermis, subcutaneous tissue, and muscle.

In severe burns, where over two-thirds of the body surface has been destroyed, complications can cause death. The three major complications are **shock**, **infection**, and **toxins**.

Shock results from water loss. Ordinarily, the skin prevents water from entering and leaving the body. However, when large amounts of skin are destroyed, water loss can be significant. Loss of fluid leads to a drop in blood pressure, resulting in reduced blood flow to vital organs, or shock.

Infection is also a significant concern in burn patients. The skin is the first line of defense against microbes. When the skin is burned, this defense is lost. Bacteria readily enter the body and can become life-threatening.

Toxins released from burned skin are also a concern because they are poisonous to the body. **Debridement** (dah-breed-**MAW**), the removal of burned skin, prevents these poisonous reactions. In extensive burns, the patient is submerged in a large tank of water called a Hubbard tank, which loosens the skin and makes debridement easier.

Treatment for burns ranges from the application of ointment for minor burns to skin grafting for major burns.

SKIN CANCER

Cancers are malignant tumors (neoplasms) within body tissues. Just as different tissues are named according to their origin (muscle tissue, osseous tissue, nervous tissue), cancers are broadly named according to their tissue of origin. **Melanoma** (mel-ah-**NOH**-mah) is a tumor arising from the melanocytes. **Carcinomas** (kar-sih-**NOH**-mahz) arise from epithelial cells. **Sarcomas** (sar-**KOH**-mahz) arise from connective tissue. One example is Kaposi's sarcoma, a type of skin cancer that is a typical complication of AIDS. **Adenocarcinomas** (**ad**-eh-no-**kar**-sih-**NOH**-mahz) arise from epithelial tissue in glands.

Carcinomas can be further classified by the type of epithelial tissue from which the cancer originated. Squamous cell carcinoma originates from epithelial tissue found in the outer layer of the epidermis. Basal cell carcinoma originates from epithelial tissue in the bottom layer of the epidermis.

6.7   Abbreviations

Abbreviation	Meaning
bx	biopsy
SC; subq, subcut	subcutaneous
UV	ultraviolet

6.8   Putting It All Together

Exercise 6-1   FILL IN THE BLANKS

1. The two layers of skin are the _____ and _____.

2. The layer under the dermis is the _____ layer.

3. The epidermis is void of _____, _____, and _____.

4. The dermis is made up of _____ tissue.

5. The main function of the epidermis is _____.

6. Hair is formed at the _____.

7. Name the glands found in the dermis and their secretions.

Exercise 6-2   MATCHING—ANATOMY

Match the term in Column A with its definition in Column B.

Column A	Column B
_____ 1. basal cell	a. The most superficial layer of the epidermis, sometimes called the horny layer.
_____ 2. epithelium	b. Tissue that lines body cavities and covers the body and body organs.
_____ 3. fibroblasts	c. A protein that makes the epidermis tough, waterproof, and resistant to bacteria.
_____ 4. keratin	d. A substance responsible for skin color.
_____ 5. keratinized cells	e. Cells producing histamine.

_____	6. mast cells	f.	Constriction and dilation of the blood vessels control inner body temperature.
_____	7. melanin	g.	Deepest layer of the epidermis.
_____	8. plasma cells	h.	Cells producing collagen.
_____	9. stratum corneum	i.	Dead epithelial cells that are filled with keratin.
_____	10. thermoregulation	j.	Cells that produce antibodies.

Exercise 6-3   DEFINING ROOTS AND COMBINING FORMS

Underline the root or the combining form in the following words, and then define each word.

1. subcutaneous _____

2. cyanotic _____

3. hypodermic _____

4. epithelial _____

5. erythematous _____

6. hyperhidrosis _____

7. leukoderma _____

8. necrotic _____

9. paronychia _____

10. seborrhea _____

11. steatoma _____

12. rhytidectomy _____

13. xeroderma _____

14. melanoma _____

15. albinism _____

Exercise 6-4   DEFINING SUFFIXES

Give the meaning of each of the following suffixes.

1. -oma _____

2. -ar _____

3. -derma _____

4. -rrhea _____

5. -genic _____

6. -ia _____

7. -ium _____

8. -osis _____

9. -cyte _____

10. -ion _____

11. -al _____

12. -logy _____

Exercise 6-5 BUILDING MEDICAL WORDS

Build the medical word for the following definitions.

1. excision of wrinkles _____

2. pertaining to a bluish discoloration of the skin _____

3. one who specializes in the study of the skin and its diseases _____

4. lack of sweat _____

5. cell that produces melanin _____

6. fungal infection of the skin _____

7. fungal infection of the nail _____

8. hardening of the skin _____

9. malignant tumor of epithelial cells _____

10. malignant tumor arising from the melanocytes _____

Exercise 6-6 MATCHING

Match the word element in Column A with its meaning in Column B.

Column A	Column B
_____ 1. albin/o	A. death
_____ 2. myc/o	B. sweat
_____ 3. hidr/o	C. hard; hornlike
_____ 4. kerat/o	D. white
_____ 5. melan/o	E. nipple-like
_____ 6. necr/o	F. fungus
_____ 7. onych/o	G. black
_____ 8. cry/o	H. cold
_____ 9. papill/o	I. dry
_____ 10. xer/o	J. nail

Exercise 6-7   ANTONYMS (OPPOSITES)

An antonym is a word of opposite meaning. Write the antonym for the following roots. Use the appendices "Word Element to Definition" and "Definition to Word Element" located at the back of the book if necessary.

1. albin/o   _____

2. scler/o   _____

3. cry/o   _____

4. necr/o   _____

Exercise 6-8   SHORT ANSWER—PATHOLOGY

1. Define the following:

   a. debridement _____

   b. adenocarcinoma _____

   c. carcinoma _____

   d. sarcoma _____

2. Describe how infection, toxins, and shock can be life-threatening to burn patients.

   _____

   _____

   _____

   _____

   _____

Exercise 6-9 MATCHING

Match the term in Column A with its definition in Column B.

Column A

_____ 1. subcutaneous

_____ 2. cyanotic

_____ 3. erythematous

_____ 4. hyperhidrosis

_____ 5. paronychia

_____ 6. seborrhea

_____ 7. periungual

_____ 8. steatoma

_____ 9. cryotherapy

_____ 10. papilloma

Column B

A. destruction of tissue by using liquid nitrogen, which freezes the tissue

B. benign epithelial tumor

C. inflammation of tissue around the nail

D. excessive secretion of sweat

E. pertaining to under the skin

F. pertaining to a bluish discoloration of the skin

G. red discoloration of the skin

H. fatty tumor of the sebaceous glands

I. increased discharge of sebum from sebaceous glands

J. pertaining to around the nail

Exercise 6-10 SPELLING PRACTICE

Circle any misspelled words in the list below. Correctly spell the misspelled words in the space provided.

1. cianotic _____

2. dermatologist _____

3. diaphoreses _____

4. epithlial _____

5. arythema _____

6. dermatomycosis _____

7. necrotic _____

8. hemangioma _____

9. cryotherapy _____

10. anhydrosis _____

....

6.9   Review of Vocabulary

In the tables following, the medical terms found in this chapter are organized into these categories: anatomy, pathology, and clinical and surgical procedures. Define each term and decide into which category the word belongs. This will help you associate the term with its purpose and help you remember its meaning.

TABLE 6-2	
ANATOMICAL TERMS	
1. adipose	
2. antibodies	
3. cerumen	
4. ceruminous glands	
5. dermatologist	
6. dermatology	
7. epidermis	
8. epithelial	
9. epithelium	
10. eponychium	
11. fibroblast	
12. histamine	
13. hypodermic	
14. keratin	
15. keratinized	
16. keratinocyte	
17. lunula	
18. macrophages	
19. mast cell	
20. melanin	

continued on page 111

Table 6-2 *continued from page 110*

21. melanocyte	
22. periungual	
23. pilosebaceous	
24. plasma cell	
25. sebaceous glands	
26. sebum	
27. stratum corneum	
28. subcutaneous	
29. sudoriferous glands	

TABLE 6-3

PATHOLOGICAL TERMS

1. adenoma	
2. albinism	
3. anhidrosis	
4. carcinoma	
5. cyanotic	
6. dermatitis	
7. dermatomycosis	
8. diaphoresis	
9. erythema	
10. erythematous	
11. erythroderma	
12. hemangioma	
13. hyperhidrosis	

continued on page 112

Table 6-3 *continued from page 111*

14. hyperkeratosis	
15. leukoderma	
16. lipoma	
17. melanoma	
18. necrotic	
19. onychomycosis	
20. papilloma	
21. paronychia	
22. pyoderma	
23. pyogenic	
24. scleroderma	
25. seborrhea	
26. steatoma	
27. xeroderma	

TABLE 6-4

CLINICAL AND SURGICAL TERMS

1. cryotherapy	
2. dermabrasion	
3. laser therapy	
4. liposuction	
5. rhytidectomy	
6. skin biopsy	

6.10 Medical Terms In Context

Read the following Medical Note and then answer the questions that follow. Use your text, medical dictionary, or other references if necessary.

MEDICAL NOTE

A 30-year-old African-American woman was admitted with a chronic inflammation involving the superficial layers of the skin, especially the hand. The skin is bright red and itchy. In addition, there are multiple ulcerations on the eponychium. As the tissue dies around the eponychium, the area becomes black.

Approximately eight years ago, the patient had large papillomas on her hand. Laser therapy successfully removed the papillomas.

When seen in the dermatology clinic, it was thought the patient has an advanced case of onychomycosis. Pieces of skin were removed and examined. The diagnosis of onychomycosis was confirmed.

QUESTIONS ON THE MEDICAL NOTE

1. How long has the patient suffered with the skin inflammation?

    a. short time

    b. prolonged time

    c. intermittently

2. Which layer of skin is involved in the inflammation?

    a. epidermis

    b. dermis

    c. subcutaneous tissue

3. What medical term describes an inflammation of the skin?

    a. papilloma

    b. dermatitis

    c. onychomycosis

4. Which of the following terms describes bright red skin?

    a. cyanotic

    b. albinism

    c. erythema

5. What is the medical term for black tissue that has formed around an ulcer?

   a. melanin

   b. necrotic

   c. scleroderma

6. Papillomas involve the:

   a. epidermis

   b. dermis

   c. connective tissue

7. What treatment was given for the papillomas?

   a. freezing the tissue

   b. destruction of tissue by electricity

   c. intense beam of light

8. What procedure was used to remove a piece of skin for examination?

   a. liposuction

   b. dermabrasion

   c. skin biopsy

9. What microorganism has infected the nail?

   a. bacteria

   b. fungus

   c. parasite

10. What body system is the specialty of a dermatology clinic?

   a. orthopedics

   b. integumentary

   c. digestive

The Skeletal System

CHAPTER ORGANIZATION

This chapter will help you understand the skeletal system. It is divided into the following sections:

7.1   Anatomy and Physiology of Bone

7.2   Description of the Skeleton

7.3   Joints

7.4   Additional Word Parts

7.5   Term Analysis and Definition

7.6   Common Diseases

7.7   Abbreviations

7.8   Putting It All Together

7.9   Review of Vocabulary

7.10   Medical Terms in Context

CHAPTER OBJECTIVES

On completion of this chapter, you will be able to do the following:

1. Describe the functions of the bones

2. Define terms relating to bone structure

3. Describe the axial and appendicular skeletons

4. Name and locate the major bones of the body

5. Analyze, define, pronounce, and spell common terms of the skeletal system

6. Describe common diseases

7. Define common abbreviations of the skeletal system

INTRODUCTION

Many people think that bones are simply solid masses of nonliving tissue. Nothing could be further from the truth. Each of the 206 bones of the body is a complex, living organ. In this chapter, you will learn the anatomy and physiology of this fascinating body system, together with the terms associated with it.

7.1   Anatomy and Physiology of Bone

BONE FUNCTION

Height, width, and the basic shape of the body are determined by the length and thickness of the bones that make up the skeleton. But bones have other important functions. They make movement possible by acting as rigid and strong levers on which the muscles can exert force. They also provide protection and support for vital inner organs. Two examples are the skull bones (the cranium), which protect and support the brain, and the ribs, which do the same for the heart and lungs. Blood cells, which are essential to life, are produced by the red bone marrow, which lies in the inner portion of bone. Bones also play an important role in regulating the amount of essential minerals in the blood, particularly calcium and phosphorus. The bones store these minerals and release them into the bloodstream when required.

> **Memory Key**   Bones provide protection and support, make movement possible, produce blood cells, and store and release calcium and phosphorus.

BONE STRUCTURE

As do all the other parts of the body, bones consist of cells. Mature bone cells are called **osteocytes** (**OS**-tee-oh-sights). They have a limited life span, because other cells, called **osteoclasts** (**OS**-tee-oh-klasts), are constantly breaking them down and reabsorbing the remaining material. New bone cells are created by a third type of cell called **osteoblasts** (**OS**-tee-oh-blasts). The process of bone formation is called **ossification** (**os**-ih-fih-**KAY**-shun) or **osteogenesis** (**os**-tee-oh-**JEN**-eh-sis). There is continual turnover of bone to ensure that bone tissue remains strong and that the bones mold themselves to match the stresses placed on them. This breakdown and renewal of bone is called **remodeling** and keeps the bones young and strong.

You may be surprised to learn that the process of remodeling changes the shape of bones, if the demands placed on the body require it. For example, if you start a weightlifting program, your bones will begin to thicken in certain areas to better cope with the new demands. Start jogging regularly, and a different change in bone shape will occur, to adjust to the unique requirements of running.

> **Memory Key**   Osteoblasts create bone; osteoclasts reabsorb it. Mature bone cells are osteocytes. The process of bone formation is ossification. Breakdown and renewal of bone is called remodeling.

7.2   Description of the Skeleton

Figure 7-1 illustrates the anterior and posterior views of the skeleton. As you work your way through the material in this section, you will find it useful to regularly refer to this figure.

FIGURE 7-1

The human skeleton: (A) anterior view; (B) posterior view. The axial skeleton is colored yellow and includes the head, vertebral column, thoracic cage, and hyoid bone.

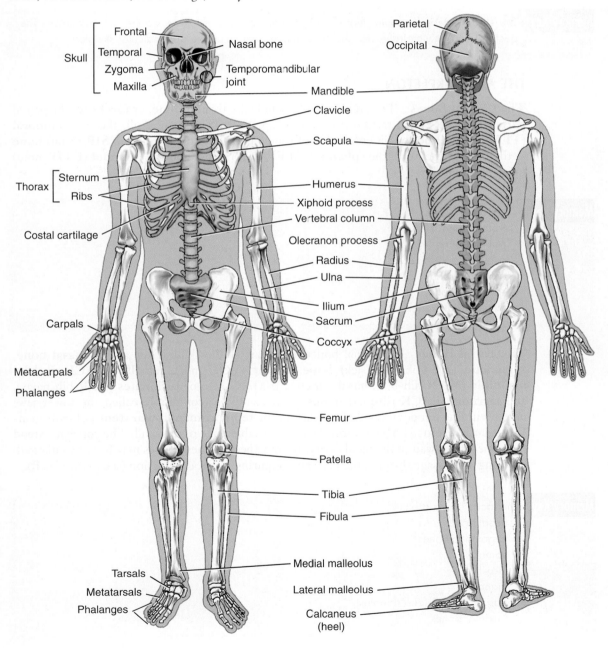

A. Anterior   **B. Posterior**

THE AXIAL AND APPENDICULAR SKELETONS

The bones related to the head and trunk make up the **axial** (**ACKS**-ee-ul) **skeleton**. It consists of the **skull**, **vertebral** (**VER**-teh-bral) **column**, **thoracic** (thoh-**RAS**-ick) **cage**, and a special bone in the throat called the **hyoid** (**HIGH**-oid) **bone**. The **appendicular** (**app**-en-**DICK**-you-lar) **skeleton** consists of the **pectoral girdle** (which connects the arms to the thoracic cage), the **pelvic girdle** (which connects the legs to the axial skeleton), and the arms and legs.

Memory Key   The skull, vertebral column, thoracic cage, and hyoid bone make up the axial skeleton. The pectoral and pelvic girdles and the arms and legs make up the appendicular skeleton.

THE AXIAL SKELETON

The Cranial Bones   The cranial bones include the **frontal bone**, or **forehead**, the paired **parietal** (pah-**RYE**-eh-tal) **bones**, making up the crown of the skull, the two **temporal** (**TEM**-poh-ral) **bones** on either side of the cranium, the **occipital** (ock-**SIP**-ih-tal) **bone** at the back of the head, the **sphenoid** (**SFEE**-noid) **bone**, and the **ethmoid** (**ETH**-moid) **bone** (see Figure 7-2A).

Memory Key   The cranial bones are the:
    frontal bone
    parietal bones
    occipital bone
    temporal bones
    sphenoid bone
    ethmoid bone

The Facial Bones   The facial bones form part of the skull. They are the **nasal bone**, **zygomatic** (zye-goh-**MAT**-ick) **bone**, **vomer** (**VOH**-mer), **maxilla** (**MACK**-sih-lah), **mandible** (**MAN**-dih-bul), **nasal conchae** (**KONG**-kee) or **turbinates** (**TER**-bih-nayts), and **lacrimal** (**LACK**-rih-mal) **bones**. The mandible (commonly called the lower jaw) unites with the temporal bone of the skull at the **temporomandibular** (tem-poh-roh-man-**DIB**-you-lar) **joint** (**TMJ**) to form the only movable bone of the skull. The conchae extend from the lateral wall of the nasal cavity. In some people, these bones may become enlarged, blocking air passage through the nose and requiring surgical reduction (see Figure 7-2B).

Memory Key   The facial bones are the:
    nasal bones
    zygomatic bones
    vomer
    maxilla
    mandible
    nasal conchae (or turbinates)
    lacrimal bones

FIGURE 7-2
Bones of the skull: (A) lateral view; (B) frontal view

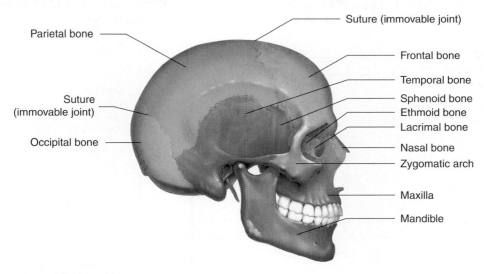

Parietal bone
Suture (immovable joint)
Frontal bone
Temporal bone
Sphenoid bone
Ethmoid bone
Lacrimal bone
Suture (immovable joint)
Nasal bone
Occipital bone
Zygomatic arch
Maxilla
Mandible

A. Lateral View

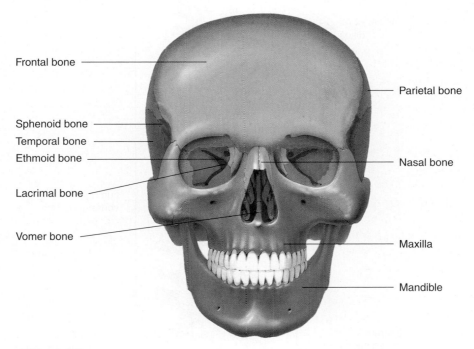

Frontal bone
Parietal bone
Sphenoid bone
Temporal bone
Ethmoid bone
Nasal bone
Lacrimal bone
Vomer bone
Maxilla
Mandible

B. Frontal View

The Vertebral Column   Figure 7-3 illustrates the spine. The spine consists of 33 bones called **vertebrae** and thus is often referred to as the vertebral column. The vertebrae are named by location. Just below the skull are the seven **cervical** (**SER**-vih-kal) vertebrae. Next in the chest area are 12 **thoracic** vertebrae (also called **dorsal** vertebrae), followed by five **lumbar** (**LUM**-bar) vertebrae in the lower back. Below that is the **sacrum** (**SAY**-krum), which consists of five fused bones, and the **coccyx** (**KOCK**-sicks), or tailbone, consisting of four fused bones. Except for the coccyx, the vertebrae are referred to by a letter followed by a number. The cervical vertebrae are C1–C7; the thoracic are T1–T12 (if dorsal is used, they are D1–D12); the lumbar are L1–L5; and the sacrum is S1–S5.

FIGURE 7-3
Vertebral column,
anterior view

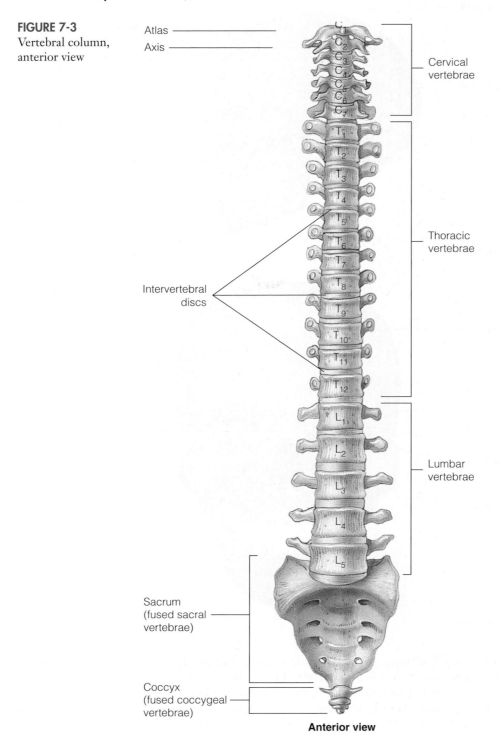

Atlas

Axis

Cervical
vertebrae

Thoracic
vertebrae

Intervertebral
discs

Lumbar
vertebrae

Sacrum
(fused sacral
vertebrae)

Coccyx
(fused coccygeal
vertebrae)

Anterior view

Between the vertebrae are little round shock absorbers called **intervertebral discs**. Together, they absorb much of the shock of movement and jumping. The discs are made of cartilage. The tough outer layer is called the **annulus fibrosus** (**AN**-you-lus figh-**BROH**-sus). The soft, gel-like inner portion is called the **nucleus pulposus** (**NEW**-klee-us pul-**POH**-sus). The common, painful condition called a slipped or herniated (**HER**-nee-ay-ted) **disc** occurs when some of the gel material pushes the outer layer out of its normal position. When the layer is out of position, nerves are pinched, causing pain messages to be sent to the brain. Also, nerve impulses are sent to back muscles, causing them to painfully contract. This contraction is called a muscle spasm and contributes to the discomfort of a herniated disc (see Figure 7-4).

Memory Key
- There are 33 vertebrae.
- The number of vertebrae in each segment of the vertebral column can be remembered by the following: eat breakfast at 7 A.M. (7 cervical), lunch at 12 noon (12 thoracic), and dinner at 5 P.M. (5 lumbar).
- A slipped disc is a herniated disc.

The Thoracic Cage   Figure 7-1 illustrates the thoracic cage. Included are the breastbone, or **sternum** (**STER**-num), 12 pairs of ribs, **costal cartilage**, and thoracic vertebrae. Posteriorly, all of the ribs attach to the 12 thoracic vertebrae. Anteriorly, the top 10 pairs of ribs are connected by costal cartilage to the sternum. The other two pairs do not attach to the sternum and are therefore called **floating ribs**.

Memory Key   The thoracic cage consists of the sternum, 12 pairs of ribs, costal cartilage, and thoracic vertebrae.

FIGURE 7-4
Herniated disc

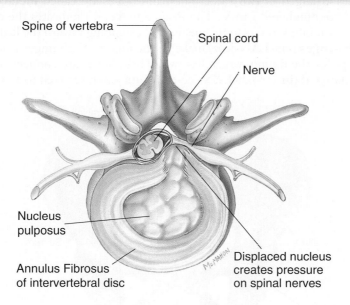

Spine of vertebra

Spinal cord

Nerve

Nucleus pulposus

Annulus Fibrosus of intervertebral disc

Displaced nucleus creates pressure on spinal nerves

THE APPENDICULAR SKELETON

Pectoral Girdle   The collarbones or **clavicles** (**KLAV**-ih-kulz), and shoulder blades or **scapulae** (**SKAP**-you-lee) make up the pectoral girdle. Refer to Figure 7-1 to view the clavicles and scapulae and their relationship to the thoracic cage.

> **Memory Key**   The pectoral girdle consists of the clavicles and scapulae.

Pelvic Girdle   The pelvic girdle protects the pelvic organs. It consists of the two hip, or **coxal** (**KOCKS**-al), bones. Each hip bone contains three segments that become fused: the **ilium** (**ILL**-ee-um), **ischium** (**ISS**-kee-um), and **pubis** (**PYOO**-bis). Figure 7-5 illustrates the pelvis. The **acetabulum** (**ass**-eh-**TAB**-yoo-lum), or hip socket, allows the head of the femur to fit into it, forming the hip joint. The right and left hip bones form a circle by joining with each other anteriorly at the **symphysis** (**SIM**-fih-sis) **pubis** and posteriorly with the sacrum to form the **sacroiliac** (**say**-kroh-**ILL**-ee-ack) joint. In females, the symphysis pubis will stretch slightly to assist delivery of a baby.

> **Memory Key**   The pelvic girdle consists of two coxal bones; joined anteriorly at the symphysis pubis and posteriorly at the sacrum.

Upper Extremity   The bones of the arm and hand make up the upper extremity. The arm bones include the upper arm or **humerus** (**HYOO**-mer-us), and the two lower arm bones, the **ulna** (**ULL**-nah) and the **radius** (**RAY**-dee-us). The humerus, ulna, and radius can be seen in Figure 7-1. The bulge on the proximal end of the ulna is the elbow, also called the **olecranon** (oh-**LEK**-rah-non) **process**, and can be seen in Figure 7-1B.

Figure 7-6 illustrates the wrist and hand. The wrist is made up of eight **carpal** (**KAR**-pal) bones arranged in two rows. The hand bones are called **metacarpals** (met-a-**KAR**-palz) and are numbered I to V. The Roman numeral I indicates the metacarpal extending toward the thumb; V refers to the metacarpal extending toward the little finger. Small bones called **phalanges** (fah-**LAN**-jeez) make up the fingers. Each finger consists of three phalanges, except for the thumb, which has two. These bones are connected to each other at the **interphalangeal** (**in**-ter-fah-**LAN**-jee-al) **joints**, often referred to as **IP joints**.

FIGURE 7-5
Pelvis, anterior view

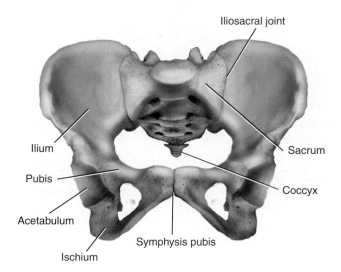

Iliosacral joint

Ilium

Sacrum

Pubis

Coccyx

Acetabulum

Symphysis pubis

Ischium

FIGURE 7-6
Bones of the distal left
arm, wrist, and hand

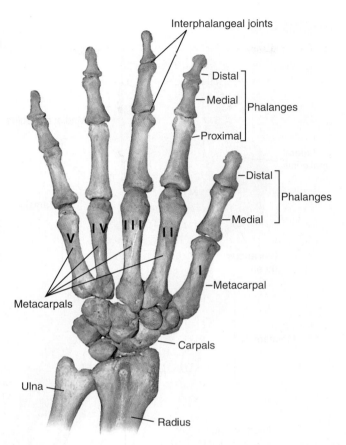

Interphalangeal joints

Distal
Medial } Phalanges
Proximal

Distal
} Phalanges
Medial

Metacarpal

Metacarpals

Carpals

Ulna

Radius

The upper extremity consists of the humerus, ulna, radius, carpals, metacarpals, and phalanges.

Lower Extremity   The bones of the leg and the foot make up the lower extremity. The bones of the leg include the thighbone, or **femur** (**FEE**-mur); the knee, or **patella** (pah-**TEL**-ah); the shin, or **tibia** (**TIB**-ee-ah); and the **fibula** (**FIB**-yoo-lah), which is the lateral bone of the lower leg. A projection (bump) on the distal tibia is called the **medial malleolus** (mal-**EE**-oh-lus); the projection on the distal fibula is called the **lateral malleolus**.

The bones of the foot are illustrated in Figure 7-7. The ankle bones are called the **tarsals** (**TAHR**-salz). The foot bones are the **metatarsals** (**met**-ah-**TAHR**-salz). Like the metacarpals, the metatarsals are numbered I to V. The toes are called the **phalanges** (fah-**LAN**-jeez). The phalanges of the toes, like those of the fingers, are joined at the IP joints. The heel is called the calcaneus (kal-**KAY**-nee-us).

The lower extremity consists of the femur, patella, tibia, fibula, tarsals, metatarsals, and phalanges.

FIGURE 7-7
Bones of the foot

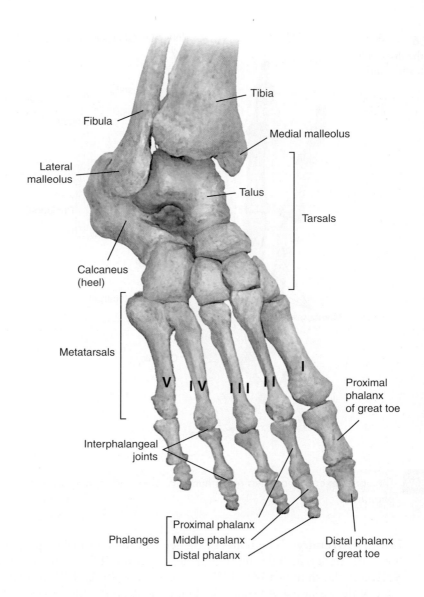

Tibia

Fibula

Medial malleolus

Lateral
malleolus

Talus

Tarsals

Calcaneus
(heel)

Metatarsals

V IV III II I

Proximal
phalanx
of great toe

Interphalangeal
joints

Phalanges

Proximal phalanx
Middle phalanx
Distal phalanx

Distal phalanx
of great toe

SUMMARY OF THE AXIAL AND APPENDICULAR SKELETONS

Table 7-1 summarizes the bones of the axial and appendicular skeletons.

TABLE 7-1

SUMMARY OF SKELETAL STRUCTURES

AXIAL SKELETON

Anatomical Name	Common Name
Cranial bones	**Skull**
• Frontal bone	Forehead
• Parietal bones	
• Temporal bones	Temples
• Occipital bone	
• Sphenoid bones (adj. sphenoidal)	
• Ethmoid bones (adj. ethmoidal)	
Facial bones	
• Zygoma (adj. zygomatic)	Cheek
• Vomer	
• Maxilla (adj. maxillary)	Upper jaw
• Mandible (adj. mandibular)	Lower jaw
• Conchae, or turbinates	
• Lacrimal bone	
Vertebral column	**Spine**
• Cervical vertebrae	
• Thoracic vertebrae	
• Lumbar vertebrae	
• Sacrum (adj. sacral)	
• coccyx (adj. coccygeal)	Tailbone
Thoracic cage (thorax)	**Chest, Torso**
• Sternum (adj. sternal)	Breastbone
• Ribs	
• Costal cartilage	

APPENDICULAR SKELETON

Anatomical Name	Common Name
Pectoral girdle	
• Clavicle (adj. clavicular)	Collarbone
• Scapula (adj. scapular)	Shoulder blade

continued on page 126

Table 7-1 *continued from page 125*

Anatomical Name	Common Name
Pelvic girdle	
• Ilium (adj. iliac)	Hip
• Ischium (adj. ischial)	
• Pubis (adj. pubic)	
Upper extremity	**Arm**
• Humerus (adj. humeral)	Upper arm
• Ulna (adj. ulnar)	Forearm
• Radius (adj. radial)	Forearm
• Olecranon (adj. olecranal)	Elbow
• Carpals	Wrist
• Metacarpals	
• Phalanges (adj. phalangeal)	Fingers
Lower extremity	**Leg**
• Femur (adj. femoral)	Thigh
• Tibia (adj. tibial)	Shin
• Fibula (adj. fibular)	
• Patella (adj. patellar)	Knee
• Tarsals	
• Malleolus (adj. malleolar)	
• Metatarsals	
• Phalanges (adj. phalangeal)	Toes
• Calcaneus (adj. calcaneal)	Heel

7.3   Joints

A joint is a place where bones unite. The most familiar joints are the movable joints, such as the shoulder and knee joints, but joints can also be stationary, as are those between the bones of the skull.

The movable joints are all similar in structure. **Articular cartilage** covers the ends of bones, preventing friction and allowing painless movement. Between the articular cartilages is the **joint cavity**. The joint cavity is lined with a **synovial membrane**, which secretes **synovial fluid** that acts as a joint lubricant. A **joint capsule**, strengthened by ligaments, encases the joint attaching bone to bone (see Figure 7-8). All of these structures work together to allow movement of body parts.

Joints are named for the bones that form the union. For example, the joint between the radius and the wrist is called the **radiocarpal** joint; the joint between the ilium and the femur is called the **iliofemoral** joint.

SUPPORTING STRUCTURES

Also at joints, but not inside the joint, are **ligaments** (**LIG**-ah-mentz), and **bursae** (**BUR**-see). Ligaments attach bone to bone. Bursae are tiny, purselike sacs lined with synovial membrane and filled with synovial fluid. The body has hundreds of bursae. Each **bursa** (**BUR**-sah) prevents friction between two structures that need to glide past each other when they move, for example, between bone and skin. The bursa can become inflamed through overuse, resulting in a condition called **bursitis** (ber-**SIGH**-tis). Golfers sometimes develop bursitis at the shoulder; tennis players often develop it in the elbow.

Memory Key	• A joint is the union between two bones.
	• Joint structures consist of: articular cartilage synovial fluid
	joint cavity joint capsule
	synovial membrane
	• Joints are named after the bones that form the union.

FIGURE 7-8
A synovial joint

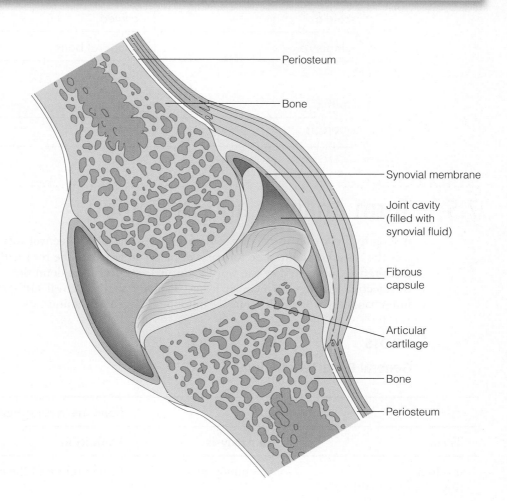

Periosteum

Bone

Synovial membrane

Joint cavity
(filled with
synovial fluid)

Fibrous
capsule

Articular
cartilage

Bone

Periosteum

Before you continue, review Sections 7.1, 7.2, and 7.3. Then complete Exercises 7-1, 7-2, and 7-3 found at the end of the chapter.

7.4   Additional Word Parts

The following roots and suffix will also be used in this chapter to build medical terms.

Root	Meaning
kyph/o	humpback
lord/o	swayback
ped/o	child
scoli/o	curved
tempor/o	temporal bone

Suffix	Meaning
-porosis	porous

7.5   Term Analysis and Definition

A lengthy list of terms follows. Whenever possible, the adjectival form is given because it is the most common. The format will help you visualize the root with different suffixes and prefixes, observe how the word is formed, and learn the definition. Notice the variety of adjectival endings. Remember from Chapter 3 that adjectival suffixes usually cannot be interchanged: for example, cranial cannot be changed to cranious.

ROOTS

General Bone Terminology

	myel/o	bone marrow; spinal cord
Term	**Term Analysis**	**Definition**
myeloma (my-el-**LOH**-mah)	-oma = tumor; mass	benign tumor of the bone marrow
osteomyelitis (**oss**-tee-oh-**my**-eh-**LYE**-tis)	-itis = inflammation **oste/o** = bone	inflammation of bone and bone marrow

Memory Key   Do not confuse **my/o**, meaning "muscle," with **myel/o**, meaning "bone marrow" or "spinal cord."

	osse/o; oste/o	bone
Term	**Term Analysis**	**Definition**
osteitis (os-tee-**EYE**-tis)	-itis = inflammation	inflammation of the bone
osteochondritis (**os**-tee-oh-kon-**DRYE**-tis)	-itis = inflammation **chondr/o** = cartilage	inflammation of bone and cartilage
osteocyte (**OS**-tee-oh-sight)	-cyte = cell	mature bone cell
osteoma (os-tee-**OH**-mah)	-oma = tumor; mass	benign tumor of bone
osteotome (**OS**-tee-oh-tohm)	-tome = instrument used to cut	instrument used to cut bone
osteotomy (oss-tee-**OT**-oh-mee)	-tomy = process of cutting; incision	process of cutting bone
endosteum (en-**DOS**-tee-um)	-um = structure endo- = within	inner lining of the shaft (long slender portion) of a long bone such as the tibia or ulna
periosteum (**per**-ee-**OS**-tee-um)	-um = structure peri- = around	the structure around the shaft of a long bone

Axial Skeleton

The axial skeleton includes bones of the skull, face, and thorax; the vertebrae; and the hyoid bone (see Figures 7-1, 7-2, and 7-3).

Skull and Facial Bones

	crani/o	skull
Term	**Term Analysis**	**Definition**
craniofacial (**kray**-nee-oh-**FAY**-shahl)	-al = pertaining to **faci/o** = face	pertaining to the skull and face
cranioplasty (**KRAY**-nee-oh-**plas**-tee)	-plasty = surgical repair or reconstruction	surgical repair of the skull

Term	Term Analysis	Definition
craniotomy (**kray**-nee-**OT**-oh-mee)	-tomy = incision; processing of cutting	incision into the skull
	mandibul/o	**mandible; lower jaw**
mandibular (man-**DIB**-yoo-lar)	-ar = pertaining to	pertaining to the lower jaw
temporomandibular joint (TMJ) (**tem**-poh-roh-man-**DIB**-yoo-lar)	-ar = pertaining to **tempor/o** = temporal bone	pertaining to the joint between the temporal bone and the lower jaw
	maxill/o	**maxilla; upper jaw**
maxillary (**MACK**-sih-**ler**-ee)	-ary = pertaining to	pertaining to the upper jaw

Memory Key To remember that *maxilla* means upper jaw, think of maximum, meaning the greatest, highest, or uppermost.

Thoracic Cage

The sternum, ribs, costal cartilage, and thoracic vertebrae make up the thoracic cage (see Figure 7-1).

	chondr/o	**cartilage**
Term	**Term Analysis**	**Definition**
achondroplasia (ah-**kon**-droh-**PLAY**-zee-ah)	-plasia = development; formation, a- = no; not; inadequate	inadequate cartilage formation resulting in a type of dwarfism
chondrocyte (**KON**-droh-sight)	-cyte = cell	cartilage cell
chondroma (kon-**DROH**-mah)	-oma = tumor; mass	benign tumor of cartilage
	cost/o	**rib**
costochondral (**kos**-toh-**KON**-drahl)	-al = pertaining to **chondr/o** = cartilage	pertaining to the ribs and cartilage

Term	Term Analysis	Definition
subcostal (sub-**KOS**-tal)	-al = pertaining to sub- = under	pertaining to under the ribs
	stern/o	**sternum; breastbone**
costosternal (**kos**-toh-**STER**-nal)	-al = pertaining to **cost/o** = ribs	pertaining to the ribs and sternum
sternotomy (ster-**NOT**-oh-mee)	-tomy = process of cutting; incision	process of cutting the sternum
	xiph/o	**sword**
xiphoid (**ZIGH**-foid)	-oid = resembling	distal portion of the sternum; literally means "resembling a sword"

Vertebrae

The vertebrae include the cervical, thoracic, lumbar, sacral, and coccygeal bones (see Figure 7-3).

Term	Term Analysis	Definition
	cervic/o	**neck**
cervical (**SER**-vih-kal)	-al = pertaining to	pertaining to the neck
	coccyg/o	**coccyx; tailbone**
coccygeal (kock-**SIJ**-ee-al)	-eal = pertaining to	pertaining to the tailbone
	lumb/o	**lower back; loins**
lumbodynia (**lum**-boh-**DIN**-ee-ah)	-dynia = pain	pain in the lower back; also known as lumbago
lumbosacral joint (**lum**-boh-**SAY**-kral)	-al = pertaining to **sacr/o** = sacrum	pertaining to the joint between L5 and the sacrum
	sacr/o	**sacrum**
sacrococcygeal joint (**say**-kro-kock-**SIJ**-ee-al)	-eal = pertaining to **coccyg/o** = tailbone	pertaining to the joint between the sacrum and the coccyx

	spondyl/o (see also vertebr/o)	vertebra
Term	**Term Analysis**	**Definition**
spondylitis (spon-dih-**LYE**-tis)	-itis = inflammation	inflammation of the vertebrae
spondylopathy (spon-dil-**OP**-ah-thee)	-pathy = disease	any disease of the vertebrae

Memory Key   **Spondyl/o** is most often used in words referring to conditions of the vertebrae. Compare with **vertebr/o**, which is most often used in words to describe structure.

	thorac/o	chest
thoracolumbar (thoh-**rack**-oh-**LUM**-bar)	-ar = pertaining to **lumbo/o** = lower back; loins	pertaining to the chest and lower back
	vertebr/o	**vertebra**
costovertebral joint (**kos**-toh-**VER**-teh-brahl)	-al = pertaining to **cost/o** = rib	pertaining to the joint between a rib and a vertebra
intervertebral (**in**-ter-**VER**-te-bral)	-al = pertaining to inter- = between	pertaining to between the vertebrae

Appendicular Skeleton

The appendicular skeleton includes the pectoral and pelvic girdles and the upper and lower extremities (see Figure 7-1).

Pectoral Girdle

	clavicul/o	clavicle; collarbone
Term	**Term Analysis**	**Definition**
sternoclavicular joint (**ster**-noh-klah-**VICK**-yoo-lar)	-ar = pertaining to **stern/o** = sternum; breastbone	pertaining to the joint between the sternum and clavicle
infraclavicular (**in**-frah-klah-**VICK**-yoo-lar)	-ar = pertaining to infra- = below, beneath	pertaining to below the collarbone

	scapul/o	**scapula**
Term	**Term Analysis**	**Definition**
subscapular (sub-**SKAP**-yoo-lar)	-ar = pertaining to sub- = under; below	pertaining to below the scapula

Upper Extremities

	brachi/o	**arm**
Term	**Term Analysis**	**Definition**
brachial (**BRAY**-kee-al)	-al = pertaining to	pertaining to the arm
brachiocephalic (**bray**-kee-oh-seh-**FAL**-ick)	-ic = pertaining to **cephal/o** = head	pertaining to the arm and head
	carp/o	**wrist**
carpectomy (kar-**PECK**-toh-mee)	-ectomy = excision; surgical removal	excision of a carpal (wrist) bone
	olecran/o	**olecranon (elbow)**
olecranal (oh-**LEK**-ran-al)	-al = pertaining to	pertaining to the olecranon, a bony projection on the ulna
	phalang/o	**phalanx; one of the bones making up the fingers or toes**
interphalangeal (IP) joint (**in**-ter-fah-**LAN**-jee-al)	-eal = pertaining to inter- = between	pertaining to the joint between the phalanges
	radi/o	**radius (one of the bones of the lower arm)**
radiocarpal joint (**ray**-dee-oh-**KAR**-pal)	-al = pertaining to **carp/o** = wrist	pertaining to the joint between the radius and wrist
	uln/o	**ulnar (one of the bones of the lower arm)**
ulnar (**UL**-nar)	-ar = pertaining to	pertaining to the ulna

Pelvic Girdle

	acetabul/o	acetabulum; hip socket
Term	**Term Analysis**	**Definition**
acetabular (**ass**-eh-**TAB**-yoo-lar)	-ar = pertaining to	pertaining to the hip socket
acetabuloplasty (**ass**-eh-**TAB**-yoo-loh-**plas**-tee)	-plasty = surgical repair or reconstruction	surgical repair of the hip socket

Memory Key   The hip socket resembles a cup that the Romans used to hold vinegar. *Acetum* is Latin for vinegar.

	ili/o	hip
iliosacral joint (**ill**-ee-oh-**SAY**-kral)	-al = pertaining to sacr/o = sacrum	pertaining to the joint between the hip and sacrum; also known as the sacroiliac (**say**-kroh-**ILL**-ee-ack) joint

Memory Key   To remember that ili/o means hip and ile/o means intestine, relate the "i" in il**i**/o to the "i" in h**i**p and the "e" in il**e**/o to the "e" in int**e**stine.

	pelv/i; pelv/o	pelvis
pelvic (**PEL**-vick)	-ic = pertaining to	pertaining to the pelvis

Lower Extremities

	calcane/o	heel
Term	**Term Analysis**	**Definition**
calcaneal (kal-**KAY**-nee-al)	-eal = pertaining to	pertaining to the heel

	femor/o	**femur; thigh bone**
iliofemoral joint (**ill**-ee-oh-**FEM**-or-al)	-al = pertaining to **ili/o** = hip	pertaining to the joint between the hip and femur
	fibul/o	**fibula**
fibulocalcaneal (**fib**-yoo-loh-kal-**KAY**- nee-al)	-eal = pertaining to **calcane/o** = heel	pertaining to the fibula and heel

Memory Key   *Fibula* is Latin for clasp or pin. The fibula is pinned to the tibia like a brooch.

	patell/a; patell/o	**patella; kneecap**
patellapexy (pa-**TEL**-ah-**peck**-see)	-pexy = surgical fixation	surgical fixation of the kneecap
infrapatellar (**in**-frah-pah-**TEL**-ar)	-ar = pertaining to infra- = below	pertaining to below the kneecap
suprapatellar (**sue**-prah-pah-**TEL**-ar)	-ar = pertaining to supra- = above	pertaining to above the kneecap
	tibi/o	**tibia; shin**
tibiofibular joint (**tib**-ee-oh-**FIB**-yoo-lar)	-ar = pertaining to **fibul/o** = fibula	pertaining to the joint between the tibia and fibula

Joints

	arthr/o; articul/o	**joint**
Term	**Term Analysis**	**Definition**
arthralgia (ar-**THRAL**-jee-ah)	-algia = pain	joint pain; also known as arthrodynia (ar-throh-**DIN**-ee-ah)

Term	Term Analysis	Definition
arthritis (ar-**THRIGH**-tis)	-itis = inflammation	inflammation of a joint *NOTE:* Types include: **osteoarthritis (OA)**, which is degeneration of the articular cartilage due to overuse and resulting in painful movement of the joint (see Figure 7-9); and **rheumatoid arthritis (RA)**, an autoimmune (protection or immunity against one's self) disease in which the body's immune system fails to recognize its own cells as normal and the body's tissues are attacked as if they were foreign invaders, resulting in the degeneration of the joint (see Figure 7-10).

FIGURE 7-9

Osteoarthritis: (A) normal joint; (B) early signs of osteoarthritis with degeneration of the articular cartilage; (C) late stages of osteoarthritis with complete breakdown of the joint, thickened bone, and exposed bone.

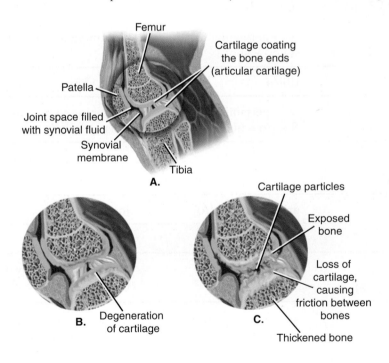

FIGURE 7-10
Rheumatoid
hand
deformity

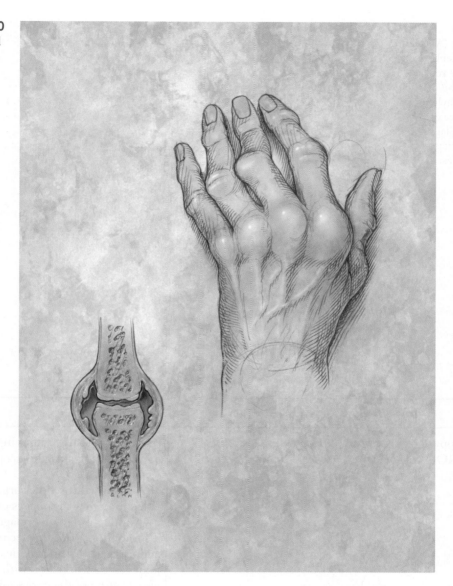

Term	Term Analysis	Definition
arthropathy (ar-**THROP**-ah-thee)	-pathy = disease	any disease of a joint
arthroplasty (**ar**-throh-**plas**-tee)	-plasty = surgical repair or reconstruction	surgical repair of a joint; usually refers to the total or partial replacement of the knee or hip joints with a **prosthetic** (artificial) device (see Figure 7-11)

FIGURE 7-11
Arthroplasty: (A) total
hip replacement;
(B) total knee replace-
ment. A strong plastic
called polyethylene
takes the place of
articular cartilage,
preventing friction
between bones.

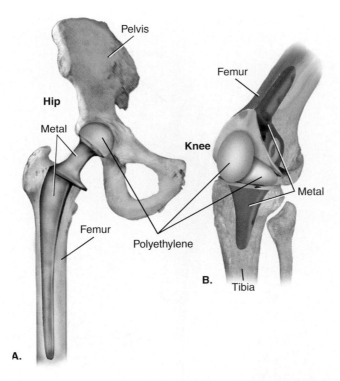

Term	Term Analysis	Definition
arthroscopy (ar-**THROS**-koh-pee)	-scopy = process of visual examination	process of visually examining the joint cavity by using an arthroscope (see Figure 7-12) *NOTE:* In arthroscopic surgery, a video camera takes images of a joint cavity and displays the images on a TV monitor. With this technique, and using a local anesthetic, the joint can be worked on with good visualization of the entire joint. Recovery time is minimal and hospital stay is reduced.

FIGURE 7-12
(A) Arthroscopic surgery; (B) a picture of the inside of the knee joint as seen through an arthroscope

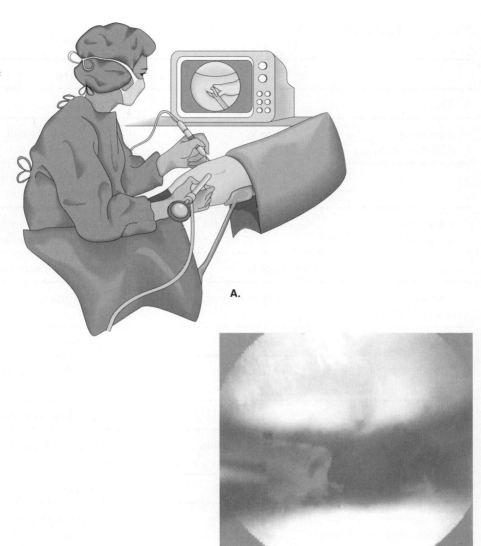

A.

B.

Term	Term Analysis	Definition
interarticular (**in**-ter-ar-**TICK**-yoo-lar)	-ar = pertaining to inter- = between	pertaining to between the joints
	burs/o	**bursa (sac filled with synovial fluid located around joints)**
bursitis (ber-**SIGH**-tis)	-itis = inflammation	inflamed bursa
bursectomy (ber-**SECK**-toh-mee)	-ectomy = excision; surgical removal	excision of the bursa

SUFFIXES

Term	Term Analysis	Definition
	-blast	immature
osteoblast (**OS**-tee-oh-blast)	**oste/o** = bone	immature bone cell
	-centesis	**surgical puncture to remove fluid; aspiration**
arthrocentesis (**ar**-throh-sen-**TEE**-sis)	**arthr/o** = joint	surgical puncture of a joint to remove fluid; aspiration of a joint cavity
	-clasis	**surgical fracture or refracture**
osteoclasis (**os**-tee-**OCK**-lah-sis)	**oste/o** = bone	surgical fracture or refracture of bone
	-clast	**breakdown**
osteoclast (**OS**-tee-oh-clast)	**oste/o** = bone	bone cell that breaks down bone
	-desis	**surgical fusion; surgical binding**
arthrodesis (ar-throh-**DEE**-sis)	**arthr/o** = joint	surgical fusion of a joint
	-genesis	**formation**
osteogenesis (**os**-tee-oh-**JEN**-eh-sis)	**oste/o** = bone	bone formation; also known as ossification
	-malacia	**softening**
chondromalacia (**kon**-droh-mah-**LAY**-shee-ah)	**chondr/o** = cartilage	softening of cartilage
osteomalacia (**os**-tee-oh-mah-**LAY**-shee-ah)	**oste/o** = bone	softening of bone
	-osis	**abnormal condition**
kyphosis (kye-**FOH**-sis)	**kyph/o** = humpback	exaggerated posterior curvature of the thoracic spine; humpback (see Figure 7-13A)

Term	Term Analysis	Definition
lordosis (lor-**DOH**-sis)	**lord/o** = swayback	exaggerated anterior curvature of the lumbar spine; swayback (see Figure 7-13B)
scoliosis (**skoh**-lee-**OH**-sis)	**scoli/o** = curved	abnormal lateral curvature of the spine (see Figure 7-13C)
	-physis	**to grow**
diaphysis (dye-**AF**-eh-sis)	**dia-** = through	the shaft of a long bone
epiphysis (eh-**PIF**-eh-sis)	**epi-** = on; upon	the bulbous portion of a long bone on both sides of the shaft
	-porosis	**porous**
osteoporosis (**os**-tee-oh-poh-**ROH**-sis)	**oste/o** = bone	loss of bone density resulting in open spaces within bony substance
	-sarcoma	**malignant tumor of connective tissue**
chondrosarcoma (**kon**-droh-sar-**KOH**-mah)	**chondr/o** = cartilage	malignant tumor of cartilage

FIGURE 7-13

Abnormal curvatures of the spine: (A) kyphosis; (B) lordosis; (C) scoliosis

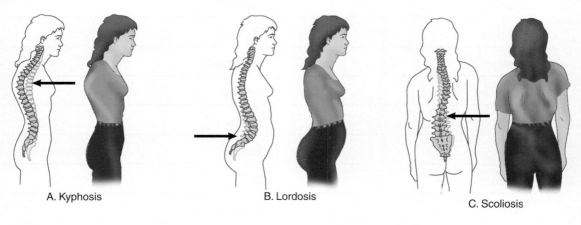

A. Kyphosis B. Lordosis C. Scoliosis

Term	Term Analysis	Definition
osteosarcoma (**os**-tee-oh-sar-**KOH**-mah)	**oste/o** = bone	malignant tumor of bone; also known as osteogenic sarcoma

PREFIXES

	ortho-	straight
Term	**Term Analysis**	**Definition**
orthopedics (**or**-thoh-**PEE**-dicks)	-ic = pertaining to **ped/o** = child	surgical specialty dealing with the correction of deformities and dysfunctions of the skeletal system

Study the names of major bones in Table 7-2 along with each name's adjectival form.

TABLE 7-2

MAJOR BONES OF THE BODY — NOUN AND ADJECTIVAL FORMS

Noun	Adjective
acetabulum	acetabular
articulation	articular
calcaneus	calcaneal
cervix	cervical
clavicle	clavicular
coccyx	coccygeal
cranium	cranial
ethmoid	ethmoidal
femur	femoral
fibula	fibular
humerus	humeral
ilium	iliac

continued on page 143

Table 7-2 *continued from page 142*

Noun	Adjective
ischium	ischial
lower back	lumbar
malleolus	malleolar
mandible	mandibular
maxilla	maxillary
olecranon	olecranal
patella	patellar
pelvis	pelvic
phalanx	phalangeal
pubis	pubic
radius	radial
ribs	costal
sacrum	sacral
scapula	scapular
sphenoid	sphenoidal
sternum	sternal
thorax	thoracic
tibia	tibial
ulna	ulnar
vertebra	vertebral
wrist bones	carpals
zygoma	zygomatic

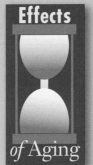

Decreased bone density and degeneration of articular cartilage are the most common problems affecting the skeletal system as people age. Decreased bone density results in osteoporosis, and articular degeneration leads to osteoarthritis (OA).

In **osteoporosis**, bone density decreases because the rate of bone formation is less than the rate of bone loss. The bone becomes thin, porous, and weak. Fractures are common. Postmenopausal reduction in estrogen is the most important cause of osteoporosis for women. Another cause is prolonged immobility. The main goal of treatment is to prevent further bone loss. This includes drug therapy, weight-bearing exercises, and increased dietary calcium.

Osteoarthritis is the degeneration of articular cartilage. Although the exact cause is unknown, joint injury and cartilage degeneration stimulate the body to form new cartilage; however, it might not be adequate to cover the articular ends of bone. With inadequate cartilage formation, the underlying bone is exposed. Because bone rubs on bone without protection from the articular cartilage, movement is painful. There is no cure for arthritis. Physical exercise improves mobility. Aspirin may be taken to reduce pain. For advanced OA, arthroplasty (surgical replacement of the joint) is the treatment of choice.

7.6 Common Disease of the Skeletal System

BONE CANCERS

Malignant bone tumors start in bone cells and metastasize quickly. Although pain and swelling are common symptoms, it is often a fracture that leads to the diagnosis of the tumor. Types of malignancies include osteosarcoma, the most common bone cancer, Ewing's tumor (occurs in children), and chondrosarcoma. Treatment includes excision of the tumor, amputation, chemotherapy, and radiotherapy.

The cancers noted in the preceding paragraph are primary bone tumors, meaning they originate from bone tissue. More commonly, bone cancers are metastatic or secondary tumors that result from the spread of cancer to bone from other locations such as the breast and lungs.

FRACTURES

A fracture is a break or crack in a bone (Figure 7-14). An **open fracture** means a bone is broken and there is an open cut in the skin. A **closed fracture** means a bone is broken but there is no open cut in the skin. A **pathological fracture** means the bone breaks because it is weak from disease. For example, osteoporosis, a disease that weakens bones, might cause the bone to fracture. Names are given to describe a fracture in one way or another. For example, **comminuted** (kom-ih-**NOOT**-id) means the bone has been splintered, greenstick means a bone is partially broken on one side and bent on the opposite side, a **Colles'** (**KOL**-eez) fracture is of the distal radius near the wrist, and an **intra-articular** fracture is on the joint surfaces of bone.

FIGURE 7-14
Fractures:
(A) Compound or
open fracture;
(B) Closed fracture;
(C) Comminuted
fracture;
(D) greenstick fracture

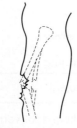
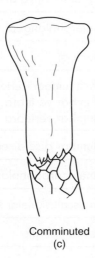

Compound / open fracture
(a)

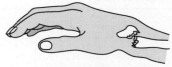

Colles' (closed fracture)
(b)

Comminuted
(c)

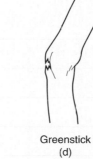

Greenstick
(d)

Fractures are caused by injury or disease. Treatment involves **reduction** (placing the bones back together) and **immobilization** (placement of a cast over the broken bone to prevent movement).

If an incision in the skin is not necessary to place the bones back together, the procedure is called **closed reduction**. If it is necessary to incise the skin to place the bones back together, under direct visualization, the procedure is called **open reduction**. When the fracture is severe and screws, nails, or pins are needed to hold the bones in place, the procedure is called **open reduction internal fixation (ORIF)**.

7.7 Abbreviations

Abbreviation	Meaning
C	cervical
C1, C2, . . . C7	first cervical vertebra, second cervical vertebra, . . . seventh cervical vertebra
DDD	degenerative disc disease
IP	interphalangeal
L	lumbar
L1, L2, . . . L5	first lumbar vertebra, second lumbar vertebra, . . . fifth lumbar vertebra
LDD	lumbar disc disease
MCP	metacarpophalangeal
MSS	musculoskeletal system
OA	osteoarthritis
ORIF	open reduction internal fixation (open reduction is the realignment of bone into its normal position under direct visualization after cutting open the skin)
ortho	orthopedics
RA	rheumatoid arthritis
S1, S2, . . . S5	first sacral vertebra, second sacral vertebra, . . . fifth sacral vertebra
T	thoracic
T1, T2, . . . T12 (also D1, D2, . . . D12 if *dorsal* is used)	first thoracic vertebra, second thoracic vertebra, . . . twelfth thoracic vertebra
TKR	total knee replacement
TMJ	temporomandibular joint

....

7.8   Putting It All Together

Exercise 7-1   SHORT ANSWER

1. The bony structure protecting the brain is the _____
   _____ .

2. Name five functions of the skeletal system _____
   _____ .

3. Two minerals found in bone are _____ and _____ .

4. Distinguish between osteoclasts, osteocytes, and osteoblasts.

Exercise 7-2   CLASSIFICATION

Classify the following bones as part of the axial or appendicular skeleton.

1. skull   _____

2. arms   _____

3. rib cage   _____

4. femur   _____

5. hyoid bone   _____

6. clavicle   _____

7. ilium   _____

Exercise 7-3   IDENTIFICATION

Identify the location of individual bones using the following list.

a. cranium   d. face   g. vertebral column
b. thoracic cage   e. upper extremity   h. lower extremity
c. pelvic girdle   f. pectoral girdle

1. maxilla   _____   8. lumbar   _____

2. carpals   _____   9. occipital bone _____

3. femur   _____   10. patella   _____

4. phalanges   _____   11. xiphoid process _____

5. parietal bone   _____   12. radius   _____

6. costal cartilage _____   13. fibula   _____

7. humerus   _____   14. zygoma   _____

continued

15. cervical _____

16. ilium _____

17. calcaneus _____

18. mandible _____

19. coccyx _____

20. ischium _____

21. metatarsals _____

22. olecranon _____

23. sternum _____

24. tarsals _____

25. ulna _____

26. clavicle _____

Exercise 7-4   BUILDING MEDICAL WORDS

I. Use **myel/o** to build medical terms for the following definitions.

   1. benign tumor of the bone marrow _____

   2. inflammation of the bone and
      bone marrow _____

II. Use **oste/o** to build medical terms for the following definitions.

   3. inflammation of bone and joints _____

   4. immature bone cell _____

   5. inflammation of bone and cartilage _____

   6. mature bone cell _____

   7. bone formation _____

   8. benign tumor of bone _____

   9. malignant tumor of bone _____

III. Use **crani/o** to build medical terms for the following definitions.

   10. incision into the skull _____

   11. surgical repair of the skull _____

   12. pertaining to the skull and face _____

IV. Use **chondr/o** to build medical terms for the following definitions.

   13. cartilage cell _____

   14. benign tumor of cartilage _____

   15. malignant tumor of cartilage _____

V. Use **cost/o** to build medical terms for the following definitions.

   16. pertaining to the ribs and cartilage _____

   17. pertaining to the rib and vertebra _____

   18. pertaining to under the ribs _____

VI. Use **arthr/o** to build medical terms for the following definitions.

19. joint pain _____

20. inflammation of a joint _____

21. any disease of a joint _____

22. surgical repair of a joint _____

23. process of visually examining a joint _____

Exercise 7-5   TERMS FOR BONES

Give the common name for the following bones.

1. thorax _____

2. clavicle _____

3. carpals _____

4. humerus _____

5. olecranon _____

6. ilium _____

7. calcaneus _____

8. femur _____

9. tibia _____

Exercise 7-6   IDENTIFY SURGICAL PROCEDURES

Mark with an **X** the terms indicating surgical procedures.

1. myeloma _____

2. osteoclasis _____

3. lordosis _____

4. arthrodesis _____

5. osteoporosis _____

6. acetabular _____

7. brachial _____

8. lumbodynia _____

9. orthopedics _____

10. cranioplasty _____

Exercise 7-7   SPELLING

Circle any misspelled words in the list below and correctly spell them in the space provided.

1. calcaneous   _____
2. tibula   _____
3. hyoid   _____
4. myloma   _____
5. temperomandibular   _____
6. ileosacral   _____
7. osteogeneses   _____
8. craniofacial   _____
9. maleolus   _____
10. coccx   _____
11. humerous   _____
12. olecranal   _____
13. parietal   _____
14. arthrodeses   _____
15. patella   _____

Exercise 7-8   ADJECTIVES

Give the adjective for each of the following.

1. cranium   _____
2. face   _____
3. ethmoid   _____
4. mandible   _____
5. maxilla   _____
6. zygoma   _____
7. sternum   _____
8. coccyx   _____
9. malleolus   _____
10. sacrum   _____
11. vertebra   _____
12. thorax   _____
13. clavicle   _____

14. scapula   _____

15. olecranon   _____

16. radius   _____

17. acetabulum   _____

18. ischium   _____

19. calcaneus   _____

20. fibula   _____

Exercise 7-9   PATHOLOGY

Answer the following questions on skeletal pathology.

1. What is the difference between the following?

   a. Primary and secondary tumors?

   _____

   _____

   _____

   b. Open and closed fractures?

   _____

   _____

   _____

   c. Comminuted and Colles' fractures?

   _____

   _____

   _____

2. What is meant by reduction and immobilization of fractures?

   _____

   _____

   _____

7.9   Review of Vocabulary

In the following tables, the medical terms found in this chapter are organized into these categories: anatomy, pathology, diagnostics, surgery, and joints. Define each term and decide in which category the word belongs. This will help you associate the term with its purpose and help you remember its meaning.

TABLE 7-3

REVIEW OF ANATOMICAL TERMS

1. acetabular	2. brachial	3. brachiocephalic
4. calcaneal	5. cervical	6. chondrocyte
7. costochondral	8. costosternal	9. craniofacial
10. infrapatellar	11. interarticular	12. interphalangeal
13. intervertebral	14. lumbosacral	15. mandibular
16. maxillary	17. olecranal	18. orthopedics
19. osteoblast	20. osteoclast	21. osteocyte
22. osteogenesis	23. pelvic	24. subcostal
25. subscapular	26. suprapatellar	27. thoracolumbar
28. ulnar	29. vertebral	30. vertebrofemoral
31. xiphoid		

TABLE 7-4

REVIEW OF PATHOLOGIC TERMS

1. achondroplasia	2. arthralgia	3. arthritis
4. arthropathy	5. chondroma	6. chondromalacia
7. chondrosarcoma	8. kyphosis	9. lordosis
10. lumbodynia	11. myeloma	12. osteoarthritis
13. osteitis	14. osteochondritis	15. osteoma
16. osteomalacia	17. osteomyelitis	18. osteoporosis
19. osteosarcoma	20. scoliosis	21. spondylitis
22. spondylopathy		

TABLE 7-5

REVIEW OF DIAGNOSTIC TERMS

1. arthrocentesis	2. arthroscopy

TABLE 7-6

REVIEW OF SURGICAL TERMS

1. acetabuloplasty	2. arthrodesis	3. arthroplasty
4. carpectomy	5. cranioplasty	6. craniotomy
7. osteoclasis	8. osteotome	9. osteotomy
10. patellapexy		

TABLE 7-7

REVIEW OF JOINT VOCABULARY

1. bursectomy	2. bursitis	3. costovertebral
4. fibulocalcaneal	5. iliofemoral	6. iliosacral; sacroiliac
7. interphalangeal	8. lumbosacral	9. radiocarpal
10. sacrococcygeal	11. sternoclavicular	12. temporomandibular
13. tibiofibular		

7.10   Medical Terms in Context

After you have read the following Medical Notes, answer the questions that follow. Use your text, medical dictionary, or other references if necessary.

MEDICAL NOTE #1

This 66-year-old man was involved in an MVA. He was stabilized at the site of the accident and brought to the hospital. On examination, he had multiple contusions and abrasions. Among his injuries is a laceration above the patella that severed the patellar tendon, a dislocated sternoclavicular joint, and, most significant, a left radial fracture and a distal ulnar fracture on the left.

QUESTIONS ON MEDICAL NOTE #1

1. MVA means:

   a. motorcycle and van accident

   b. motor vehicle accident

   c. minivan accident

2. What was the most serious injury?

   a. dislocated collarbone

   b. patellar tendon detachment

   c. radial and ulnar fractures

3. Name the injury above the patella.

   a. tear of the tissue

   b. scrape

   c. bruise

4. Name the location of the dislocated joint.

   a. breastbone and collarbone

   b. shoulder blade and collarbone

   c. shoulder blade and upper arm

5. A bruise is a(n):

   a. abrasion

   b. laceration

   c. contusion

MEDICAL NOTE #2

This 72-year-old woman was admitted because of complications from osteoporosis. She has an eight-month history of chronic, disabling back pain associated with kyphosis of the thoracolumbar spine. There is also cervical lordosis and pain in the midthoracic area.

On physical examination, the patient exhibits the previously mentioned thoracic kyphosis and cervical lordosis. There is pain over the lower thoracic and upper lumbar spine areas. There are no neurological abnormalities in the lower extremities.

X-rays of the thoracic vertebrae were done. These films showed a compression fracture of T12 and L1. These fractures are complications of severe osteoporosis.

The patient was fitted with a neck brace and prescribed analgesics. She will return to her primary care physician in six weeks for followup.

QUESTIONS ON MEDICAL NOTE #2

1. In this patient, swayback involves which vertebrae?

    a. cervical

    b. thoracic

    c. lumbar

    d. b and c only

2. A humpback abnormality appeared on which vertebrae?

    a. cervical

    b. thoracic

    c. lumbar

    d. b and c only

3. Osteoporosis means:

    a. bone formation

    b. loss of bone density

    c. surgical fracture of bone

    d. the bulbous portion of a long bone

4. Complication(s) of osteoporosis shown on x-rays is (are):

    a. fractures

    b. kyphosis

    c. lordosis

    d. all the above

5. The patient was treated with:

   a. pain killers

   b. surgery

   c. traction

   d. none of the above

8 CHAPTER

The Muscular System

CHAPTER ORGANIZATION

This chapter will help you understand the muscular system. It is divided into the following sections:

8.1 Skeletal Attachments

8.2 Major Skeletal Muscles

8.3 Additional Word Parts

8.4 Term Analysis and Definition

8.5 Common Diseases

8.6 Abbreviations

8.7 Putting It All Together

8.8 Review and Vocabulary

8.9 Medical Terms in Context

CHAPTER OBJECTIVES

On completion of this chapter, you will be able to do the following:

1. Differentiate between voluntary, involuntary, skeletal, cardiac, and visceral muscles

2. Define terms relating to skeletal attachments

3. Name and locate common skeletal muscles

4. Analyze, define, pronounce, and spell terms relating to the muscular system

5. Describe common diseases

6. Define abbreviations relating to the muscular system

INTRODUCTION

Grip your right forearm with your left hand. Move the right hand up and down, then rotate it. What you feel are the various contractions of your forearm muscles as they respond to your mental command to move. While you were doing this simple exercise, your heart continued to beat. This action, too, involves muscular contraction, but did you mentally will it to happen? Of course not. The difference is that the muscles of your forearm are known as **voluntary** muscles, because they perform movement on command. The heart is an **involuntary** muscle. It performs without conscious command.

All bodily movement—whether it involves the lifting of a skeletal part such as an arm, the beating of the heart, or the action of the diaphragm during breathing—involves the contraction and expansion of voluntary or involuntary muscle. Skeletal movement is performed by **skeletal** muscles. Heartbeats are performed by **cardiac** muscle. Breathing, digestion, and other movements involving internal organs are performed by **visceral** muscles, muscles within the organ itself.

In this chapter, you will learn the terms associated with the skeletal muscles. Cardiac and visceral muscles will be addressed in other chapters.

Memory Key   Skeletal muscle is voluntary. Cardiac and visceral muscles are involuntary.

....

8.1   Skeletal Attachments

Bones are connected to other bones by tough connective tissue called **ligaments**. Muscles are connected to bones by equally tough connective tissue called **tendons**. There are tendons on each end of skeletal muscles because they need to be attached to two bones to make movement possible. To illustrate this concept to yourself, lift your forearm, starting from a 90 degree angle with your upper arm (Figure 8-1). Do you see the similarity to a drawbridge? Just as the deck of a bridge cannot be lifted without being pulled up by something that is attached to a structure that does not move, neither can your forearm. The muscle that moves the forearm is the **biceps brachii** (**BRAY**-kee-eye). It lies over the humerus and is attached at one end to the scapula, which does not move when the biceps contracts. The other end of the biceps is attached to the radius and moves when the biceps contracts. The point of attachment of the biceps to the scapula is called the **origin**. This is the term used for muscle attachment to the bone that does not move when the muscle contracts. The point of attachment to the bone that does move, the radius in this example, is called the **insertion**. This is the term used for muscle attachment to the bone that moves when the muscle contracts.

| Memory Key | Muscles attach to the stable bone at the origin and to the moving bone at the insertion. |

FIGURE 8-1
Movement of the forearm by the biceps brachii

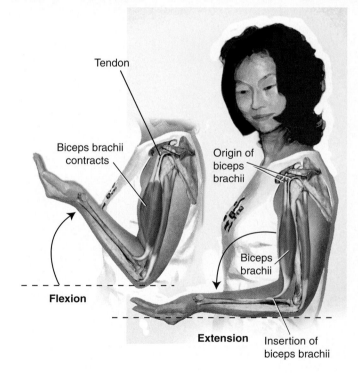

Tendon

Biceps brachii contracts

Origin of biceps brachii

Biceps brachii

Flexion

Extension   Insertion of biceps brachii

8.2   Major Skeletal Muscles

Figure 8-2 illustrates the major superficial muscles of the body.

FIGURE 8-2
Major superficial muscles of the body: (A) Anterior view; (B) Posterior view

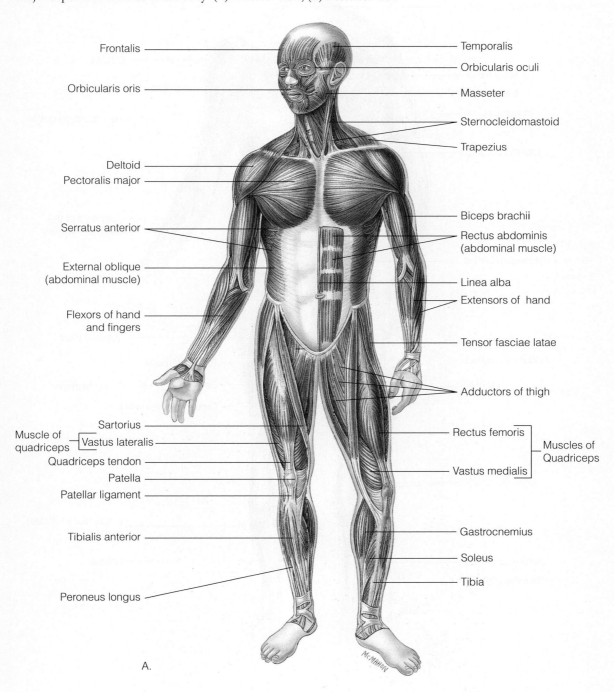

Frontalis

Orbicularis oris

Deltoid
Pectoralis major

Serratus anterior

External oblique
(abdominal muscle)

Flexors of hand
and fingers

Muscle of
quadriceps
Sartorius
Vastus lateralis
Quadriceps tendon
Patella
Patellar ligament

Tibialis anterior

Peroneus longus

Temporalis
Orbicularis oculi
Masseter
Sternocleidomastoid
Trapezius

Biceps brachii
Rectus abdominis
(abdominal muscle)

Linea alba
Extensors of hand

Tensor fasciae latae

Adductors of thigh

Rectus femoris
Muscles of
Quadriceps
Vastus medialis

Gastrocnemius
Soleus
Tibia

A.

Figure 8-2 *continued*

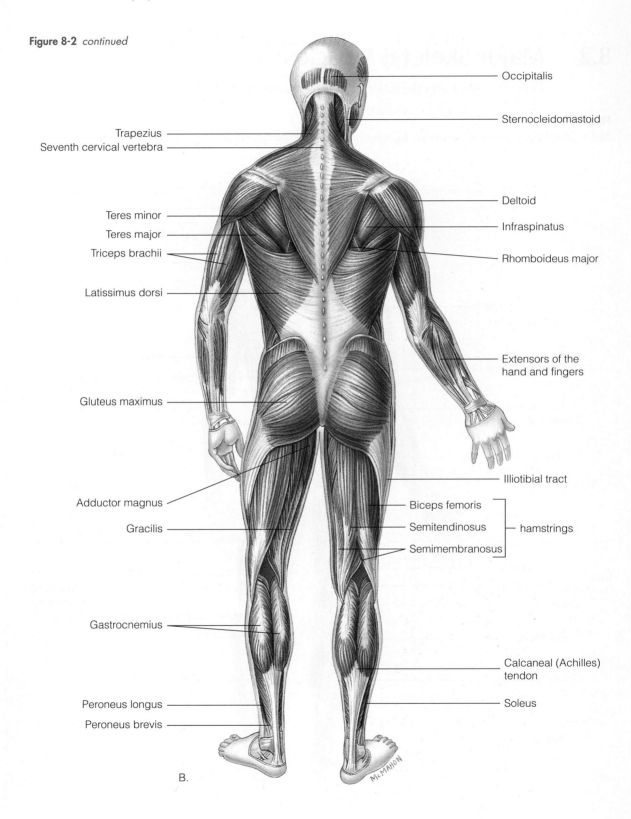

Occipitalis

Sternocleidomastoid

Trapezius

Seventh cervical vertebra

Deltoid

Teres minor

Infraspinatus

Teres major

Triceps brachii

Rhomboideus major

Latissimus dorsi

Extensors of the
hand and fingers

Gluteus maximus

Illiotibial tract

Adductor magnus

Biceps femoris

Gracilis

Semitendinosus   hamstrings

Semimembranosus

Gastrocnemius

Calcaneal (Achilles)
tendon

Peroneus longus

Soleus

Peroneus brevis

B.

Before you continue, review the Introduction and Section 8.1. Then, complete Exercise 8-1 found at the end of the chapter.

8.3   Additional Word Parts

The following roots and prefix will also be used in this chapter to build medical terms.

Root	Meaning
flex/o	bend
pronati/o	facing backward
supinati/o	facing forward
tens/o	stretch

Prefix	Meaning
dorsi-	back

8.4   Term Analysis and Definition

ROOTS

	duct/o	to draw
Term	**Term Analysis**	**Definition**
abductor (ab-**DUCK**-tor)	-or = person or thing that does something ab- = away from	muscles that move a part away from the midline
adductor (ah-**DUCK**-tor)	-or = person or thing that does something ad- = toward	muscles that move a part toward the midline

Term	Term Analysis	Definition
	electr/o	**electric**
electromyography (EMG) (ee-**leck**-troh-my-**OG**-rah-fee)	-graphy = process of recording **my/o** = muscle	process of recording the electrical activity of muscle *NOTE:* Electrical activity is produced in a muscle when it is stimulated by a nerve.
	fasci/o	**fascia (band of tissue surrounding the muscle)**
fascial (**FASH**-ee-al)	-al = pertaining to	pertaining to the fascia
fasciectomy (**fash**-ee-**ECK**-toh-mee)	-ectomy = excision; surgical removal	excision of fascia
fasciitis; fascitis (fas-ee-**EYE**-tis); (fah-**SIGH**-tis)	-itis = inflammation	inflammation of fascia
fasciorrhaphy (**fash**-ee-**OR**-ah-fee)	-rrhaphy = suture	suturing the fascia
	kinesi/o	**movement**
kinesiology (kih-**nee**-see-**OL**-oh-jee)	-logy = study of	study of movement
kinesimeter (**kin**-eh-**SIM**-eh-ter)	-meter = instrument movement	instrument used to measure used to measure
	lei/o	**smooth**
leiomyoma (**lye**-oh-my-**OH**-mah)	-oma = tumor; mass **my/o** = muscle	benign tumor of smooth muscle *NOTE:* The visceral muscles are smooth, whereas the skeletal and cardiac muscles are striated. They appear striped under the microscope. Striated means striped.
leiomyosarcoma (**lye**-oh-**my**-oh-sar-**KOH**-mah)	-sarcoma = malignant tumor of connective tissue **my/o** = muscle	malignant tumor of smooth muscle *NOTE:* Muscle is composed of connective tissue.
	muscul/o **(see also my/o)**	**muscle**
muscular (**MUS**-kyoo-lar)	-ar = pertaining to	pertaining to muscle

Term	Term Analysis	Definition
musculoskeletal (**mus**-kyoo-loh-**SKEL**-eh-tal)	-al = pertaining to **skelet/o** = skeleton	pertaining to the muscle and skeleton
	my/o	**muscle**
electromyogram (ee-**leck**-troh-**MY**-oh-gram)	-gram = record **electr/o** = electric	record of the electrical currents in a muscle
fibromyalgia (**figh**-broh-my-**AL**-jee-ah)	-algia = pain **fibr/o** = fiber	pain in fibrous tissues such as muscles, tendons, and ligaments
myalgia (my-**AL**-jee-ah)	-algia = pain	muscle pain
myopathy (my-**OP**-ah-thee)	-pathy = disease	any muscular disease
	myos/o	**muscle**
myositis (**my**-oh-**SIGH**-tis)	-itis = inflammation	inflammation of muscle
polymyositis (**pol**-ee-**my**-oh-**SIGH**-tis)	-itis = inflammation poly- = many	inflammation of many muscles
	rhabd/o	**rod-shaped; striped; striated**
rhabdomyoma (**rab**-doh-my-**OH**-mah)	-oma = tumor; mass **my/o** = muscle	benign tumor of striated muscle
rhabdomyosarcoma (**rab**-doh-**my**-oh-sar-**KOH**-mah)	-sarcoma = malignant tumor of connective tissue **my/o** = muscle	malignant tumor of striated muscle tissue
rhabdomyolysis (**rab**-doh-my-**OL**-ih-sis	-lysis = destruction; breakdown **my/o** = muscle	breakdown of striated muscle tissue
	tendin/o; ten/o	**tendon**
tendinitis (**ten**-dih-**NIGH**-tis)	-itis = inflammation	inflammation of a tendon
tendinous (**TEN**-dih-nus)	-ous = pertaining to	pertaining to a tendon

Term	Term Analysis	Definition
tenodesis (ten-**ODD**-eh-sis)	-desis = surgical fixation	surgical fixation of a tendon
tenotomy (teh-**NOT**-oh-me)	-tomy = to cut	cutting of a tendon
	tenosynovi/o	**tendon sheath (covering of a tendon)**
tenosynovitis (**teh**-noh-**sin**-oh-**VIGH**-tis)	-itis = inflammation	inflammation of a tendon sheath
	ton/o	**tone; tension**
atonic (a-**TON**-ick)	-ic = pertaining to a- = no; not; lack of	pertaining to a muscle that has no tone or tension; atony
dystonia (dis-**TOH**-nee-ah)	-ia = condition dys- = bad; difficult; painful	abnormal muscle tone or tension
myotonia (**my**-oh-**TOH**-nee-ah)	-ia = condition **my/o** = muscle	inability of the muscle to relax after increased muscular contraction
tonic (**TON**-ick)	-ic = pertaining to	pertaining to tone; tension

SUFFIXES

	-asthenia	**no strength**
Term	Term Analysis	Definition
myasthenia (**my**-as-**THEE**-nee-ah)	**my/o** = muscle	no muscle strength
	-clonus	**turmoil**
myoclonus (**my**-oh-**KLOH**-nus) (my-**OCK**-loh-nus)	**my/o** = muscle	alternate muscular relaxation and contraction in rapid succession

Term	Term Analysis	Definition
	-ion	**process of**

The following terms are used when describing muscle action (see Figure 8-3).

Term	Term Analysis	Definition
abduction (ab-**DUCK**-shun)	ab- = away from **duct/o** = to draw	process of drawing away from; opposite of adduction
adduction (ah-**DUCK**-shun)	ad- = toward **duct/o** = to draw	process of drawing toward; opposite of abduction
circumduction (**ser**-kum-**DUCK**-shun)	circum- = around **duct/o** = to draw	process of drawing a part in a circular motion
dorsiflexion (**door**-see-**FLECK**-shun)	dorsi- = back **flex/o** = bend	bending the ankle joint so that the foot bends backward (upward); opposite of plantar flexion
plantar flexion (**PLAN**-tar **FLECK**-shun)	**flex/o** = bend plantar = the sole of the foot	bending the ankle joint so that the top the foot bends toward the sole of the foot
extension (eck-**STEN**-shun)	ex- = out **tens/o** = stretch	to stretch out; stretching out a limb; increasing the angle between two bones; opposite of flexion
flexion (**FLECK**-shun)	**flex/o** = bend	bending a limb; decreasing the angle between two bones; opposite of extension
pronation (pro-**NAY**-shun)	**pronati/o** = facing backward	as applied to the hand, process of turning the palm backward; opposite of supination
supination (**soo**-pih-**NAY**-shun)	**supinati/o** = facing forward	as applied to the hand, the process of turning the palm forward; opposite of pronation

FIGURE 8-3
Types of muscle action

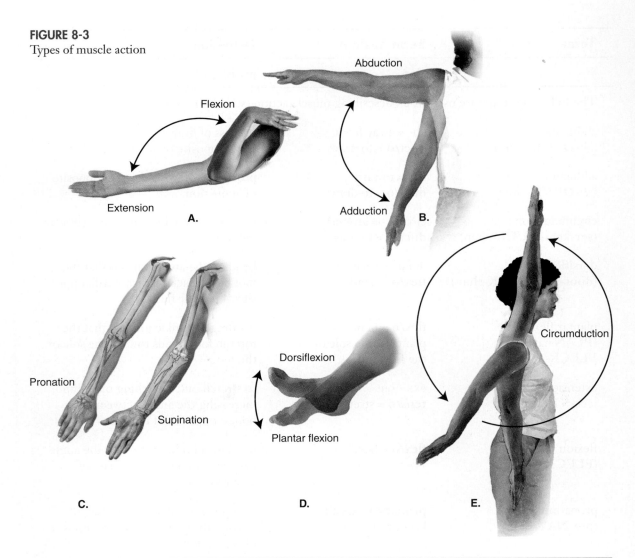

	-kinesia	movement; motion
Term	**Term Analysis**	**Definition**
bradykinesia (**brad**-ee-kih-**NEE**-zee-ah) (**brad**-ee-kih-**NEE**-shuh)	brady- = slow	slow movement
dyskinesia (**dis**-kih-**NEE**-zee-ah)	dys- = bad; difficult; painful; poor	impairment of muscle movement
hyperkinesia (**high**-per-kye-**NEE**-zee-ah)	hyper- = excessive; above normal	excessive movement

Term	Term Analysis	Definition
	-trophy	**nourishment; growth**
atrophy (**AH**-troh-fee)	a- = no; not	wasting away of the muscle
dystrophy (**DIS**-troh-fee)	dys- = poor; bad; difficult; painful	abnormal development, especially muscular dystrophy
hypertrophy (high-**PER**-troh-fee)	hyper- = excessive; above normal	enlargement of an organ due to an increase in the size of cells
	-thermy	**heat**
diathermy (**DYE**-ah-**ther**-mee)	dia- = complete;	heat applied to deep tissues through *NOTE:* A treatment for muscle soreness.

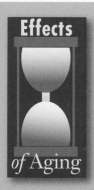

Effects

of Aging

Age-related muscle atrophy results from disuse and decreased levels of testosterone (hormone responsible for male characteristics), estrogen (hormone responsible for female characteristics), and the growth hormone. Also known as sarcopenia (sarc/o = flesh; -penia = deficient), **atrophy** is the wasting away of muscle tissue. Atrophy, along with changes in nervous control to muscles, results in muscle weakness that accompanies increasing age. Atrophy occurs most commonly in people who do not keep physically active.

8.5 Common Diseases

CARPAL TUNNEL SYNDROME (CTS)

The carpal tunnel is a small passageway in the wrist on the palmar side of the forearm. This passageway is made of ligaments. It protects the median nerve and tendons on the palmar side of the wrist. When the tendons and ligaments in this area are overused, they become inflamed, putting pressure on the median nerve. This causes numbness, pain, and weakness.

Treatment involves exercise, analgesics (pain killers), steroids, ergonomic improvements such as changing computer keyboards, and surgery to reduce the compression on the median nerve.

MUSCULAR DYSTROPHY (MD)

Muscular dystrophy is a broad term that includes a number of inherited disorders of the skeletal muscles. The main features are muscular weakness and degeneration of muscle tissue. The most common type is **Duchenne's** (doo-**SHENZ**) muscular dystrophy. There is no cure for the disease.

STRAIN

Commonly called a pulled muscle, a strain is the tearing, twisting, overstretching, or overextension of muscles and tendons. Rest, ice, compression, and elevation (RICE) is the most common treatment.

8.6   Abbreviations

Abbreviation	Meaning
EMG	electromyography
IM	intramuscular
ROM	range of motion (Degree to which a joint can be moved. Range is measured in degrees. Full range is 360 degrees. Limited movement may be 60 degrees.)
RICE	rest, ice, compression, elevation
SLR	straight leg raising

8.7   Putting It All Together

Exercise 8-1   SHORT ANSWER

1. Differentiate between the following terms in each group.

   (a) voluntary and involuntary muscles

   (b) cardiac, skeletal, and visceral muscles

(c) origin and insertion

_____

(d) ligaments and tendons

_____

Exercise 8-2   BUILDING TERMS

I. Use **my/o** or **myos/o** to build terms for the following definitions.

1. record of the electric currents in
   a muscle   _____

2. muscle pain   _____

3. inflammation of a muscle   _____

4. any muscle disease   _____

5. inflammation of many muscles   _____

II. Use the suffix -kinesia to build terms for the following definitions.

6. slow movement   _____

7. impaired movement   _____

8. excessive movement   _____

III. Use the suffix -trophy to build terms for the following definitions.

9. wasting away of the muscle   _____

10. abnormal development   _____

11. enlargement of an organ (due to an
    increase in the size of cells)   _____

IV. Use the suffix -or to build medical terms for muscles that:

12. move a part away from the midline   _____

13. move a part toward the midline   _____

14. bend a joint   _____

15. extend a joint   _____

16. turn the palm backward   _____

17. turn the palm forward   _____

Exercise 8-3   IDENTIFICATION

Identify the location of individual muscles using the following list:

    a. head

    b. upper extremities

    c. shoulder

    d. abdomen

    e. lower extremities

    f. back

  1. masseter _____

  2. trapezius _____

  3. serratus anterior _____

  4. external oblique _____

  5. biceps brachii _____

  6. vastus lateralis _____

  7. soleus _____

  8. semimembranosus _____

  9. latissimus dorsi _____

10. deltoid _____

11. semitendinosus _____

12. adductor magnus _____

13. triceps brachii _____

14. gastrocnemius _____

15. orbicularis oris _____

16. frontalis _____

17. gracilis _____

18. teres major _____

19. rhomboideus major _____

20. biceps femoris _____

Exercise 8-4   SPELLING PRACTICE

Circle any misspelled words in the list below and correctly spell them in the space provided.

  1. maseter _____

  2. sternocliedomastoid _____

3. serratus _____

4. rectus abdominis _____

5. transversus _____

6. trapezious _____

7. latisimus dorsi _____

8. terres major _____

9. rhomdoideus _____

10. semitendinosus _____

11. gastrocnemius _____

12. Achiles _____

Exercise 8-5   OPPOSITES

State the opposite muscle action in the space provided.

1. abduction _____

2. extension _____

3. plantar flexion _____

4. supination _____

8.8   Review of Vocabulary

In the following tables, the medical terms found in this chapter are organized into these categories: anatomy, pathology, diagnostics, surgery, and muscle movements. Define each term and decide in which category the word belongs. This will help you associate the term with its purpose and help you remember its meaning.

TABLE 8-1

REVIEW OF ANATOMICAL TERMS

1. abductor	2. adductor	3. fascial
4. kinesiology	5. ligaments	6. muscular
7. musculoskeletal	8. tendinous	9. tonic

TABLE 8-2

REVIEW OF PATHOLOGIC TERMS

1. atonic	2. atrophy	3. bradykinesia
4. carpal tunnel syndrome	5. dyskinesia	6. dystonia
7. dystrophy	8. fasciitis/fascitis	9. fibromyalgia
10. hyperkinesia	11. hypertrophy	12. leiomyoma
13. leiomyosarcoma	14. myalgia	15. myasthenia
16. myoclonus	17. myopathy	18. myositis
19. myotonia	20. polymyositis	21. rhabdomyoma
22. rhabdomyolysis	23. rhabdomyosarcoma	24. strain
25. tendinitis	26. tenosynovitis	

TABLE 8-3

REVIEW OF DIAGNOSTIC TERMS

1. electromyogram	2. electromyography	3. kinesimeter

TABLE 8-4

REVIEW OF CLINICAL AND SURGICAL TERMS

1. bursectomy	2. diathermy	3. fasciectomy
4. fasciorrhaphy	5. tenodesis	6. tenotomy

TABLE 8-5

REVIEW OF MUSCULAR MOVEMENTS

1. abduction	2. adduction	3. circumduction
4. dorsiflexion	5. extension	6. flexion
7. plantar flexion	8. pronation	9. supination

....

8.9   MEDICAL TERMS IN CONTEXT

After you have read the following Discharge Summary, answer the questions that follow it. Use your text, medical dictionary, or other references if necessary.

DISCHARGE SUMMARY

The patient is a 10-year-old boy whose first signs of weakness were noticed at age 2 to 3 years. The diagnosis of muscular dystrophy was confirmed by abnormalities found in his blood work. Muscular degeneration was confirmed on biopsy. He was started on drug therapy and is still ambulatory.

On examination, the patient is a pleasant young boy. He has proximal muscle weakness. He has calf hypertrophy and some deformity of the heel tendons. Otherwise, the general physical examination is within normal limits.

Based upon laboratory findings and biopsy, a diagnosis of muscular dystrophy was confirmed.

QUESTIONS ON THE DISCHARGE SUMMARY

1. Signs and symptoms of muscular dystrophy include:

   a. abnormalities found in blood work

   b. muscle weakness

   c. muscular degeneration

   d. all the above

2. The medical term for heel tendon is:

   a. Achilles tendon

   b. patellar tendon

   c. quadriceps tendon

   d. sartorius

3. Which muscle was enlarged?

   a. hamstrings

   b. gastrocnemius

   c. quadriceps

   d. none of the above

4. Muscular weakness of the leg was demonstrated at the point:

   a. away from the midline

   b. farthest away from the point of attachment to the trunk

   c. nearest the point of attachment to the trunk

   d. toward the midline

The Nervous System

CHAPTER ORGANIZATION

This chapter will help you understand the nervous system. It is divided into the following sections:

9.1   Divisions of the Nervous System

9.2   Functions of the Nervous System

9.3   Nerve Cells

9.4   Synapses

9.5   The Central Nervous System

9.6   The Peripheral Nervous System

9.7   Additional Word Parts

9.8   Term Analysis and Definition

9.9   Common Diseases

9.10   Abbreviations

9.11   Putting It All Together

9.12   Review of Vocabulary

9.13   Medical Terms in Context

CHAPTER OBJECTIVES

On completion of this chapter, you will be able to do the following:

1. Name and describe the divisions of the nervous system

2. State the major functions of the nervous system

3. Name and state the function of nerve cells

4. Differentiate between the cell body, the axon, and dendrites

5. Define *synapse*

6. List and describe the major portions of the brain

7. Describe the spinal cord

8. Name the protective covering of the brain and spinal cord

9. Differentiate between the somatic and autonomic nervous systems

10. Analyze, define, pronounce, and spell common terms of the nervous system

11. Describe common diseases

12. Define common abbreviations of the nervous system

INTRODUCTION

The nervous system allows the body to adjust to the requirements of internal and external environments. As soon as a change in the environment is sensed, the brain is notified. It then formulates an appropriate response and sends signals to the body to bring about the needed change. This is not a simple task. A vastly complex system is required to maintain bodily equilibrium. In fact, the human nervous system is far more complex than the most complicated computer. In this chapter, you will learn the terms associated with this amazing system.

9.1   Divisions of the Nervous System

As you study this section, you will find it helpful to refer to Figure 9-1, which diagrammatically represents the divisions of the nervous system.

There are two parts to the nervous system: the **central nervous system** (CNS) and the **peripheral nervous system** (PNS). The CNS consists of the spinal cord, which is the body's information superhighway, and the brain, which is the information-processing center. The PNS is mostly made up of nerve tissue, commonly referred to as **nerves**. Like all body tissues, nerves are made up of cells. The cells of the nerves are called **neurons** (**NEW**-ronz).

The PNS is made up of both **sensory** and **motor neurons**. Sensory neurons detect external and internal environmental influences and carry **sensory impulses** about those influences to the brain. Motor neurons carry messages called **motor impulses** from the brain to various parts of the body. These messages result in some type of movement.

Memory Key	• The CNS consists of the spinal cord and brain. • The PNS consists of the sensory and motor nerves. • Neurons are the cells that make up nerves.

9.2   Functions of the Nervous System

The nervous system has three functions: **sensory**, **integrative** (**IN**-teh-gray-tiv), and **motor**.

The sensory function detects changes inside and outside the body. Information about these changes is transmitted to the spinal cord and brain.

The integrative function is performed by the brain. It receives incoming information from the sensory system, processes it, and initiates the proper response through the motor system.

The motor function takes over when the brain has decided that a response is needed. A mot or impulse is sent through the motor neurons to the skeletal muscles, to an organ such as the heart, or to a gland such as the adrenal gland. These motor impulses stimulate the muscle, organ, or gland to initiate some needed change. The muscle, organ, or gland involved is called an **effector**, because it effects the required change.

Memory Key   The nervous system has sensory, integrative, and motor functions.

FIGURE 9-1
Divisions of the
central nervous
system and peripheral
nervous system

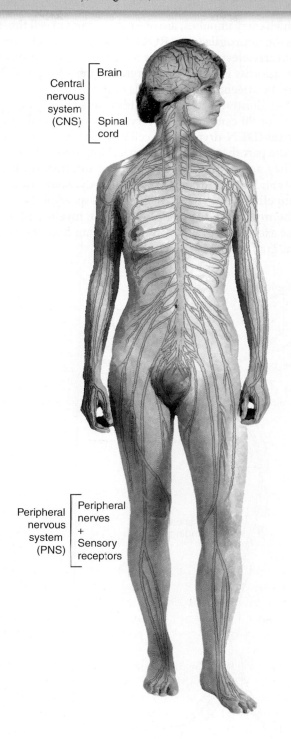

Central
nervous
system
(CNS)

Brain

Spinal
cord

Peripheral
nervous
system
(PNS)

Peripheral
nerves
+
Sensory
receptors

9.3   Nerve Cells

Neurons, which carry impulses, are one of two types of cell that make up nervous tissue. The other type is the **neuroglia** (new-**ROG**-lee-ah). These cells are found between the neurons. They do not carry electrical impulses but protect the neurons by engulfing unwanted substances. This process is called **phagocytosis** (**fag**-oh-sigh-**TOH**-sis). Neuroglia also provide nutrients by attaching blood vessels to the neurons.

Figure 9-2 illustrates a neuron. Although neurons vary greatly in size (some are as long as 3 feet, or 90 centimeters), every neuron has a **cell body**, an **axon** (**ACK**-son), and many **dendrites** (**DEN**-drytes). The cell body performs the work of maintaining the neuron. The axon is the part that transmits electrical impulses. The dendrites look like the branches of a tree. They are responsible for receiving information from the internal and external environments and transmitting it to the cell body. Some axons, but not all, are covered by a white fatty **myelin sheath**, which increases the speed of the electrical impulse. These axons are said to be **myelinated** (Figure 9-2). These myelinated axons are referred to as white matter. Some axons look gray because they do not have the myelin sheath. Those axons are referred to as gray matter.

FIGURE 9-2
Structures of the neuron. The neuron (nerve cell) includes the dendrites, axon, and cell body

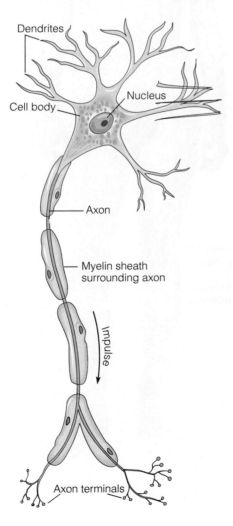

> **Memory Key**
> * Nervous tissue consists of neurons and neuroglia.
> * Neuroglia protect neurons through phagocytosis and attach blood vessels to neurons.
> * Every neuron has a cell body, an axon, and many dendrites.

9.4   Synapses

Neurons need a way to transmit electrical impulses to another neuron or to a muscle. This transmission is done at a junction called a **synapse** (**SIN**-apps). A synapse is a gap between a neuron and a muscle or between two neurons. When an electrical impulse travels down the neuron and reaches the synapse, a chemical referred to as a **neurotransmitter** (**new**-roh-trans-**MIT**-er) is released from a little sac at the end of the neuron. The neurotransmitter travels across the synapse and acts on the muscle, causing it to generate its own electrical impulse that produces muscle movement. Figure 9-3 illustrates a synapse.

FIGURE 9-3
Synapse between a
nerve cell and a muscle

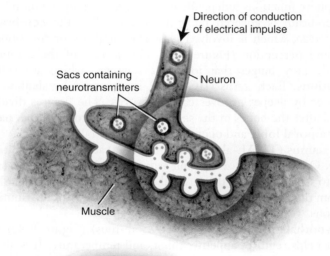

Direction of conduction
of electrical impulse

Sacs containing
neurotransmitters

Neuron

Muscle

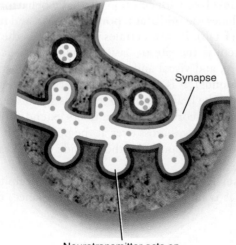

Synapse

Neurotransmitter acts on
the muscle, causing movement

| Memory Key | Synapses transmit impulses from neuron to neuron or from neuron to muscle. |

9.5 The Central Nervous System

THE BRAIN

The central nervous system (CNS) consists of the brain and the spinal cord. The structures of the brain are illustrated in Figure 9-4.

The **cerebrum** (seh-**REE**-brum) is the largest part of the brain. It receives sensory impulses from the peripheral nerves and initiates motor impulses to the viscera, especially muscles. It is the site of higher intellectual functioning. The cerebrum is divided into right and left **hemispheres** by a deep gap known as the **longitudinal fissure** (Figure 9.5). Bundles of nerve fibers called the **corpus callosum** (**KOR**-pus kah-**LOH**-sum) connect the two hemispheres, allowing them to share information. If the corpus callosum is severed, each hemisphere functions independently because the only communication link is gone.

The cerebrum is covered by gray matter called the **cerebral cortex** (seh-**REE**-bral **KOR**-tecks), which is involved in sensory and motor functions as well as thought, judgment, and perception (Figure 9-5). The surface of the cerebrum has the appearance of little gray bulges that look like sausages, which are called **gyri** (**JIGH**-rye) or **convolutions**. Each gyrus (**JIGH**-rus) is separated by shallow grooves called **sulci** (**SUL**-sigh) or by deeper grooves called **fissures**. The fissures divide the cerebrum into lobes named after the bones of the skull above them: **frontal lobe**, **parietal** (pah-**RYE**-eh-tal) **lobe**, **temporal lobe**, and **occipital** (ock-**SIP**-ih-tal) **lobe**.

The **thalamus** (**THAL**-ah-mus) (Figure 9-4a) acts as a relay station for incoming sensory stimuli. Once it recognizes stimuli as pain, temperature, touch, and so on, it transmits the stimuli to specific areas of the cerebral cortex for interpretation and then transmits motor impulses from the different cortex areas to the spinal cord for distribution to the appropriate motor neurons.

The **hypothalamus** (**high**-poh-**THAL**-ah-mus) (Figure 9-4a) is located below the thalamus. It helps regulate appetite, thirst, and temperature. It is also associated with the endocrine system and is involved with emotion and basic behavior patterns.

The **brain stem** includes the **midbrain**, **pons** (**PONZ**), and **medulla oblongata** (meh-**DULL**-ah ob-long-**GAH**-tah). It is sometimes referred to as the ancient brain or the animal brain. The brain stem is the site of basic life functions such as arousal, respiration, heart rate, blood pressure, and visual and auditory reflexes (moving the eyes and head to view objects or to hear sounds). It is also the center for nonvital reflexes such as coughing, sneezing, and swallowing. The brain stem also serves as a pathway for impulses traveling to and from the brain and spinal cord. The nerve fibers extend through the midbrain, pons, and medulla oblongata. The nerves cross over at the pons. Therefore, the right side of the brain controls the left side of the body, and the left side of the brain controls the right side of the body.

The **cerebellum** (ser-eh-**BELL**-um) lies under the occipital lobe of the cerebrum and protrudes dorsally. It is important in maintaining balance, muscle coordination, and equilibrium.

FIGURE 9-4
Lateral view of the
brain: (A) internal
brain structures;
(B) external brain
structures

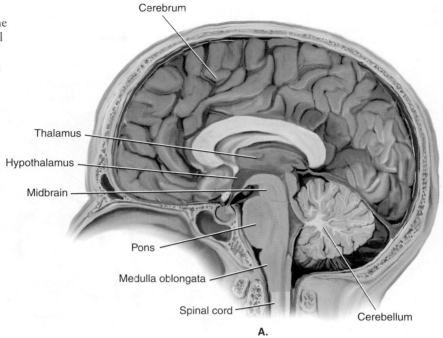

Cerebrum

Thalamus

Hypothalamus

Midbrain

Pons

Medulla oblongata

Spinal cord

Cerebellum

A.

Cerebral cortex

Parietal lobe

Frontal lobe

Occipital lobe

Temporal lobe

Medulla oblongata

Cerebellum

B.

FIGURE 9-5
Anatomical structures
of the cerebrum

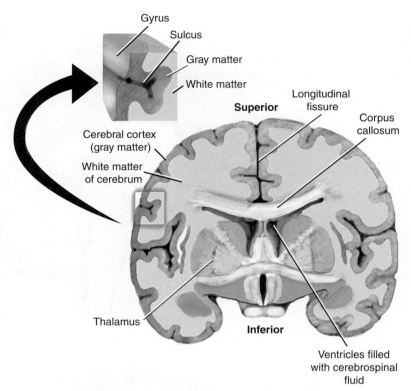

• The brain consists of the:
  cerebrum
  thalamus (a relay station for sensory and motor impulses)
  hypothalamus (helps regulate appetite, thirst, emotions, and basic behavior patterns)
  brain stem (midbrain, pons, medulla oblongata; involved with visual and auditory
    reflexes, respiration, heart rate, blood pressure, and arousal)
  cerebellum (involved with maintaining balance, muscle coordination, and
    equilibrium)

• The lobes of the cerebrum are:
  frontal
  parietal
  temporal
  occipital

• The cerebrum is covered by the cerebral cortex, which is divided into right and left hemispheres by the longitudinal fissures but is joined by the corpus callosum.

THE SPINAL CORD

The **spinal cord** consists of nerves. It is encased within the vertebrae for protection, extending from the medulla oblongata to the second lumbar vertebra and ending in a cone-shaped structure called the **conus medullaris** (**KO**-nus med-you-**LAR**-is). The nerves extend downward from the conus medullaris, looking somewhat like a horse's tail. This is referred to as the **cauda equina** (**KAW**-dah ee-**KWI**-nah).

The spinal cord branches into 31 pairs of spinal nerves. Each pair extends from the spinal cord bilaterally throughout its entire length. Eight pairs are cervical, 12 pairs are thoracic, 5-pairs are lumbar, 5 pairs are sacral, and 1 pair is coccygeal (Figure 9-6).

> **Memory Key** The spinal cord starts at the medulla oblongata, extends through the vertebrae, and ends at the conus medullaris, from which the nerves extend (cauda equina). Thirty-one pairs extend from the spinal cord (8 cervical, 12 thoracic, 5 lumbar, 5 sacral, and 1 coccygeal).

PROTECTIVE COVERINGS

The most obvious protection for the brain and spinal cord are the skull bones and the vertebrae. However, three membranes called **meninges** (meh-**NIN**-jeez) also serve as protective coverings. The outermost covering is the tough and thick **dura mater** (**DOO**-rah **MAY**-ter). The middle layer is the **arachnoid membrane** (ah-**RACK**-noid **MEM**-brain), and the inner one the **pia mater** (**PEE**-yah **MAY**-ter). Figure 9-7 shows the meninges. Note also the **subdural space** below the dura mater and the **subarachnoid space** below the arachnoid membrane.

Another form of protection is the **cerebrospinal fluid (CSF)**, a colorless liquid that continually circulates within the subarachnoid space around the brain and spinal cord, in the central canal inside the spinal cord, and in hollow cavities inside the brain called **ventricles** (see Figure 9-5). Because the brain and spinal cord float in the CSF, the central nervous system is cushioned, absorbing shocks.

The brain has a third type of protection, the **blood-brain barrier** (BBB), which is a protective mechanism that prevents toxic substances from entering the brain, while allowing necessary substances such as oxygen and glucose to enter.

> **Memory Key** The CNS is protected by bone, meninges, CSF, and the BBB.

FIGURE 9-6
Spinal cord,
posterior view

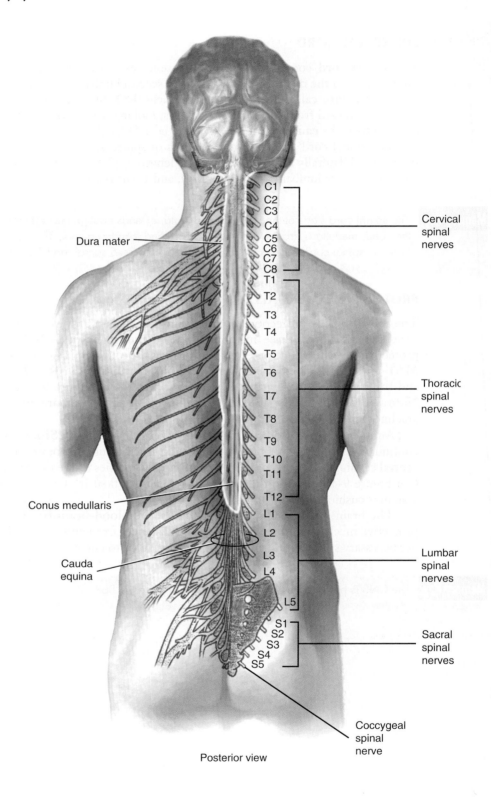

C1
C2
C3
C4
C5
C6
C7
C8

Cervical
spinal
nerves

Dura mater

T1
T2
T3
T4
T5
T6
T7
T8
T9
T10
T11
T12

Thoracic
spinal
nerves

Conus medullaris

L1
L2
L3
L4
L5

Lumbar
spinal
nerves

Cauda
equina

S1
S2
S3
S4
S5

Sacral
spinal
nerves

Coccygeal
spinal
nerve

Posterior view

FIGURE 9-7
Meninges: Dura mater,
arachnoid mater, and
pia mater

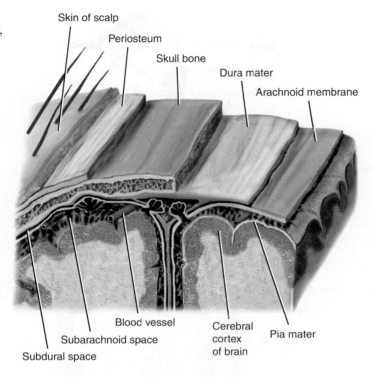

Skin of scalp
Periosteum
Skull bone
Dura mater
Arachnoid membrane
Blood vessel
Subarachnoid space
Subdural space
Cerebral cortex of brain
Pia mater

9.6   The Peripheral Nervous System

Twelve pairs of **cranial nerves** emerge bilaterally from the base of the skull, carrying nerve impulses to the muscles of the upper regions of the body, such as the tongue, larynx, thorax, abdominal viscera, eyes, face, pharynx, and mouth. Thirty-one pairs of **spinal nerves** emerge from the spinal cord bilaterally, carrying nerve impulses to a variety of organs. Figure 9-8 illustrates some spinal nerves as they extend from the spinal cord to peripheral sites. The names given to these nerves as they extend through the body reflect the artery closest to them or the organ or structure the nerve serves. For example, the radial nerve stimulates the muscles attaching to the radius bone of the arm.

Memory Key   There are 12 pairs of cranial nerves and 31 pairs of spinal nerves in the PNS.

FIGURE 9-8
Peripheral nerves

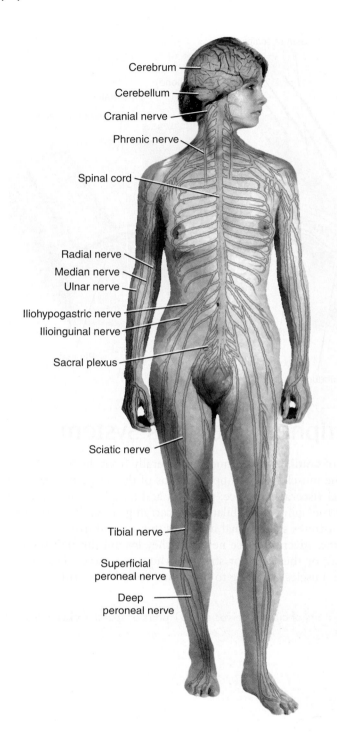

Cerebrum

Cerebellum

Cranial nerve

Phrenic nerve

Spinal cord

Radial nerve

Median nerve

Ulnar nerve

Iliohypogastric nerve

Ilioinguinal nerve

Sacral plexus

Sciatic nerve

Tibial nerve

Superficial
peroneal nerve

Deep
peroneal nerve

Before you continue, review sections 9–1 to 9–6. Then complete Exercises 9–1 and 9–2 found at the end of the chapter.

9.7 Additional Word Parts

The following roots, suffixes, and prefixes will also be used in this chapter to build medical terms.

Root	Meaning
gli/o	glue
myelin/o	myelin sheath
tom/o	to cut

Suffix	Meaning
-schisis	cleft; splitting
-us	condition; thing

Prefix	Meaning
para-	abnormal
polio-	gray
tetra-	four

9.8 Term Analysis and Definition

ROOTS

	cerebell/o	cerebellum
Term	**Term Analysis**	**Definition**
cerebellar (**ser**-eh-**BEL**-ar)	-ar = pertaining to	pertaining to the cerebellum

Term	Term Analysis	Definition
cerebellitis (**ser**-eh-bel-**EYE**-tis)	-itis = inflammation	inflammation of the cerebellum
	cerebr/o (see also encephal/o)	**brain**
cerebral (seh-**REE**-bral)	-al = pertaining to	pertaining to the brain
cerebrospinal (**ser**-eh-broh-**SPYE**-nal)	-al = pertaining to **spin/o** = spinal cord	pertaining to the brain and spinal cord *NOTE:* In this example, spin/o means spinal cord.
cerebrovascular (**ser**-eh-broh-**VAS**-kyoo-lar)	-ar = pertaining to **vascul/o** = vessel	pertaining to the brain and blood vessels
	cortic/ o	**cortex; outer covering**
cortical (**KOR**-tih-kal)	-al = pertaining to	pertaining to the cortex
corticospinal (**kor**-ti-koh-**SPYE**-nal)	-al = pertaining to **spin/o** = spine	pertaining to the cerebral cortex and spine
	dur/o	**dura mater (one of the membranes surrounding the brain)**
epidural (**ep**-ih-**DOO**-ral)	-al = pertaining to epi- = on; upon; above	upon the dura mater
subdural (sub-**DOO**-ral)	-al = pertaining to sub- = below; under	under the dura mater
	encephal/o	**brain**
electroencephalogram (ee-**leck**-troh-en-**SEF**-ah-loh-gram)	-gram = record **electr/o** = electric	record of the electrical activity of the brain (brain waves) *NOTE:* Brain waves can be **alpha waves** (typical of the awake person at rest), **beta waves** (typical of increased activity), or **delta waves** (typical of deep sleep). In conditions such as **seizure disorders** (**epilepsy**), the brain waves are abnormal in that they are uncoordinated and unorganized (see Figure 9-9).

FIGURE 9-9

Brain waves:
(A) normal brain waves
are usually consistent
in height and width;
(B) abnormal brain
waves. Note the in-
consistent height and
width of the brain
waves as seen in
patients with seizure
disorders (epilepsy)

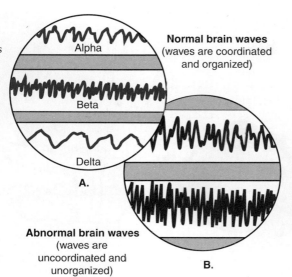

Normal brain waves
(waves are coordinated
and organized)

Alpha

Beta

Delta

A.

Abnormal brain waves
(waves are
uncoordinated and
unorganized)

B.

Term	Term Analysis	Definition
electroencephalograph (ee-**leck**-troh-en-**SEF**-ah-loh-graf)	-graph = instrument **electr/o** = electric	instrument used to record the used to record the electrical activity of the brain
encephalitis (en-**sef**-ah-**LYE**-tis)	-itis = inflammation	inflammation of the brain
encephalomalacia (en-**sef**-ah-loh-mah-**LAY**-see-ah)	-malacia = softening	softening of the brain
encephalopathy (en-**sef**-ah-**LOP**-ah-thee)	-pathy = disease	any disease of the brain
	hydr/o	**water**
hydrocephalus (**high**-droh-**SEF**-ah-lus)	-us = condition; thing **cephal/o** = head	accumulation of fluid in the brain (see Figure 9-10)
	magnet/o	**magnet**
magnetic resonance imaging (MRI) (mag-**NET**-ik **RES**-oh-nance)	-tic = pertaining to resonance = magnification imaging = a picture	a picture of the brain produced by using magnetic waves (see Figure 9-11) *NOTE:* Radiation is not used to produce an image.

FIGURE 9-10
Hydrocephalus.
*(Courtesy of
Dr. Russell Cox,
Gastonia, NC)*

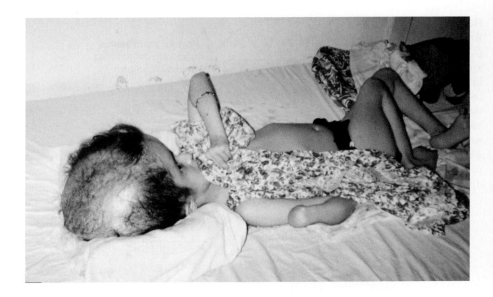

FIGURE 9-11
Schematic drawing of
magnetic resonance
imaging

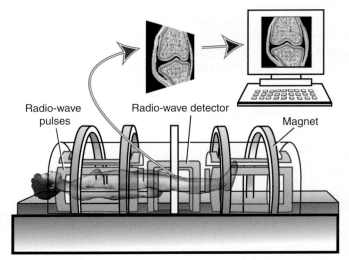

Term	Term Analysis	Definition
	mening/o	**meninges; membrane**
meningitis (**meh**-nin-**JIGH**-tis)	-itis = inflammation	inflammation of the meninges
meningoencephalitis (meh-**NING**-goh-en-sef-ah-**LYE**-tis)	-itis = inflammation **encephal/o** = brain	inflammation of the meninges and brain

	myel/o	spinal cord, bone marrow
Term	**Term Analysis**	**Definition**
myelogram (**MY**-eh-loh-gram)	-gram = record	record of the spinal cord
myeloschisis (**my**-eh-**LOS**-kih-sis)	-schisis = cleft; splitting	splitting of the spinal cord
poliomyelitis (**poh**-lee-oh-my-eh-**LYE**-tis)	-itis = inflammation polio- = gray	inflammation of the gray matter of the spinal cord
	neur/o	**nerve**
myoneural (**my**-oh-**NEW**-ral)	-al = pertaining to **my/o** = muscle	pertaining to the muscle and nerve; also known as neuromuscular
neuralgia (new-**RAL**-jee-ah)	-algia = pain	nerve pain
neurology (new-**ROL**-oh-jee)	-logy = study of	the study of the nervous system including diseases and treatment
neurologist (new-**ROL**-oh-jist)	-logist = a specialist in the study of	a specialist in the study of the diagnosis and treatment of nervous system disorders
neurolysis (new-**ROL**-is-is)	-lysis = destruction, breakdown; separation	nerve destruction
polyneuritis (**pol**-ee-new-**RYE**-tis)	-itis = inflammation poly- = many	inflammation of many nerves
	radicul/o	**nerve roots**
myeloradiculitis (**my**-eh-loh-rah-**dick**-you-**LYE**-tis)	-itis = inflammation **myel/o** = spinal cord	inflammation of the spinal cord and nerve roots

	spin/o	spine
Term	**Term Analysis**	**Definition**
spinal tap (**SPYE**-nal)	-al = pertaining to tap = draining of fluid	insertion of a needle into the subarachnoid space below the third lumbar vertebra to withdraw cerebrospinal fluid for diagnostic purposes; also known as lumbar puncture (see Figure 9-12)
	thalam/o	**thalamus**
thalamocortical (**thal**-ah-moh-**KOR**-tih-kal)	-al = pertaining to **cortic/o** = cortex	pertaining to the thalamus and cerebral cortex
	ventricul/o	**ventricles**
ventriculostomy (ven-**trick**-yoo-**LOS**-toh-me)	-stomy = new opening	new opening in the ventricles; used to treat hydrocephalus

FIGURE 9-12
Lumbar puncture

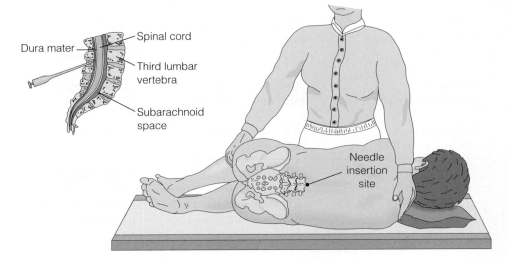

SUFFIXES

	-cele	hernia (protrusion)
Term	**Term Analysis**	**Definition**
meningocele (meh-**NING**-goh-**seel**)	**mening/o** = meninges; membrane	hernia of the meninges; displacement of the meninges from its normal position (see Figure 9-13A)
myelomeningocele (**my**-eh-loh-meh-**NING**-goh-**seel**)	**myel/o** = spinal cord **mening/o** = meninges; membrane	hernia of the spinal cord and meninges; displacement of the spinal cord and meninges from their normal position (see Figure 9-13B)
	-esthesia	**sensation**
anesthesia (**an**-es-**THEE**-zee-ah)	an- = no; not	loss of sensation
hypoesthesia (**high**-poh-es-**THEE**-zee-ah)	hypo- = below; under; decrease	decreased sensation

FIGURE 9-13
Meningocele and myelomeningocele

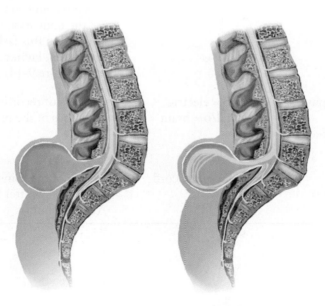

A. Meningocele   **B. Myelomeningocele**

Term	Term Analysis	Definition
hyperesthesia (**high**-per-es-**THEE**-zee-ah)	hyper- = excessive; above	increased sensation
dysesthesia (**dis**-es-**THEE**-zee-ah)	dys- = bad; painful difficult	irritating sensation in response to normal stimuli
paresthesia (**par**-es-**THEE**-zee-ah)	para- = abnormal	abnormal sensation such as numbness and tingling
	-graphy	**process of recording; process of producing images**
cerebral angiography (**SER**-eh-bral an-jee-**OG**-rah-fee)	**angi/o** = vessel -al = pertaining to **cerebr/o** = brain	the cerebral arteries are visualized after injection of a contrast medium (a dye used to highlight structures being studied) (to see an angiogram, refer to Figure 12-10)
computed tomography (CT scan) (toh-**MOG**-rah-fee)	**tom/o** = to cut	x-ray beam rotates around the patient, detailing the structure at various depths. The information is computer analyzed and converted to a picture of the body part. Common body parts studied in this fashion include the abdomen, kidneys, brain, and chest (see Figure 9-14)
electroencephalography (EEG) (ee-**leck**-troh-en-**sef**-ah-**LOG**-rah-fee)	**electr/o** = electric **encephal/o** = brain	process of recording the electrical impulses of the brain
myelography (**my**-eh-**LOG**-rah-fee)	**myel/o** = spinal cord	image of the spinal cord is produced using x-rays after injection of a contrast medium

FIGURE 9-14
Computed tomography and conventional x-ray procedure

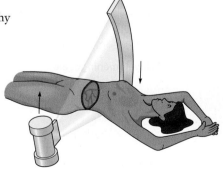

A. Computed tomography

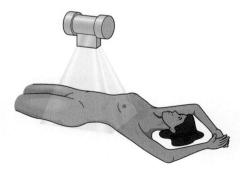

B. Conventional x-ray

	-kinesia;-kinesis	movement; motion
Term	**Term Analysis**	**Definition**
hyperkinesis (**high**-per-kih-**NEE**-sis)	hyper- = excessive; above	excessive motion; hyperactivity
dyskinesia (**dis**-kih-**NEE**-zee-ah)	dys- = bad; difficult	impaired movement
bradykinesia (**brad**-ee-kih-**NEE**-zee-ah) (**brad**-ee-kih-**NEE**-zhuh)	brady- = slow	slow movement
	-oma	**tumor; mass**
hematoma (**hem**-ah-**TOH**-mah)	**hemat/o** = blood	accumulation of blood in a space, organ, or tissue due to a break in a blood vessel; examples are epidural and subdural hematomas *NOTE:* Unlike other tumors, a hematoma is not an abnormal growth of tissue but a mass or accumulation of blood in tissues after a hemorrhage.
glioma (glye-**OH**-mah)	**gli/o** = glue	tumor of neuroglial cells
meningioma (men-**in**-jee-**OH**-mah)	**mening/o** = meninges; membrane	benign tumor of meninges
	-phasia	**speech**
aphasia (ah-**FAY**-zee-ah)	a- = no; not	no speech
dysphasia (dis-**FAY**-zee-ah)	dys- = bad; difficult	difficult speech
	-plegia	**paralysis (loss or impairment of motor function)**
diplegia (dye-**PLEE**-jee-ah)	di- = two	paralysis of like extremities on both sides of the body
hemiplegia (**hem**-ee-**PLEE**-jee-ah)	hemi- = half	paralysis of either the right or the left half of the body
monoplegia (**mon**-oh-**PLEE**-jee-ah)	mono- = one	paralysis of one extremity

Term	Term Analysis	Definition
paraplegia (**par**-ah-**PLEE**-jee-ah)	para- = beside; near	paralysis of the lower part of the body and legs
tetraplegia (**TET**-rah-**PLEE**-jee-ah	tetra- = four	paralysis of all four limbs; quadriplegia
	-taxia	**order; coordination**
ataxia (ah-**TACK**-see-ah)	a- = no; not	no muscular coordination (often due to cerebellar dysfunction)

PREFIXES

Term	Term Analysis	Definition
	de-	**lack of; removal**
demyelination (dee-**my**-eh-lih-**NAY**-shun)	-ion = process **myelin/o** = myelin sheath	lack of myelin sheath *NOTE:* Demyelination occurs in a condition called multiple sclerosis (MS), in which loss of the myelin sheath results in a variety of disorders such as muscle weakness, paralysis, visual disturbances, and urinary dysfunction.
	pachy	**thick**
pachymeningitis (pack-ee-**men**-in-**JYE**-tis)	-itis = inflammation **mening/o** = meninges; membrane	inflammation of the pachymeninges *NOTE:* Pachymeninges is another name for dura mater.

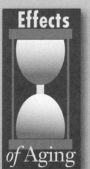

Effects *of* **Aging**

As we age, there is a steady loss of myelin sheath around the axon. Because the myelin sheath keeps the electrical impulse on course as it travels to its destination, significant loss may cause impaired coordination, which is relatively common in the elderly.

The number of neuroglia also diminishes with age. Because neuroglia provide support and nutrition to the neuron, the ability of the neuron to perform its function decreases as the number of neuroglia decrease. This contributes to neuron loss. This loss of neurons can contribute to muscle weakness, impaired coordination and reflexes, verbal and learning dysfunction, and short-term memory loss.

The destruction and deterioration of brain neurons causes Alzheimer's disease. This causes dementia, which is the loss of brain function that affects specific behaviors, normal daily routines, and intellectual abilities. It is more common in people older than 65 years.

9.9   Common Diseases

BRAIN TUMOR

A brain tumor is a neoplasm (new growth) in the brain tissue or the meninges. There are two types of brain tumors: **gliomas** and **meningiomas**.

Gliomas are malignant tumors. They can be fast or slow growing. They do not metastasize because the cells cannot pass through the cranium. However, tumors from elsewhere in the body (lungs and breasts) can spread to the brain.

Meningiomas are benign tumors. They are located outside the brain tissue but still within the cranium. They are slow growing, encapsulated (surrounded by a capsule), and do not tend to spread.

Because brain tumors place pressure on surrounding tissues, the symptoms will vary depending on the tumor's location.

Treatment involves the surgical removal of the, tumor followed by chemotherapy (killing of cancer cells using drugs) and radiotherapy (killing of cancer cells using radiation.)

MULTIPLE SCLEROSIS (MS)

Multiple sclerosis (**MUL**-tih-pul skler-**OH**-sis) is a condition in which the myelin sheath covering the axons in the brain and spinal cord is destroyed. This is called demyelination. It prevents impulses from being transmitted through the axon. This results in muscle weakness, paresthesia, dysesthesia, visual problems, tremors, paralysis, and other physical disabilities.

PARKINSON'S DISEASE (PD)

Parkinson's is a disease that results in slow movement (bradykinesia), muscular rigidity, and resting tremors (shaking). Parkinson's is a chronic, progressive condition.

The cause is unknown. However, the abnormal movements are due to a decrease of dopamine in the brain. Dopamine is a neurotransmitter necessary for normal brain function. Treatment includes drugs that replace dopamine and brain surgeries to reduce the tremors.

SEIZURE DISORDER; EPILEPSY

Disorganized, uncoordinated, and excessive electrical impulses in the brain can be caused by a seizure disorder, or epilepsy. This results in cerebral dysfunction, which in turn causes abnormal movement and sensations. The patient may or may not lose consciousness. Each attack is called an epileptic seizure. Refer to Figure 9-9, which illustrates normal and abnormal brain waves. Normal brain waves are the same in height and width. Abnormal brain waves, as seen in seizure disorder, have unequal height and width.

Most seizures are **idiopathic**, which means that their origin is unknown. Known causes include **pyrexia** (high fevers), brain tumors, and infections of the central nervous system. Seizures can be effectively controlled, but not cured, by drugs. A commonly used drug is Dilantin (dih-**LAN**-tin).

9.10 Abbreviations

Abbreviation	Meaning
ALS	amyotrophic lateral sclerosis (death of nerve cells in the brain and spinal cord results in muscular degeneration; typically fatal within 3 to 5 years), also known as Lou Gehrig's disease
BBB	blood-brain barrier
CNS	central nervous system
CSF	cerebrospinal fluid
CTS	carpal tunnel syndrome (pressure on a nerve in the lower forearm near the wrist results in pain and disuse of the hand)
CT	computed tomography
EEG	electroencephalography
HNP	herniated nucleus pulposus
LP	lumbar puncture
MRI	magnetic resonance imaging
MS	multiple sclerosis
PD	Parkinson's disease
PET	positron emission tomography (a diagnostic imaging procedure)
PNS	peripheral nervous system

9.11   Putting It All Together

Exercise 9-1   SHORT ANSWER

1. Define a neuron and state its function.

   _____

2. Differentiate between the sensory and motor neurons.

   _____

   _____

   _____

3. Name the meninges.

   _____

4. Write the name and number of the spinal nerves, in order from superior to inferior.

   _____

   _____

5. Describe the location of the cerebral cortex.

   _____

   _____

Exercise 9-2   MATCHING

Match Column A with Column B.

Column A	Column B
_____ 1. cell body	A. divides the cerebrum into right and left hemispheres
_____ 2. axon	B. maintains homeostasis of appetite, thirst, and temperature
_____ 3. dendrites	C. part of neuron containing organelles
_____ 4. cerebral cortex	D. acts as a relay station for incoming sensory stimuli
_____ 5. neuroglia	E. part of neuron that transmits impulses
_____ 6. longitudinal fissure	F. part of neuron that looks like branches of a tree
_____ 7. thalamus	G. gray matter covering the cerebrum
_____ 8. hypothalamus	H. protects the nervous system

Exercise 9-3 WORD BUILDING

Build the word for each of the following definitions.

1. nerve pain _____

2. a specialist in the study of the nervous system and its diseases _____

3. nerve destruction _____

4. inflammation of many nerves _____

5. record of the electrical activity of the brain _____

6. hernia of the meninges _____

7. hernia of the spinal cord and meninges _____

8. loss of sensation _____

9. decreased sensation _____

10. increased sensation _____

11. irritating sensation in response to normal stimuli _____

12. abnormal sensation such as numbness and tingling _____

13. paralysis of like extremities on both sides of the body _____

14. paralysis of either the right half or the left half of the body _____

15. paralysis of one extremity _____

16. paralysis of the lower part of the body and legs _____

17. paralysis of all four limbs _____

18. inflammation of the brain _____

19. softening of the brain _____

20. any disease of the brain _____

Exercise 9-4 ADJECTIVAL FORMS

Give the adjectival form for the following.

1. cerebellum _____

2. cerebrum _____

3. cortex   _____

4. nerve   _____

5. dura   _____

Exercise 9-5   SPELLING PRACTICE

Circle any misspelled words in the list below and correctly spell them in the space provided.

1. thalmus   _____

2. medula   _____

3. corpus callosum   _____

4. encephalomalasia   _____

5. cerrebelum   _____

6. epidurral space   _____

7. myeloschises   _____

8. ventricalostomy   _____

9. disphasia   _____

10. quadraplegia   _____

Exercise 9-6   PATHOLOGY

In the space provided, write the name of the disease described.

1. A disease characterized by the demyelination of axons in the central nervous system.

   _____

2. A disease that might be due to pyrexia, brain tumors, or infections of the central nervous system.

   _____

3. The main symptoms of this disease are tremors, bradykinesia, and muscular rigidity.

   _____

4. Treatment includes chemotherapy and radiotherapy.

   _____

5. This disease can be treated with Dopamine.

   _____

9.12 Review of Vocabulary

In the following tables, the medical terms found in this chapter are organized into these categories: anatomy, pathology, diagnostics, and clinical and surgical procedures. Define each term and decide into which category the word belongs. This will help you associate the term with its purpose, and help you remember its meaning.

TABLE 9-1

REVIEW OF ANATOMICAL TERMS

1. cerebellar	2. cerebral	3. cerebrospinal
4. cerebrovascular	5. conus medullaris	6. corpus callosum
7. cortical	8. corticospinal	9. dendrites
10. epidural	11. myoneural	12. nerve
13. neuroglia	14. neurologist	15. neurology
16. neuron	17. subdural	18. thalamocortical

TABLE 9-2

REVIEW OF PATHOLOGIC TERMS

1. aphasia	2. ataxia	3. bradykinesia
4. cerebellitis	5. demyelination	6. diplegia
7. dysesthesia	8. dyskinesia	9. dysphasia
10. encephalitis	11. encephalomalacia	12. encephalopathy
13. glioma	14. hematoma	15. hemiplegia
16. hydrocephalus	17. hyperesthesia	18. hyperkinesis
19. hypoesthesia	20. meningioma	21. meningitis
22. meningocele	23. meningoencephalitis	24. monoplegia
25. multiple sclerosis	26. myelomeningocele	27. myeloradiculitis
28. myeloschisis	29. neuralgia	30. pachymeningitis
31. paraplegia	32. Parkinson's disease	33. paresthesia

continued on page 204

Table 9-2 *continued from page 203*

34. poliomyelitis	35. polyneuritis	36. tetraplegia
37. seizure disorder		

TABLE 9-3

REVIEW OF DIAGNOSTIC TERMS

1. cerebral angiography	2. computed tomography	3. electroencephalogram
4. electroencephalograph	5. electroencephalography	6. myelogram
7. myelography	8. magnetic resonance imaging	

TABLE 9-4

REVIEW OF CLINICAL AND SURGICAL TERMS

1. anesthesia	2. neurolysis	3. spinal tap; lumbar puncture
4. ventriculostomy		

9.13   Medical Terms in Context

After you read the following Medical Note, answer the questions that follow. Use your text, medical dictionary, or other references if necessary.

MEDICAL NOTE

This gentleman is admitted with cervical spondylosis. He presents with progressive muscle weakness in his upper and lower extremities with evidence of spinal cord compression on his MRI. This is complicated by the presence of motor neuropathy confirmed on EMG nerve-conduction studies.

The influence of cervical spondylosis of future activities has been discussed with this gentleman in view that return to normalcy is unlikely.

QUESTIONS ON THE MEDICAL NOTE

1. Spondylosis is a disease affecting the:

   a. brain

   b. spinal cord

   c. nerve roots

   d. vertebrae

2. Compression means to:

   a. deteriorate

   b. press together

   c. displacement

   d. widen

3. The electromyogram confirmed:

   a. cord compression

   b. motor neuropathy

   c. spondylosis

4. Tests revealed the patient had problems:

   a. detecting changes inside and outside the body

   b. moving his muscles

   c. mentally processing the incoming information

5. The medical term for muscle weakness is:

    a. bradykinesia

    b. hypesthesia

    c. myasthenia

    d. myotonia

The Eyes and Ears

CHAPTER ORGANIZATION

This chapter will help you understand eyes and ears. It is divided into the following sections:

10.1   Eye

10.2   Additional Word Parts

10.3   Term Analysis and Definition Pertaining to the Eye

10.4   Common Diseases of the Eye

10.5   Abbreviations Pertaining to the Eye

10.6   Ear

10.7   Term Analysis and Definition Pertaining to the Ear

10.8   Common Diseases of the Ear

10.9   Abbreviations Pertaining to the Ear

10.10 Putting It All Together

10.11 Review of Vocabulary Pertaining to the Eye

10.12 Review of Vocabulary Pertaining to the Ear

10.13 Medical Terms in Context

CHAPTER OBJECTIVES

On completion of this chapter, you will be able to do the following:

1. Describe the structure, function, and location of the internal and external structures of the eye

2. Analyze, pronounce, define, and spell the medical terms common to the eye

3. Describe the structure, function, and location of the external, middle, and inner ear

4. Analyze, define, pronounce, and spell the medical terms common to the ear

5. Describe common diseases of the eye and ear

6. Give meanings for abbreviations common to the eyes and ears

INTRODUCTION

Our eyes and ears are the windows that let in the light and sound of the outer world. Light waves and sound waves are transformed by these organs into nerve impulses. Impulses from the eye are sent to the occipital lobe of the brain for processing, and those from the ear are sent to the temporal lobe. The results are what we experience as vision and hearing.

10.1   Eye

It is the job of the eye to let in light, focus it, transform it into nerve impulses, and send those impulses to the brain. Light enters the eye through an adjustable opening, the pupil, which regulates the amount of light allowed in. The lens, which lies behind the pupil, must focus the light much like the lens of eyeglasses. The difference is that the lens of the eye is not rigid like glass or plastic. It can adjust its shape to adapt to near and far objects. The light focused by the lens then goes to the back of the eyeball, where it strikes the retina. It is the retina that transforms the focused image into nerve impulses, which then travel along the optic nerve to the occipital lobe for processing.

The eye consists of the inner eye (the eyeball) and the outer eye (the facial structures and eye muscles surrounding the eye). As you read the following sections, refer to Figure 10-1, which illustrates the inner and outer eye.

INNER EYE

The inner eye consists of outer, middle, and inner layers. The outer layer consists of the **cornea** (**KOR**-nee-ah) and the **sclera** (**SKLEHR**-ah). The cornea is the transparent anterior portion, which allows light into the eye and participates in the focusing of light onto the back of the eye. The sclera is the white of the eye. It is a tough protective covering for most of the eyeball.

The middle layer is called the **uvea** (**YOU**-vee-ah), and consists of the **choroid** (**KOH**-roid), **ciliary body** (**SIL**-ee-ahr-ee), and **iris** (**EYE**-ris). The choroid is the inner lining of the sclera and contains blood vessels to nourish the eye. The ciliary body lies at the anterior edges of the choroid body and consists of the **ciliary muscles** and the **ciliary process**. The ciliary muscles adjust the shape of the lens for focusing. The ciliary process produces a watery substance, **aqueous humor**, which bathes the anterior region of the eye. The iris is the circular, colored portion of the eye. The central opening in the iris, called the **pupil**, regulates the amount of light that enters the eye. In bright light, certain muscle fibers of the iris that encircle the pupil contract, **constricting** the pupil. When these circular muscles relax in dimmer light, the pupil resumes normal size. Other muscles of the iris, called radial muscles, dilate (enlarge) the pupil beyond normal size when the person is stressed or excited.

The inner layer of the eye is the **retina** (**RET**-ih-nah). It has several layers of nervous tissue containing **cones** and **rods**, which are the cells that transform light into nerve impulses. The cones are responsible for central and bright-light vision and are concentrated in a small depression at the center of the retina called the **fovea centralis** (**FOH**-vee-ah sen-**TRAH**-lis), which lies within a small yellowish area called the **macula lutea** (**MACK**-you-lah **LOO**-tee-ah). The rods are responsible for peripheral and low-light vision and are

FIGURE 10-1
Structures of the eye:
(A) inner eye;
(B) anterior view
of eye

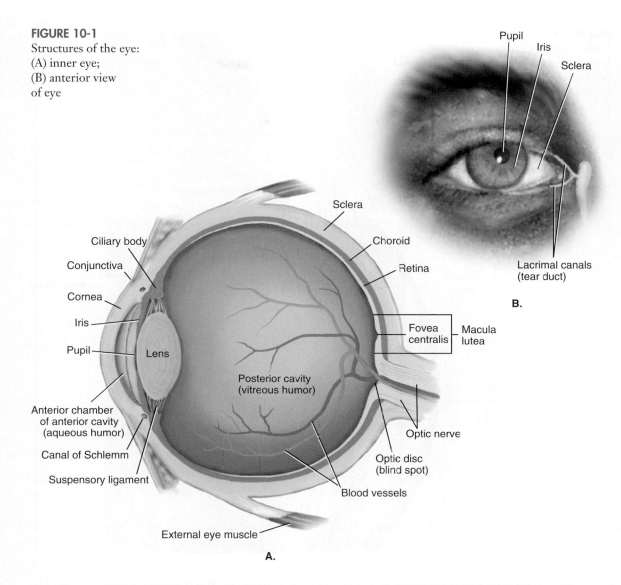

A.

B.

concentrated in the periphery of the retina, away from the macula lutea. One small area of the retina, medial to the fovea centralis, has no rods or cones, and thus does not produce a visual image. It is called the **optic disc**, or **blind spot**. It is the point at which the optic nerve begins, and the entry point for the major blood vessels of the eye. Ordinarily, you are not aware of the blind spot, but it is easy to observe. As you read this, close your left eye and place your index finger on the page. Move your finger to the right while keeping your eye focused on the left margin of the page. You may have to also move your finger up or down a little, but eventually you will find a spot where you cannot see the tip of your finger, because it is in the blind spot of your visual field.

The **lens** is illustrated in Figure 10-2. It is not considered to be part of one of the layers of the eye. It is located posterior to the iris and is held in place by ligaments called **suspensory ligaments**. As light passes through the lens, it is bent. This bending is called **refraction** (see Figure 10-6). The refracted light must be precisely focused on the

FIGURE 10-2

Uvea (choroid, ciliary body, iris); the lens and other structures of the eye

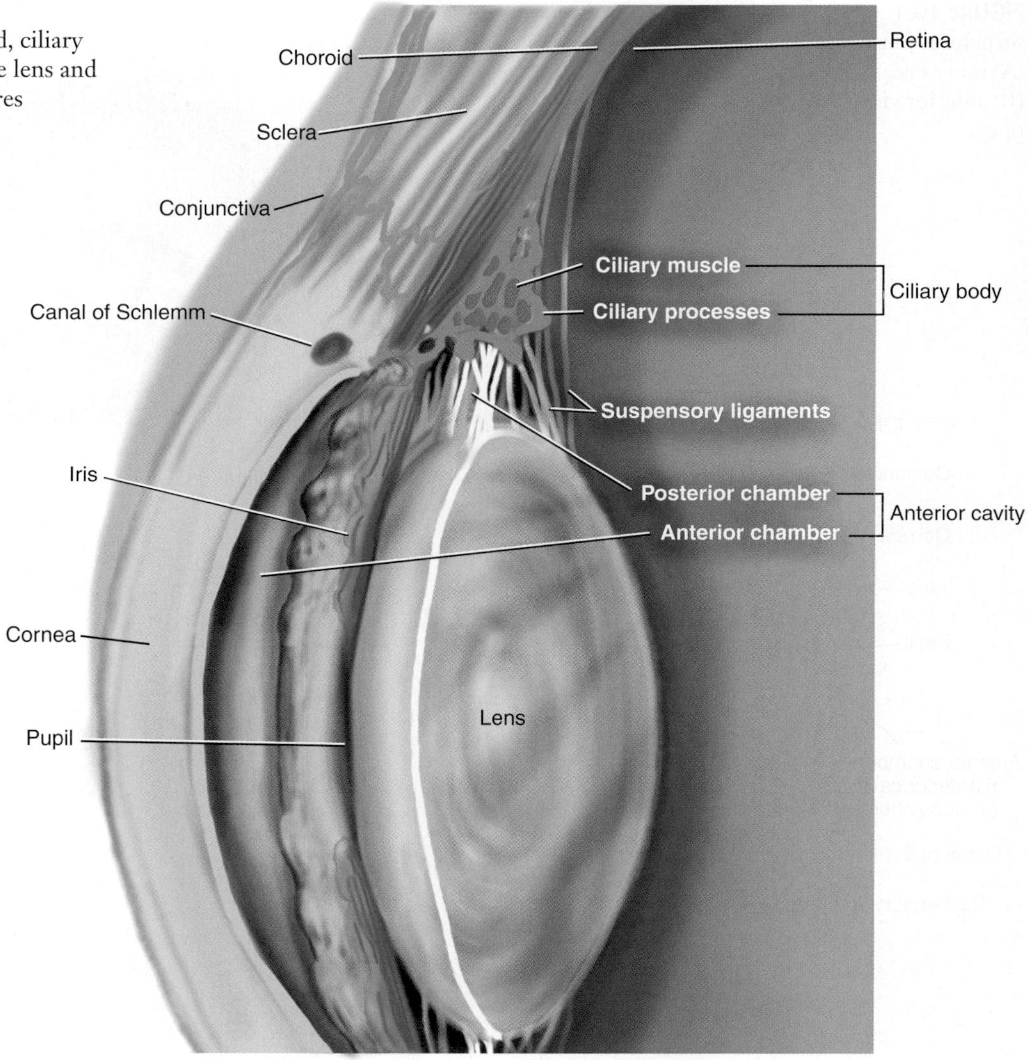

Choroid

Sclera

Conjunctiva

Canal of Schlemm

Iris

Cornea

Pupil

Retina

Ciliary muscle

Ciliary processes

Ciliary body

Suspensory ligaments

Posterior chamber

Anterior chamber

Anterior cavity

Lens

retina for a clear image to be formed. To focus the light, the lens must change shape. The ciliary muscles change the shape of the lens to allow clear vision of near and far objects. This lens-shape changing is called **lens accommodation** (ah-**kom**-oh-**DAY**-shun). Light from distant objects does not need to be bent much to focus on the retina, whereas light from near objects does. As we reach our forties, the lenses lose some of their elasticity, and we have difficulty focusing light from near objects. Reading glasses furnish the additional refraction the lenses can no longer provide.

Anterior and posterior to the lens are two cavities. The anterior cavity contains aqueous humor, a watery fluid produced by the ciliary processes. This fluid flows freely from the posterior chamber through the pupil to the anterior chamber. As this substance is produced and secreted, an equal amount is constantly drained through a lattice-type or meshwork structure called the **trabecula** (trah-**BECK**-you-lah) into the **canal of Schlemm** (shlem) and into the venous system (see Figure 10-2). Inability to drain aqueous humor causes increased intraocular pressure. This condition is called **glaucoma** (glaw-**KOH**-mah). For more detail, see Section 10.4, Common Diseases of the Eye. The equality between production and drainage helps maintain the equilibrium of the **intraocular pressure** (**IOP**).

The posterior cavity of the eye is filled with clear, jelly-like material called **vitreous** (**VIT**-ree-us) **humor**. It maintains the spherical shape of the eyeball, holds the retina firmly against the choroid, and transmits light.

Memory Key
- The inner eye consists of the: outer layer (cornea and sclera); middle layer or uvea (choroid, ciliary body, and iris); and inner layer (retina, containing rods and cones in the fovea centralis).
- The lens is not part of any of the layers. It is located posterior to the iris, and held in place by suspensory ligaments. It refracts light to focus the image on the retina, through a process called lens accommodation.
- The pupil is an opening in the center of the iris. The pupil regulates the amount of light entering the eye.
- The anterior cavity contains aqueous humor. The posterior cavity contains vitreous humor.

OUTER EYE

The outer eye is illustrated in Figure 10-3. It consists of the **orbital cavity**, **extrinsic ocular muscles**, **eyelids**, **conjunctival** (kon-junk-**TYE**-val) **membrane**, and **lacrimal** (**LACK**-rih-mal) **apparatus**. The orbital cavity is the bony depression into which the eyeball fits, providing protection. The six extrinsic ocular muscles attached to the sclera of each eye can move the eye in any direction. They are named according to their location and orientation: **rectus** means "straight," and **oblique** means "slanted." They are the superior rectus, inferior rectus, medial rectus, lateral rectus, superior oblique, and inferior oblique. The eyelids shield the eye from light, dust, and trauma. The conjunctival membrane is a thin mucous membrane lining the eyelids and the anterior part of the eye exposed to the air, providing protection and lubrication. The lacrimal apparatus produces, delivers, and drains tears from the eyes, thereby cleaning and lubricating them. The **lacrimal glands** produce the tears, which are continuously delivered to the eyes by the **lacrimal ducts**. Small openings called **punctae** (**PUNK**-tee) drain tears from the eyes into a system of canals in the nose. This is why your nose runs when you cry. Tears not only clean and lubricate the eyes; they also fight infectious microorganisms with an antibacterial enzyme called **lysozyme** (**LIGH**-so-zime).

Memory Key   The outer eye consists of the:

orbital cavity	conjunctival membrane
extrinsic ocular muscles	lacrimal apparatus
eyelids	

FIGURE 10-3

External anatomy of the eye: (A) eyebrow, conjunctiva, orbit, ocular muscles, optic nerve; (B) lacrimal apparatus

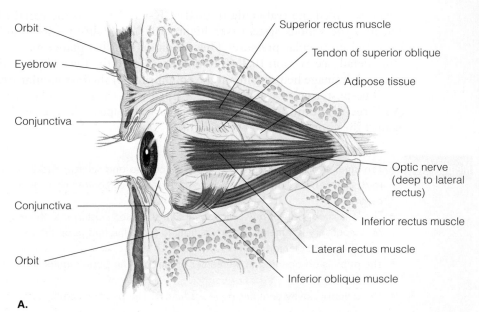

Orbit

Eyebrow

Conjunctiva

Conjunctiva

Orbit

Superior rectus muscle

Tendon of superior oblique

Adipose tissue

Optic nerve (deep to lateral rectus)

Inferior rectus muscle

Lateral rectus muscle

Inferior oblique muscle

A.

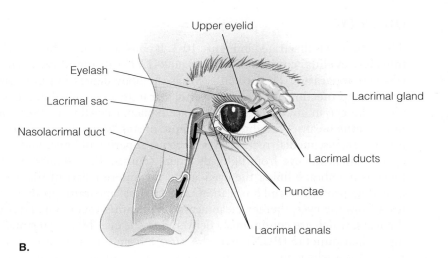

Upper eyelid

Eyelash

Lacrimal sac

Nasolacrimal duct

Lacrimal gland

Lacrimal ducts

Punctae

Lacrimal canals

B.

Before you continue, review Section 10.1. Then, complete Exercise 10-1 found at the end of the chapter.

10.2   Additional Word Parts

The following roots, suffixes, and prefixes will also be used in this chapter to build medical terms.

Root	Meaning
ambly/o	dull; dim
coagulati/o	to condense; to clot
dipl/o	double
emmetr/o	in proper measure
is/o	equal

Suffix	Meaning
-conus	cone-shaped
-edema	accumulation of fluid
-iasis	abnormal condition; process
-metrist	specialist in the measurement of
-ory	pertaining to

Prefix	Meaning
myein-	to shut
presby-	old age
pseudo-	false

10.3 Term Analysis and Definition Pertaining to the Eye

ROOTS

	aque/o	water
Term	**Term Analysis**	**Definition**
aqueous humor (**AY**-kwee-us **HYOO**-mer)	-ous = pertaining to humor = body fluid	pertaining to a watery fluid found in the anterior cavity
	blephar/o	**eyelid**
blepharopexy (**blef**-ar-oh-**PECK**-see)	-pexy = surgical fixation	surgical fixation of the eyelid
blepharoplasty (**blef**-ah-roh-**PLAS**-tee)	-plasty = surgical reconstruction	surgical reconstruction of the eyelid
symblepharon (sim-**BLEF**-ah-ron)	sym- = together; with	adhesion of the eyelid to the eyeball

Memory Key **Blephar/o** is most commonly used to indicate pathologic conditions of the eyelid.

	chori/o	choroid
chorioretinitis (**koh**-ree-oh-**ret**-in-**EYE**-tis)	-itis = inflammation **retin/o** = retina	inflammation of the choroid and retina
	choroid/o	**choroid; membrane**
choroiditis (**koh**-roid-**EYE**-tis)	-itis = inflammation	inflammation of the choroid
	conjunctiv/o	**conjunctiva**
conjunctivitis (kon-**junk**-tih-**VYE**-tis)	-itis = inflammation	inflammation of the conjunctiva

	core/o	pupil
Term	**Term Analysis**	**Definition**
anisocoria (**an**-ih-so-**KOH**-ree-ah)	-ia = condition an- = no; not **is/o** = equal	inequality in the size of the pupil
coreometer (**koh**-ree-**OM**-eh-ter)	-meter = instrument used to measure	instrument used to measure the pupil
	corne/o (see also kerat/o)	**cornea**
corneal (**KOR**-nee-al)	-eal = pertaining to	pertaining to the cornea
	cycl/o	**ciliary body**
cycloplegia (**sigh**-kloh-**PLEE**-jee-ah)	-plegia = paralysis	paralysis of the ciliary body
	-dacry/o (see also lacrim/o)	**tears**
dacryogenic (**dack**-ree-oh-**JEN**-ick)	-genic = producing	producing tears
	dacryocyst/o	**lacrimal sac**
dacryocystostenosis (**dack**-ree-oh-**SIS**-toh-steh-**NOH**-sis)	-stenosis = narrowing	narrowing of a lacrimal sac
	goni/o	**angle (of the anterior chamber)**
gonioscopy (**goh**-nee-**OS**-koh-pee)	-scopy = process of visual examination	process of visually examining the angle of the anterior chamber with the aid of a gonioscope *NOTE:* A diagnostic tool for glaucoma.
	irid/o; ir/o	**iris**
iridocyclitis (**ir**-ih-doh-seh-**KLYE**-tis)	-itis = inflammation **cycl/o** = ciliary body	inflammation of the iris and ciliary body
iritis (eye-**RYE**-tis)	-itis = inflammation	inflammation of the iris
iridectomy (**ir**-ih-**DECK**-toh-mee)	-ectomy = excision; surgical removal	excision of the iris

	kerat/o	cornea
Term	**Term Analysis**	**Definition**
keratoconjunctivitis (**ker**-ah-toh-kon-**junk**-tih-**VYE**-tis)	-itis = inflammation **conjunctiv/o** = conjunctiva	inflammation of the cornea and conjunctiva
keratoconus (**ker**-ah-toh-**KOH**-nus)	-conus = cone-shaped	abnormal, cone-shaped protrusion of the cornea *NOTE:* Keratoconus is a degenerative disease causing blurred vision. It can be corrected by wearing glasses or contact lenses.
keratomycosis (**ker**-ah-toh-my-**KOH**-sis)	-osis = abnormal condition **myc/o** = fungus	fungal infection of the cornea
keratoplasty (**KER**-ah-toh-**plas**-tee)	-plasty = surgical reconstruction; surgical repair	surgical repair of the cornea; corneal transplant *NOTE:* This operation, usually done under local anesthesia, includes the transplantation of a donor cornea from a cadaver into the eye of a recipient.
	lacrim/o	**tears**
nasolacrimal (**nay**-zoh-**LACK**-rih-mal)	-al = pertaining to **nas/o** = nose	pertaining to the nose and lacrimal apparatus
	mi/o	**contraction; less**
miosis (my-**OH**-sis)	-osis = abnormal condition	abnormal contraction of the pupil
miotic (my-**OT**-ick)	-tic = pertaining to	a drug used to constrict the pupil
	mydri/o	**wide; dilation; dilatation**
mydriasis (mih-**DRYE**-ah-sis)	-iasis = abnormal condition	dilation of the pupil
mydriatic (**mid**-ree-**AT**-ick)	-tic = pertaining to	pertaining to a drug used to dilate the pupil

	ocul/o	eye
Term	**Term Analysis**	**Definition**
extraocular (**ecks**-trah-**OCK**-yoo-lar)	-ar = pertaining to extra- = outside	pertaining to the outside of the eye
intraocular (**in**-trah-**OCK**-yoo-lar)	-ar = pertaining to intra- = within	pertaining to within the eye
	ophthalm/o	**eye**
exophthalmia (**eck**-sof-**THAL**-mee-ah)	-ia = condition ex- = outward	outward protrusion of the eyeball
ophthalmologist (**ahf**-thal-**MOL**-eh-jist)	-logist = specialist	a specialist in the study of the diagnosis and medical and surgical treatment of eye disorders
ophthalmology (**ahf**-thal-**MOL**-eh-jee)	-logy = study of	study of the eye, including diseases and treatment
ophthalmoscopy (**ahf**-thal-**MOS**-koh-pee)	-scopy = process of visual examination with the aid of an instrument	process of visual examination of the eye; also known as **funduscopy** (Figure 10-4) *NOTE*: The fundus is the back portion of the eye. It includes the retina, and macula lutea.

FIGURE 10-4
Ophthalmoscopy

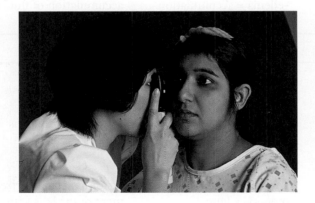

	opt/o	vision; sight
Term	**Term Analysis**	**Definition**
optic (**OP**-tick)	-ic = pertaining to	pertaining to vision or sight
optician (op-**TISH**-an)	-ician = specialist; one who specializes; expert	expert who fills prescriptions for eyeglasses and contact lenses *NOTE:* Opticians are not physicians and do not carry out medical and surgical treatment of eye conditions.
optometrist (op-**TOM**-eh-trist)	-metrist = specialist in the measurement of	specialist in the testing of visual function and in the diagnosis and nonsurgical treatment of eye conditions *NOTE:* Optometrists prescribe eyeglasses and contact lenses and are licensed in some areas to prescribe medication. They do not have a degree in medicine.
	palpebr/o	**eyelid**
palpebral (**PAL**-peh-bral)	-al = pertaining to	pertaining to the eyelid
	papill/o	**optic disc**
papilledema (**pap**-ill-eh-**DEE**-mah)	-edema = accumulation of fluid	accumulation of fluid in the optic disc
	phac/o; phak/o	**lens**
aphakia (ah-**FAY**-kee-ah)	a- = no; not; lack of	absence of lens
phacomalacia (**fack**-oh-mah-**LAY**-shee-ah)	-malacia = softening	softening of the lens
pseudophakia (**soo**-doh-**FAY**-kee-ah)	-ia = condition pseudo- = false	condition characterized by replacement of the lens with connective tissue

	phot/o	light
Term	**Term Analysis**	**Definition**
cyclophotocoagulation (**sigh**-kloh-**foh**-toh-koh-**ag**-yoo-**LAY**-shun)	-ion = process **cycl/o** = ciliary body **coagulati/o** = to condense; to clot	destruction of a portion of the ciliary body using a laser
photocoagulation (**foh**-toh-koh-**ag**-yoo-**LAY**-shun)	-ion = process **coagulati/o** = to condense; to clot	a beam from a laser is aimed at the site of injury to condense the retinal tissue, thus repairing any retinal tears or detachment (see under retin/o and Figure 10-5 for a description of retinal detachment)
photophobia (**foh**-toh-**FOH**-bee-ah)	-phobia = fear	intolerance or sensitivity to light
	pupill/o	**pupil**
pupillary (**PYOO**-pih-lar-ee)	-ary = pertaining to	pertaining to the pupil

FIGURE 10-5
Retinal detachment

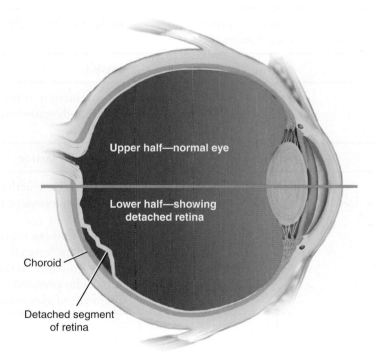

Upper half—normal eye

Lower half—showing detached retina

Choroid

Detached segment of retina

	retin/o	retina
Term	**Term Analysis**	**Definition**
retinal detachment (**RET**-ih-nal)	-al = pertaining to	separation of the retina from underlying tissue *NOTE:* The detachment might develop as a result of diabetes or because the vitreous humor shrinks with age, pulling on and separating the retina from the underlying tissue (see Figure 10-5).
retinopathy (**ret**-ih-**NOP**-ah-thee)	-pathy = disease	any disease of the retina *NOTE:* The most common retinopathy is due to diabetes.
retinopexy (**RET**-ih-noh-**peck**-see)	-pexy = surgical fixation	surgical fixation of the retina
retinoschisis (**ret**-ih-**NOS**-kih-sis)	-schisis = splitting; cleft	splitting of the retina
	scler/o	**sclera**
sclerectomy (skleh-**RECK**-toh-mee)	-ectomy = excision; surgical removal	excision of the sclera
	ton/o	**tension**
tonometry (toh-**NOM**-eh-tree)	-metry = process of measuring	measurement of intraocular pressure *NOTE:* A diagnostic tool for glaucoma.
	trabecul/o	**meshwork; lattice**
trabeculoplasty (trah-**BECK**-yoo-loh-**plas**-tee)	-plasty = surgical reconstruction; surgical repair	surgical reconstruction of the trabecular meshwork of the canal of Schlemm *NOTE:* This operation is done by laser and increases the outflow of aqueous humor, thereby reducing intraocular pressure; used in the treatment of glaucoma.

	uve/o	uvea (includes the choroid, ciliary body, and iris)
Term	**Term Analysis**	**Definition**
uveitis (**yoo**-vee-**EYE**-tis)	-itis = inflammation	inflammation of the uvea
	vitre/o	**glasslike; gel-like**
vitrectomy (vih-**TRECK**-toh-mee)	-ectomy = surgical removal	removal of some or all of the vitreous humor and its replacement with a clear fluid *NOTE:* This operation is necessary when scar tissue accumulates due to diabetic retinopathy.
vitreous humor (**VIT**-ree-us **HYOO**-mer)	-ous = pertaining to humor = body fluid	a gel-like, glassy substance in the posterior cavity

SUFFIXES

	-chalasis	relaxation
Term	**Term Analysis**	**Definition**
blepharochalasis (**blef**-ar-oh-**KAL**-ah-sis)	**blephar/o** = eyelid	relaxation of the eyelid
	-opia; -opsia	**visual condition; vision**
amblyopia (**am**-blee-**OH**-pee-ah)	**ambly/o** = dull; dim	dimness of vision
diplopia (dih-**PLOH**-pee-ah)	**dipl/o** = double	double vision
hemianopsia; hemianopia (**hem**-ee-an-**OP**-see-ah); (hem-ee-ah-**NOH**-pee-ah)	hemi- = half an- = no; not; lack of	lack of vision in half the visual field
presbyopia (**pres**-bee-**OH**-pee-ah)	presby- = old age	impaired vision due to advanced age

Term	Term Analysis	Definition
hyperopia (**high**-per-**OH**-pee-ah)	hyper- = above; beyond; excessive	light rays focus behind the retina; farsightedness (see Figure 10-6B)
myopia (my-**OH**-pee-ah)	myein- = to shut *NOTE: My* comes from the Greek word *myein*, which means "to shut."	light rays are focused in front of the retina; nearsightedness (see Figure 10-6C)

FIGURE 10-6
(A) Normal eye; (B) hyperopia (farsightedness); (C) myopia (nearsightedness)

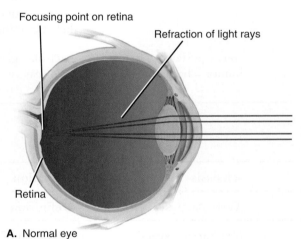

A. Normal eye
Light rays focus on the retina

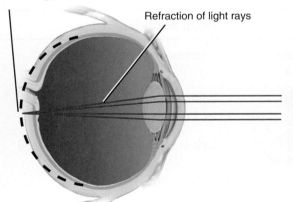

B. Hyperopia (farsightedness)
Light rays focus beyond the retina

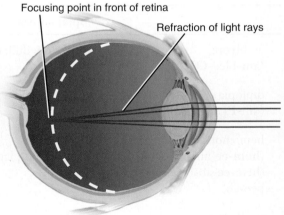

C. Myopia (nearsightedness)
Light rays focus in front of the retina

	-tropia	turning
Term	**Term Analysis**	**Definition**
emmetropia (**em**-eh-**TROH**-pee-ah)	**emmetr/o** = in proper measure	normal vision (see Figure 10-7A)
esotropia (**es**-oh-**TROH**-pee-ah)	eso- = inward	turning inward of the eyeball (see Figure 10-7B)
exotropia (**eck**-soh-**TROH**-pee-ah)	exo- = outward	turning outward of the eyeball (see Figure 10-7C)
hypertropia (**high**-per-**TROH**-pee-ah)	hyper- = above	upward turning of the eyeball
hypotropia (**high**-poh-**TROH**-pee-ah)	hypo- = below	downward turning of the eyeball

	-tropion	turning
ectropion (eck-**TROH**-pee-on)	ec- = out	outward turning of the eyelid
entropion (en-**TROH**-pee-on)	en- = inward	inward turning of the eyelid

FIGURE 10-7
Esotropia and
exotropia

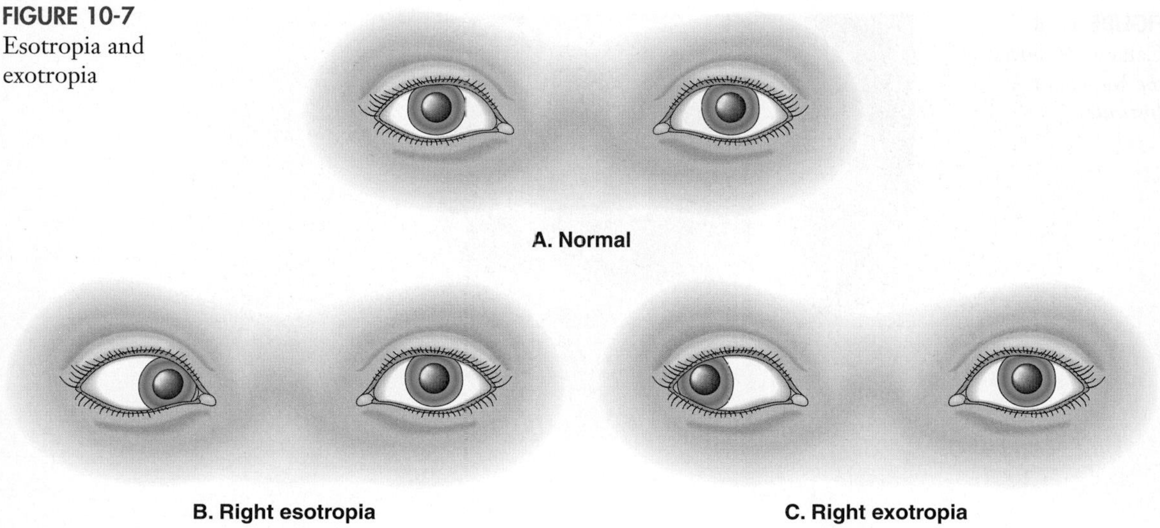

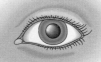

A. Normal

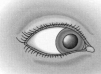 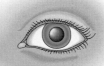

B. Right esotropia

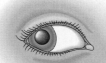 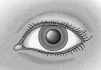

C. Right exotropia

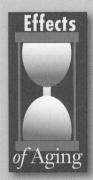

Effects of Aging on the Eye

From about age 40, the lens of the eye gradually becomes denser, harder, and thicker. Because this change in constitution makes the lens less flexible and elastic, it is difficult for the lens to change its shape, which is necessary to accommodate for distance. As a result, the majority of people 40 and older need reading glasses. This age-related condition is called presbyopia.

As we age, there also are changes in the way photoreceptors and pupils receive and transmit light. This means older adults require more light to see.

10.4 Common Diseases of the Eye

CATARACTS

A common age-related eye condition is cataracts (Figure 10-8). With age, the lens loses its transparent quality. It becomes thick and dense, progressing to a lens that is opaque and cloudy, thus interfering with the refraction of light rays. Cataracts were once a leading cause of serious vision loss but are now routinely removed surgically. One surgical technique is **phacoemulsification** (fack-oh-ee-**MUL**-sih-fih-kay-shun), which destroys the cataract by means of ultrasonic sound waves. Any fragments left are removed by suction. Another technique, **extracapsular cataract extraction** (**ECCE**), is the removal of the clouded lens, in one piece, through an incision (Figure 10-9). In both procedures, the capsule is left intact, and the defective lens is replaced with a prosthetic (artificial) implant called an **intraocular lens**.

FIGURE 10-8
Cataract (*Courtesy of the National Eye Institute*)

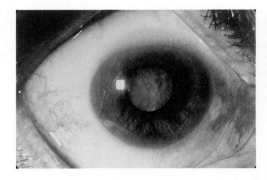

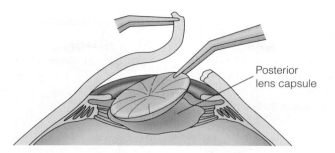

FIGURE 10-9
Extracapsular cataract extraction: lens is removed with its anterior capsule, leaving posterior capsule intact

Posterior
lens capsule

ERRORS OF REFRACTION

This category of disease refers to the way light rays bend (refract) and focus on the retina. The light rays coming into the eye must focus simultaneously on a single point on the retina. If the light rays focus before or after the retina instead of on the retina, vision will be impaired. Hyperopia (farsightedness) and myopia (nearsightedness) are two common refractive errors. In hyperopia, light rays focus behind the retina. In myopia, light rays focus in front of the retina. A third type is **astigmatism** (ah-**STIG**-mah-tizm), which is blurred vision because the curve of the cornea is uneven, thus preventing light rays from reaching a point of focus on the retina. Glasses must be worn to correct vision problems from refractive errors.

Laser surgery is a surgical procedure to correct the way the cornea refracts light. A laser is used to sculpt the cornea and change its shape. Following the surgery, light rays will focus on the same point on the retina. Vision is clear; glasses are not needed. Types of laser surgery are PRK (photorefractive keratectomy), LASIK (laser-assisted in-situ keratomileusis), and LASEK (laser epithelial keratomileusis). The type of surgery performed depends on the degree and type of refractive error the patient has.

GLAUCOMA

Glaucoma (glaw-**KOH**-mah) is defined as damage to the retina and optic nerve due to increased intraocular pressure. The intraocular pressure increases because the aqueous humor produced by the ciliary body is greater than the amount that flows out of the eye via the canal of Schlemm (Figure 10-10). Thus, aqueous humor builds up inside the anterior cavity, distorts the shape of the eye, and reduces vision. Glaucoma can result in blindness because of damage to the retina and optic nerve caused by the extra pressure.

FIGURE 10-10
Glaucoma

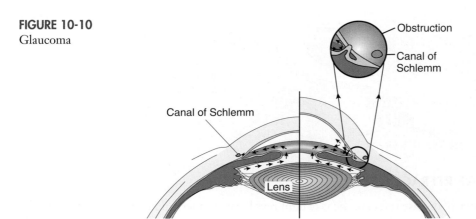

MACULAR DEGENERATION

Macular (**MAK**-yoo -ler) degeneration is deterioration of the macula (**MAK**-yoo-lah) lutea. It is also known as age-related macular degeneration (ARMD) because in some people, deterioration of the macula comes with the aging process. There is loss of central vision, progressing to blindness.

10.5   Abbreviations Pertaining to the Eye

Abbreviation	Meaning
accom	accommodation
ARMD	age-related macular degeneration
OD (oculus dextra)	right eye
OS (oculus sinistra)	left eye
OU (oculus unitas)	both eyes
PERLA	pupils equal, react to light and accommodation
PERRLA	pupils equal, round, regular, react to light and accommodation
PRK	photorefractive keratectomy
EOM	extraocular movement
IOL	intraocular lens
IOP	intraocular pressure

Abbreviation	Meaning
LASEK	laser epithelial keratomileusis
LASIK	laser-assisted in situ keratomileusis
VA	visual acuity
VF	visual field

10.6   Ear

The ear consists of the external ear, the middle ear, and the inner ear, as illustrated in Figure 10-11. The ear is responsible for hearing and plays an important role in the maintenance of balance. The hearing process consists of detection and **transduction** (tranz-**DUCK**-shun). Detection involves receiving the sound stimulus. Transduction involves converting the detected sound into a nerve impulse, which is then sent to the temporal lobe of the brain for processing. Balance is maintained through the interaction of visual signals and the balance mechanisms of the inner ear, discussed in this section.

Memory Key	The ear consists of the:
	    external ear
	    middle ear
	    inner ear
	It is responsible for hearing and plays a prominent role in maintaining balance.

EXTERNAL EAR

The external ear is composed of the **auricle** (**AW**-rick-ul), or pinna, the **external auditory meatus** (mee-**AY**-tus), and the **eardrum** or **tympanic** (tim-**PAN**-ik) **membrane** (Figure 10-11). The auricle is the part of the ear external to the head. Sound travels down the external auditory meatus, which is the canal that leads to the eardrum. When sound reaches the eardrum, it vibrates. The waves from this vibration then travel into the middle ear.

Memory Key	The external ear is composed of the:
	    auricle
	    external auditory meatus
	    eardrum (tympanic membrane)

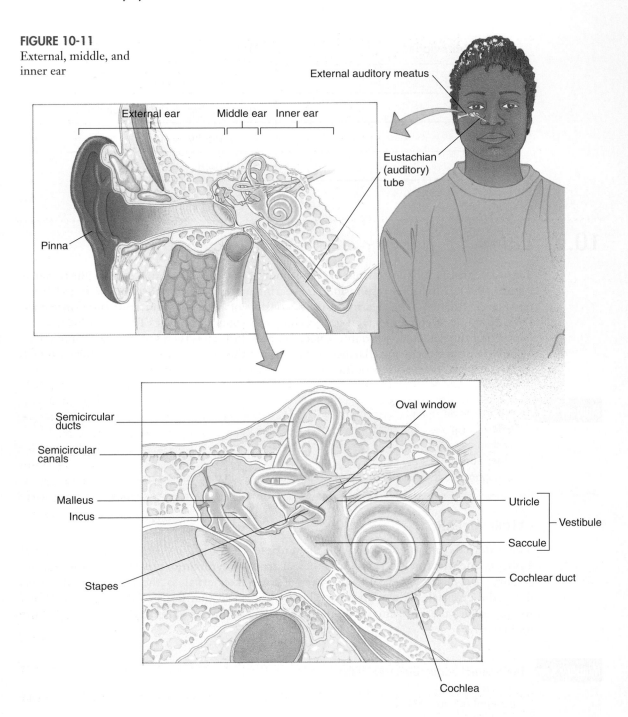

FIGURE 10-11
External, middle, and
inner ear

MIDDLE EAR

The middle ear includes three tiny bones collectively called the ossicles: the individual bones are the **malleus** (**MAL**-ee-us), **incus** (**ING**-kus), and **stapes** (**STAY**-peez), known also as the hammer, anvil, and stirrup, respectively (Figure 10-11). Sound is transmitted from the eardrum, to the malleus, to the incus, and then to the stapes. The stapes vibrates against the oval window (discussed below), which transmits the amplified sound to the inner ear, where it is changed to electrical impulses that the brain can detect and interpret.

Air pressure on each side of the eardrum is equalized by the **eustachian** (yoo-**STAY**-shun) **tube,** which connects the middle ear to the throat. When the eustachian tube is blocked, a sense of pressure is felt in the inner ear, and hearing ability is temporarily reduced. Often, pressure balance is restored with an audible popping sound. Sometimes, infectious material is transported up the eustachian tube from the throat, causing a middle ear infection (**otitis media**) (oh-**TYE**-tis **ME**-dee-ah), commonly seen in children.

> **Memory Key**   The middle ear consists of three ossicles called the malleus, incus, and stapes.

INNER EAR (LABYRINTH)

If you have ever looked at a sponge, you will have a good image of what the inner ear is like: a twisting series of canals and larger spaces (**sacs**). The canals and sacs of the inner ear are encased in bone and are thus referred to as the **bony labyrinth** (**LAB**-ih-rinth). They are filled with fluid called **perilymph** (**PEAR**-ih-limf). Within the bony labyrinth are tubes called the membranous labyrinth, filled with a fluid called **endolymph** (**EN**-do-limf).

The bony labyrinth consists of the **vestibule** (**VES**-tib-yool), **semicircular canals**, and **cochlea** (**KOCK**-lee-ah). The vestibule consists of the **utricle** (**YOO**-trih-kul) and **saccule** (**SACK**-yool), which are membranous sacs that are important in maintaining balance. Behind the vestibule are the semicircular canals, which house the **semicircular ducts**, also involved in balance. The cochlea contains the **cochlear duct**, a membranous structure responsible for hearing. Figure 10-11 illustrates all of the structures of the inner ear.

Sound is transmitted to the inner ear by the action of the stapes vibrating against an opening on the inner ear called the **oval window**. Lying within the cochlear duct is the **organ of Corti** (**KOR**-tye). It contains sensitive hair cells that react to the vibrations of the stapes by moving, much as tall grass sways in the wind. The movement of the hair cells stimulates underlying nerve cell fibers that create nerve impulses, which travel to the temporal lobe of the brain.

> **Memory Key**
> - The inner ear contains the:
>   bony labyrinth (vestibule, semicircular canals, and cochlea)
>   membranous labyrinth (utricle, saccule, semicircular ducts, and cochlear ducts)
> - Sound is transmitted by the vibration of the stapes against the oval window, causing the hair cells in the organ of Corti to sway and stimulate the underlying nerve fibers that create nerve impulses, which travel to the temporal lobe of the brain.

Before you continue, review Section 10.6. Then, complete Exercise 10-2 found at the end of the chapter.

10.7 Term Analysis and Definition Pertaining to the Ear

ROOTS

	audi/o (see also audit/o)	**hearing**
Term	**Term Analysis**	**Definition**
audiogram (**AW**-dee-oh-gram)	-gram = record	record of patient's hearing ability
audiometry (aw-dee-**OM**-eh-tree)	-metry = process of measuring	measurement of a patient's hearing ability
	audit/o	**hearing**
auditory (**AW**-dih-tor-ee)	-ory = pertaining to	pertaining to hearing
	aur/o (see also ot/o)	**ear**
aural (**AW**-ral)	-al = pertaining to	pertaining to the ear
	cochle/o	**cochlea**
cochlear (**KOCK**-lee-ar)	-ear = pertaining to	pertaining to the cochlea
electrocochleography (ee-**leck**-troh-**kock**-lee-**OG**-rah-fee)	-graphy = process of recording **electr/o** = electric	process of recording the electrical activity of the cochlea
	labyrinth/o	**inner ear; labyrinth**
labyrinthitis (**lab**-ih-rin-**THIGH**-tis)	-itis = inflammation	inflammation of the inner ear *NOTE:* Often accompanied by **vertigo** (dizziness) and a loss of balance.

	myring/o (see also tympan/o)	tympanic membrane; eardrum
Term	**Term Analysis**	**Definition**
myringotomy (**mir**-in-**GOT**-oh-mee)	-tomy = process of cutting; incision	process of cutting into the eardrum to remove fluid from the middle ear
	ossicul/o	**ossicles (malleus, incus, and stapes, collectively)**
ossiculoplasty (oss-**ICK**-yoo-loh-**plas**-tee)	-plasty = surgical repair	surgical reconstruction of the ossicles
	ot/o	**ear**
otalgia (oh-**TAL**-gee-ah)	-algia = pain	earache
otitis media (oh-**TYE**-tis **ME**-dee-ah)	-itis = inflammation media = middle	inflammation of the middle ear. If the inflammation results in a buildup of watery fluid, it is known as **serous** otitis media. If there is a buildup of pus, the condition is known as **purulent** (**PYOO**-roo-lent) otitis media (see Figure 10-12).
otorrhea (**oh**-toh-**REE**-ah)	-rrhea = discharge; flow	discharge from the ear
otosclerosis (**oh**-toh-skleh-**ROH**-sis)	-sclerosis = hardening	fusion of stapes onto the oval window *NOTE:* A common disease of the middle ear. Otosclerosis results in conductive deafness because the stapes is immobilized from the buildup of excess bone. Treatment includes the removal of the stapes and replacing it with a prosthesis.

FIGURE 10-12
(A) Normal tympanic membrane is translucent, shiny, smooth, and pearly gray; (B) serous otitis media;
(C) purulent otitis media.

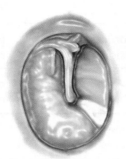

A. Normal tympanic membrane

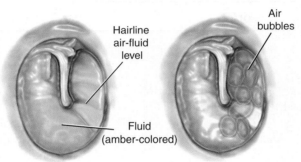

Hairline
air-fluid
level

Air
bubbles

Fluid
(amber-colored)

B. Serous otitis media

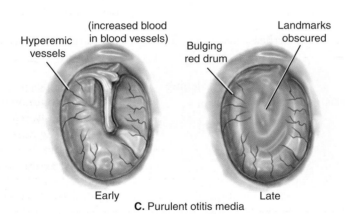

Hyperemic
vessels

(increased blood
in blood vessels)

Landmarks
obscured

Bulging
red drum

Early

Late

C. Purulent otitis media

Term	Term Analysis	Definition
otoscope (**OH**-toh-skope)	-scope = instrument used to visually examine	instrument used to visually examine the ear (see Figure 10-13)
	salping/o	**eustachian tube**
salpingoscope (sal-**PING**-goh-skohp)	-scope = instrument used to visually examine	instrument used to visually examine the eustachian tube

FIGURE 10-13
An otoscope is used to
examine the ear canal
and eardrum

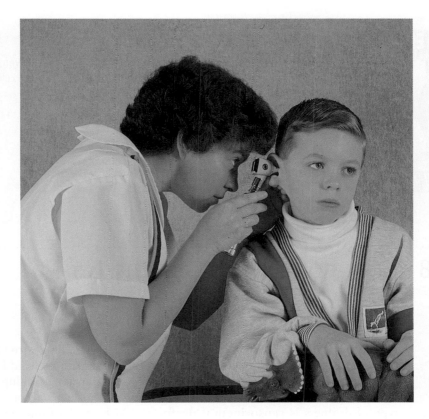

	staped/o	stapes
Term	**Term Analysis**	**Definition**
stapedectomy (**stay**-peh-**DECK**-toh-me)	-ectomy = excision; surgical removal	removal of the stapes. *NOTE:* This is procedure performed through the ear canal with a high-powered microscope.
	tympan/o	**tympanic membrane; eardrum**
tympanoplasty (**tim**-pah-no-**PLAS**-tee)	-plasty = surgical repair; surgical reconstruction	surgical reconstruction of the eardrum; myringoplasty

SUFFIXES

	-cusis	hearing
Term	**Term Analysis**	**Definition**
presbycusis (**pres**-beh-**KOO**-sis)	presby- = old age	diminished hearing due to old age. *NOTE:* Presbycusis is often accompanied by **tinnitus**, a ringing in the ears.

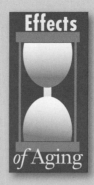

Effects of Aging on the Ear

Aging is accompanied by structural changes to the ear that prevent sound waves from reaching the inner ear. The result is age-related loss of hearing called presbycusis.

The sense of balance can also deteriorate. This is caused by a loss of inner-ear cells responsible for balance.

10.8   Common Diseases of the Ear

DEAFNESS

Deafness is defined as diminished or total loss of hearing. There are two types of deafness. **Conductive deafness** is caused by obstruction of the path traveled by sound waves from the external ear to the inner ear. Examples of obstruction are a buildup of earwax (cerumen) or a foreign body, such as popcorn, lodged in the external auditory meatus. The second type of deafness is **sensorineural deafness**, which results from damage to the auditory nerve or cochlea, causing failure of nerve stimuli to be sent to the brain from the inner ear. Sensorineural deafness is irreversible and can occur with age. It can also be caused by loud noises from machinery or music, tumors, infections, and injury.

Conductive deafness is treated by removing the obstruction. If this treatment does not help, hearing aids can be used to amplify the sound; however, hearing aids will help only if the nerve and brain structures allowing the patient to hear function normally. Hearing aids might be helpful in treating sensorineural deafness; however, if a hearing aid is not successful, cochlear implants might be needed to restore hearing.

MENIERE'S DISEASE

Meniere's (men-ee-**AYRZ**) is a condition of the inner ear that includes hearing loss, a feeling of pressure in the ear, **vertigo** (**VER**-tih-goh), meaning dizziness, and **tinnitus** (**TIN**-ih-tus), meaning ringing in the ears. The cause of the disease is unknown.

10.9   Abbreviations Pertaining to the Ear

Abbreviation	Meaning
AC	air conduction
AD (auris dextra)	right ear
AS (auris sinistra)	left ear
AU (auris unitas)	both ears
BC	bone conduction
EENT	eyes, ears, nose, throat
ENT	ears, nose, throat
HD	hearing distance
Hz	hertz (a unit of frequency, equal to one cycle per second; measurement used in audiograms)
NIHL	nerve-induced hearing loss
TM	tympanic membrane

10.10 Putting It All Together

Exercise 10-1   MATCHING—ANATOMY OF THE EYE

Match Column A with Column B.

Column A	Column B
_____ 1. cornea	A. white of the eye
_____ 2. iris	B. regulates amount of light entering the eye
_____ 3. lens	C. holds lens in place

_____ 4. conjunctiva   D. ciliary body, choroid, and iris

_____ 5. sclera   E. responsible for refraction and accommodation

_____ 6. suspensory ligament F. colored portion of the eye

_____ 7. pupil   G. adjusts shape of lens

_____ 8. ciliary muscle   H. produces aqueous humor

_____ 9. ciliary process   I. anterior portion of the eye, refracting light rays

_____ 10. uvea   J. lines the eyelid

Exercise 10-2   MATCHING

Match the anatomical term in Column A with its description in Column B. Descriptions in Column B can be used more than once.

Column A   **Column B**

_____ 1. malleus   A. function is balance

_____ 2. utricle   B. also known as the inner ear

_____ 3. tympanic membrane   C. located within the membranous labyrinth

_____ 4. perilymph   D. vibrates with sound waves

_____ 5. endolymph   E. transmits sound waves to the inner ear

_____ 6. labyrinth   F. located within the bony labyrinth

_____ 7. incus

_____ 8. vestibule

Exercise 10-3   ANALYSIS OF TERMS

Analyze the word into its component parts, and then define the term.

Example: cycloplegia

            -plegia = paralysis

            cycl/o = ciliary body

            paralysis of the ciliary body

 1. gonioscopy

_____

_____

_____

2. anisocoria

_____

_____

_____

3. miosis

_____

_____

_____

4. mydriatic

_____

_____

_____

5. optician

_____

_____

_____

6. tonometry

_____

_____

_____

7. retinoschisis

_____

_____

_____

8. hyperopia

_____

_____

_____

9. presbyopia

_____

_____

_____

10. entropion

_____

_____

_____

11. electrocochleography

_____

_____

_____

12. presbycusis

_____

_____

_____

13. otitis media

_____

_____

_____

14. audiometry

_____

_____

_____

15. aural

_____

_____

_____

Exercise 10-4   BUILDING MEDICAL TERMS

Build the medical term for the following definitions.

1. surgical fixation of the eyelid   _____

2. drooping of the eyelid   _____

3. sudden, involuntary contraction of
   the eyelid   _____

4. adhesion of the eyeball to the eyelid   _____

5. inflammation of the iris
   and ciliary body

   _____

6. excision of the iris

   _____

7. inflammation of the cornea
   and conjunctiva

   _____

8. abnormal, cone-shaped protrusion
   of the cornea

   _____

9. fungal infection of the cornea

   _____

10. surgical repair of the cornea

    _____

11. earache

    _____

12. discharge from the ear

    _____

13. surgical repair of the eardrum

    _____

14. process of cutting the eardrum

    _____

15. removal of the stapes

    _____

Exercise 10-5   DIFFERENCES IN TERMS

Distinguish between the following pairs.

1. amblyopia and diplopia

   _____

2. esotropia and exotropia

   _____

3. presbyopia, emmetropia, and presbycusis

   _____

4. hypertropia and hypotropia

   _____

5. ectropion and entropion

   _____

6. optician, optometrist, and ophthalmologist

   _____

7. vertigo and tinnitus

   _____

Exercise 10-6   ADJECTIVAL FORMS

Write the adjectival form for the following. Use the dictionary if necessary.

1. cornea   _____

2. retina   _____

3. pupil   _____

4. cochlea   _____

Exercise 10-7   SPELLING PRACTICE

Circle any misspelled words in the following list and correctly spell them in the space provided.

1. synblepharon   _____

2. goneoscopy   _____

3. miosis   _____

4. exopthalmia   _____

5. papilledema   _____

6. retinoschsis   _____

7. uveitis   _____

8. labyrinthitis   _____

9. otalgia   _____

10. presbycusis   _____

Exercise 10-8   PLURALS

Write the plural form for the following terms. Use your dictionary if necessary.

1. iris   _____

2. palpebra   _____

3. retina   _____

4. sclera   _____

Exercise 10-9   PATHOLOGY

Define the following terms relating to pathology.

1. tinnitus   _____

2. vertigo   _____

3. sensorineural deafness   _____

4. conductive deafness   _____

5. Meniere's disease   _____

6. cataracts   _____

7. astigmatism   _____

8. PRK, LASIK, and LASEK   _____

10.11 Review of Vocabulary Pertaining to the Eye

In the following tables, the medical terms are organized into these categories: anatomy, physiology, pathology, diagnostics, and surgical procedures. Define each term and decide in to which category the word belongs. This will help you associate the term with its purpose, and help you remember it.

TABLE 10-1		
REVIEW OF ANATOMICAL AND PHYSIOLOGICAL TERMS PERTAINING TO THE EYES		
1. accommodation	2. aqueous humor	3. corneal
4. emmetropia	5. extraocular	6. intraocular
7. lens	8. miotic	9. nasolacrimal
10. ophthalmologist	11. ophthalmology	12. optic
13. optic disc	14. optician	15. optometrist
16. palpebral	17. punctae	18. pupillary
19. trabeculae	20. vitreous humor	

TABLE 10-2

REVIEW OF PATHOLOGIC TERMS PERTAINING TO THE EYES

1. amblyopia	2. anisocoria	3. aphakia
4. blepharochalasis	5. blepharoptosis	6. blepharospasm
7. chorioretinitis	8. choroiditis	9. conjunctivitis
10. cycloplegia	11. dacryostenosis	12. diplopia
13. ectropion	14. entropion	15. esotropia
16. exophthalmia	17. exotropia	18. glaucoma
19. hemianopsia	20. hyperopia	21. hypertropia
22. hypotropia	23. iridocyclitis	24. iritis
25. keratoconjunctivitis	26. keratoconus	27. keratomycosis
28. miosis	29. mydriasis	30. myopia
31. papilledema	32. phacomalacia	33. photophobia
34. presbyopia	35 . pseudophakia	36. retinal detachment

continued on page 245

Table 10-2 *continued from page 244*

37. retinopathy	38. retinoschisis	39. symblepharon
40. trabeculoplasty	41. uveitis	42. vitrectomy

TABLE 10-3

REVIEW OF DIAGNOSTIC TERMS PERTAINING TO THE EYES

1. coreometer	2. funduscopy	3. gonioscopy
4. ophthalmoscopy	5. tonometry	

TABLE 10-4

REVIEW OF SURGICAL TERMS PERTAINING TO THE EYES

1. blepharopexy	2. cyclophotocoagulation	3. iridectomy
4. keratoplasty	5. phacoemulsification	6. photocoagulation
7. retinopexy	8. sclerectomy	

10.12 Review of Vocabulary Pertaining to the Ear

In the following tables, the medical terms are organized into the following categories: anatomy, pathology, diagnostics, and surgical procedures. Define each term and decide into which category the word belongs. This will help you associate the term with its purpose, and thus help you remember it.

TABLE 10-5

REVIEW OF ANATOMICAL TERMS PERTAINING TO THE EARS

1. audiometer	2. auditory	3. aural
4. cochlear	5. endolymph	6. incus
7. malleus	8. perilymph	9. stapes

TABLE 10-6

REVIEW OF PATHOLOGIC TERMS PERTAINING TO THE EARS

1. labyrinthitis	2. otalgia	3. otitis media
4. otorrhea	5. presbycusis	

TABLE 10-7

REVIEW OF DIAGNOSTIC TERMS PERTAINING TO THE EARS

1. audiogram	2. audiometry	3. electrocochleography
4. otosclerosis	5. otoscope	6. salpingoscope

TABLE 10-8

REVIEW OF SURGICAL TERMS PERTAINING TO THE EARS

1. myringoplasty	2. myringotomy	3. stapedectomy
4. tympanoplasty		

10.13 Medical Terms in Context

After you read the Discharge Summary and Operative Report, answer the questions that follow it. Use your text, medical dictionary, or other references if necessary.

DISCHARGE SUMMARY

HISTORY: Mrs. Lubetz noted progressive deteriorating vision, OS, over several years. A cataract was diagnosed. Her visual acuity deteriorated in the left eye. Her optic discs and peripheral retinae are within normal limits.

In April, glaucoma, OD, was suspected. Gonioscopy showed narrowing of the angle of the anterior chamber, OD. Her intraocular pressures were slightly elevated, and she was placed on miotics. In May, she underwent an iridotomy, OD, for glaucoma.

COURSE IN HOSPITAL: On June 21, Mrs. Lubetz underwent left phacoemulsification cataract extraction with insertion of an intraocular lens. On the first postoperative day, she was discharged home.

QUESTIONS ON DISCHARGE SUMMARY

1. The cataract was diagnosed in the:

    a. left eye

    b. right eye

2. Visual acuity means:

    a. accommodation to near and far objects

    b. clearness of vision

    c. range of vision

    d. refraction of light rays

3. On examining the eye, the patient's _____ was within normal limits.

    a. blind spot

    b. fovea centralis

    c. optic nerve

    d. macula lutea

4. Glaucoma was diagnosed in the:

    a. left eye

    b. right eye

5. The intraocular pressure was decreased by:

    a. drugs used to constrict the pupil

    b. drugs used to dilate the pupil

    c. incision of the iris

    d. A and C

6. Glaucoma can be diagnosed by a procedure called:

    a. gonioscopy

    b. intraocular pressure

    c. iridotomy

    d. phacoemulsification

7. Removal of the cataract was performed using:

    a. drugs

    b. laser

    c. radiation

    d. ultrasound

OPERATIVE REPORT

PREOPERATIVE DIAGNOSIS: OTITIS MEDIA

OPERATION PROPOSED: BILATERAL MYRINGOTOMY AND TUBE INSERTION

POSTOPERATIVE DIAGNOSIS: RECURRENT OTITIS MEDIA

OPERTION PERFORMED: BILATERAL MYRINGOTOMY WITH TUBE INSERTION

OPERATIVE NOTE: The patient was brought to the operating room, placed in the supine position, and given a general anesthetic. Using the operative microscope, the right external auditory meatus was cleaned of a small amount of cerumen, revealing an abnormal tympanic membrane with a buildup of purulent material behind it. A myringotomy was performed and the purulent material suctioned. A tube was inserted. The procedure was then performed on the left side with a similar technique, and a finding of serous otitis media was noted. The patient was then taken to the recovery room in good condition.

QUESTIONS ON OPERATIVE REPORT

1. The patient is diagnosed with otitis media involving:

   a. both ears

   b. left ear

   c. right ear

2. During the operation, the patient's position was:

   a. lying on the abdomen, face down

   b. lying on the back, face up

   c. lying on the side, face lateral

   d. toward the midline

3. There was a buildup of pus in the:

   a. external auditory canal

   b. labyrinth

   c. middle ear

   d. B and C

4. The purpose of the myringotomies were to:

   a. drain pus

   b. drain watery fluid

   c. mobilize the stapes

   d. remove wax

   e. A and B

5. There was a buildup of wax in the:

   a. external auditory meatus

   b. labyrinth

   c. middle ear

   d. B and C

6. Purulent and serous:

   a. are two types of otitis media

   b. mean pus-filled and watery fluid, respectively

   c. mean pus-filled and severe, respectively

   d. A and B

The Endocrine System

CHAPTER ORGANIZATION

This chapter will help you learn the endocrine system. It is divided into the following sections:

11.1   Central Endocrine Glands

11.2   Peripheral Endocrine Glands

11.3   Additional Word Parts

11.4   Term Analysis and Definition

11.5   Common Diseases

11.6   Abbreviations

11.7   Putting It All Together

11.8   Review of Vocabulary

11.9   Medical Terms in Context

CHAPTER OBJECTIVES

On completion of this chapter, you will be able to do the following:

1. Define hormones and homeostasis

2. Differentiate between exocrine and endocrine glands

3. Name the central and peripheral glands of the endocrine system

4. Define and name five tropic hormones

5. Name the hormones secreted by the anterior and posterior pituitary, and describe their functions

6. Name the hormones secreted by the pancreas, thyroid, parathyroid, pineal, and adrenal glands, and describe their functions

7. Analyze, define, pronounce, and spell terms related to the endocrine system

8. Describe common diseases

9. Define abbreviations common to the endocrine system

INTRODUCTION

When your body needs water, you feel a sense of thirst and take a drink. This is an example of one of the many ways the body maintains internal balance, or **homeostasis** (**hoh**-mee-oh-**STAY**-sis). The **endocrine** (**EN**-doh-krin) **system** is also involved with the maintenance of homeostasis. Endocrine glands secrete powerful chemicals called **hormones**, which are essential for the proper functioning of bodily processes. Just as your body tells you to drink when you are thirsty, these hormones are produced and secreted when the body signals a need for them. When proper levels within the blood have been reached, the signals cease, and hormone secretion stops. This is an example of a feedback mechanism.

The endocrine system consists of several glands: the **hypothalamus** (**high**-poh-**THAL**-ah-mus), **pituitary** (pih-**TOO**-ih-tar-ee), **thyroid** (**THIGH**-roid), **parathyroids** (par-ah-**THIGH**-roidz), **adrenals** (ah-**DREE**-nalz), **pineal** (**PIN**-ee-al), and **pancreas** (**PAN**-kree-as). These glands secrete hormones into the bloodstream for delivery to the target organ. This distinguishes the endocrine glands from the **exocrine** (**ECK**-soh-krin) **glands**, such as sweat glands (Figure 11-1). Exocrine glands secrete chemicals into ducts, which then deliver the secretions to the target site. With the exception of the pancreas, which has both exocrine and endocrine function, the endocrine glands have no ducts.

There are two categories of endocrine glands: the **central** and the **peripheral**. The central consists of two adjacent glands in the brain, the hypothalamus and pituitary, which

FIGURE 11-1
Exocrine and endocrine glands

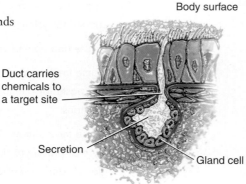

Body surface

Duct carries chemicals to a target site

Secretion

Gland cell

A. Exocrine gland (has duct)

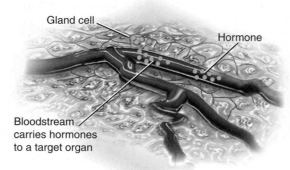

Gland cell

Hormone

Bloodstream carries hormones to a target organ

B. Endocrine gland (ductless)

coordinate to regulate body functions such as water and salt balance, growth, reproduction, and metabolism. The peripheral endocrine glands include the thyroid, parathyroids, adrenals, pineal, and pancreas. The first four have only one function, the production of hormones. The pancreas not only produces hormones, but also has important digestive system functions. In this way, the pancreas is similar to a host of mixed-function organs, such as the kidneys, small intestine, liver, heart, ovaries, testes, thymus, and placenta. In addition to their regular systemic functions, these organs secrete hormones. The function of these organs, except for the pancreas, will be covered in their respective chapters. The endocrine glands are illustrated in Figure 11-2; the hypothalamus in Figure 11-3.

Memory Key	• The central endocrine glands are the hypothalamus and pituitary.

- The central endocrine glands are the hypothalamus and pituitary.
- The peripheral glands are the:
thyroid	pineal
parathyroids	pancreas
adrenals	
- An endocrine function does not involve ducts. Hormones are secreted into the bloodstream, to be received by target organs.
- An exocrine function involves the secretion of fluids into ducts for delivery to a site.

FIGURE 11-2
Endocrine glands

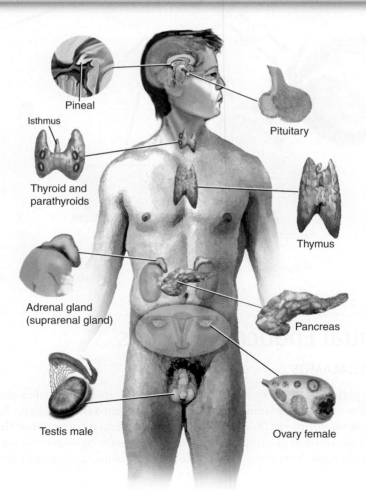

Pineal

Isthmus

Pituitary

Thyroid and
parathyroids

Thymus

Adrenal gland
(suprarenal gland)

Pancreas

Testis male

Ovary female

FIGURE 11-3
Pituitary gland and its hormonal secretions

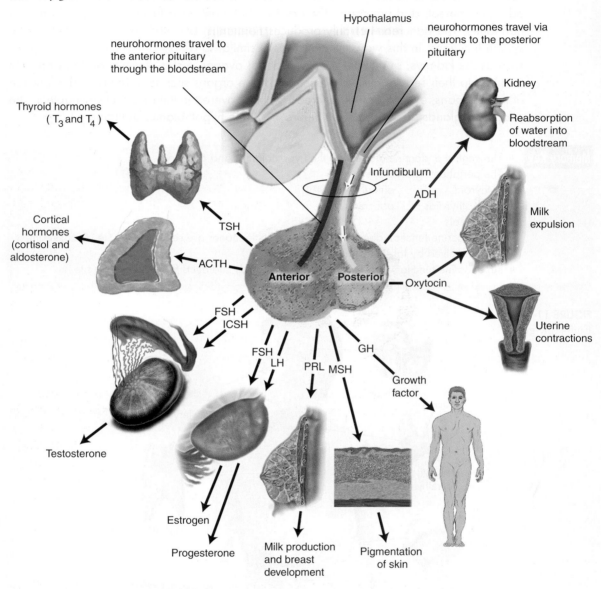

11.1   Central Endocrine Glands

HYPOTHALAMUS

The hypothalamus works in tandem with the pituitary, which lies deep within the brain and below the hypothalamus (Figure 11-2). The neurons of the hypothalamus produce and secrete neurohormones (hormones secreted from neural tissue rather than glandular tissue). Some neurohormones stimulate the anterior pituitary to secrete its own hormones. These are called **tropic** hormones. Often, the suffixes -tropic and -tropin are used in relation to substances that stimulate other organs to secrete hormones. The hypothalamus also produces **antidiuretic** (**an**-tih-**dye**-yoo-**RET**-ick) **hormone** and **oxytocin** (**ock**-see-**TOH**-sin). These neurohormones are transported via neurons to the posterior pituitary (Figure 11-3). They are stored in the posterior pituitary and released when required. These are not tropic hormones; they do not cause the posterior pituitary to release other hormones.

Memory Key	• The hypothalamus secretes tropic hormones, which have an effect on pituitary activity. • The hypothalamus secretes two other hormones that are stored in the pituitary for later release.

PITUITARY GLAND

The pea-sized pituitary gland hangs from the hypothalamus by a stalk called the **infundibulum** (**in**-fun-**DIB**-yoo-lum), as illustrated in Figure 11-3. The pituitary gland is divided into **anterior** and **posterior lobes**.

The **anterior pituitary** secretes seven hormones, triggered by neurohormones from the hypothalamus (Figure 11-3). Five of the anterior pituitary hormones are stimulating (tropic) hormones, inducing other glands to release hormones. These five are:

1. **Adrenocorticotropic** (ah-**dree**-noh-**kor**-tih-koh-**TROP**-ick) **hormone** (**ACTH**), which stimulates the adrenal cortex to produce and secrete **cortisol** (**KOR**-tih-sol), and **aldosterone** (al-**DOS**-ter-own), and sex hormones.

2. **Growth hormone** (**GH**), or **somatotropin** (**soh**-ma-toh-**TROH**-pin), which stimulates growth in all body cells and controls the release of the hormone somatomedin from the liver

3. **Thyroid-stimulating hormone** (**TSH**), or **thyrotropin** (thi-**ROT**-roh-pin), which stimulates the thyroid gland to produce and secrete its own hormones **thyroxine** (thigh-**ROCK**-sin) (T_4) and **triiodothyronine** (**try**-eye-**oh**-doh-**THIGH**-roh-nen) (T_3)

4. **Follicle-stimulating hormone** (**FSH**), a **gonadotropin** (**gon**-ah-doh-**TROH**-pin), which stimulates the development of the gonads (ovaries and testes). In males, this hormone promotes sperm formation, and in females, it promotes monthly development of the ovum (egg) and stimulates the secretion of the female hormones estrogen and progesterone.

5. **Luteinizing** (**LOO**-tee-in-eye-zing) **hormone** (**LH**), another gonadotropin that triggers ovulation in females. In males, it regulates testosterone secretion and is called **interstitial cell-stimulating hormone** (**ICSH**).

Prolactin (pro-**LACK**-tin) (**PRL**) and **melanocyte-stimulating hormone** (**MSH**) are the sixth and seventh hormones produced by the anterior pituitary. These two hormones do not stimulate the production of other hormones and are therefore not tropic hormones. PRL stimulates breast development and milk production. MSH stimulates melanocytic activity in the skin.

The **posterior pituitary** stores and secretes two neurohormones produced by the hypothalamus. The first is antidiuretic hormone (ADH), also known as **vasopressin** (**vay**-zoh-**PRESS**-in), and the second is oxytocin (OT), produced by the hypothalamus. Antidiuretic hormone prevents excessive loss of water, and oxytocin stimulates uterine contractions to assist childbirth. Oxytocin also regulates the flow of milk from the mammary glands.

Figure 11-4 summarizes all of the anterior pituitary hormones.

Memory Key
- The anterior pituitary secretes several hormones critical to life: ACTH, GH, TSH, FSH, LH (ICSH) in males), PRL, and MSH.
- The posterior pituitary stores and releases two hormones produced by the hypothalamus: ADH and OT.

FIGURE 11-4
Summary of tropic hormones from the pituitary gland

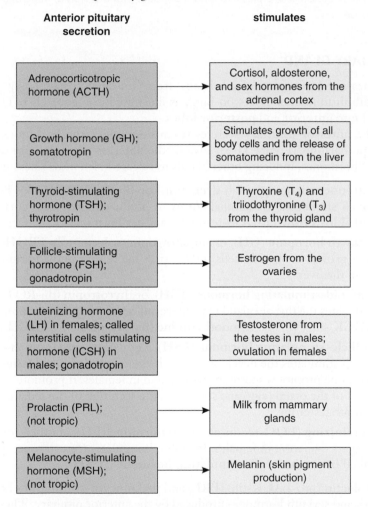

Anterior pituitary secretion — **stimulates**

Adrenocorticotropic hormone (ACTH)	→	Cortisol, aldosterone, and sex hormones from the adrenal cortex
Growth hormone (GH); somatotropin	→	Stimulates growth of all body cells and the release of somatomedin from the liver
Thyroid-stimulating hormone (TSH); thyrotropin	→	Thyroxine (T_4) and triiodothyronine (T_3) from the thyroid gland
Follicle-stimulating hormone (FSH); gonadotropin	→	Estrogen from the ovaries
Luteinizing hormone (LH) in females; called interstitial cells stimulating hormone (ICSH) in males; gonadotropin	→	Testosterone from the testes in males; ovulation in females
Prolactin (PRL); (not tropic)	→	Milk from mammary glands
Melanocyte-stimulating hormone (MSH); (not tropic)	→	Melanin (skin pigment production)

11.2 Peripheral Endocrine Glands

THYROID GLAND

Figure 11-2 illustrates the thyroid. It is located in the neck below the larynx and consists of right and left lobes connected by a structure called the **isthmus** (**ISS**-mus). The thyroid produces, stores, and secretes the two thyroid hormones: triiodothyronine (T_3) and thyroxine (T_4). These hormones regulate metabolic rate and increase the production of energy from food. Also produced by the thyroid is the hormone **calcitonin** (cal-sih-**TOH**-nin), which regulates blood calcium levels.

Memory Key	• The thyroid is in the throat area and produces T_3 and T_4, which regulate metabolic rate and increase energy production.
	• The thyroid also secretes calcitonin, which regulates blood calcium levels.

PARATHYROID GLANDS

As shown in Figure 11-2, there are four parathyroid glands, two on each of the thyroid lobes. These egg-shaped glands secrete **parathyroid** (par-ah-**THIGH**-roid) **hormone**, also called **parathormone** (par-ah-**THOR**-mohn). This hormone, referred to as **PTH**, contributes to the regulation of calcium and phosphorus.

Memory Key	• There are four parathyroids located on the thyroid.
	• The parathyroids secrete PTH, which regulates calcium and phosphorus levels.

ADRENAL GLANDS

The adrenal glands sit on top of the kidneys, as shown in Figure 11-2. Functionally and structurally, there are two parts: the adrenal cortex and the adrenal medulla.

The adrenal cortex secretes three groups of hormones:

1. **Mineralocorticoids** (**min**-er-ahl-oh-**KOR**-tih-koidz), of which aldosterone is the most important. It plays a central role in the regulation of sodium and potassium levels.
2. **Glucocorticoids** (**gloo**-koh-**KOR**-tih-koidz), of which cortisol (hydrocortisone) is the most important. Cortisol is necessary for antibody production; it plays a key role in the body's response to stress; and is necessary for the utilization of carbohydrates, fats, and proteins.
3. **Sex hormones**, called estrogens and androgens. Although these hormones are primarily secreted by the ovaries and testes, the adrenal cortex secretes small amounts, which play a role in the development of secondary sex characteristics such as the growth of pubic and facial hair and breast development.

The adrenal medulla produces **adrenaline** (ah-**DREN**-ah-len) and **noradrenaline** (**nor**-ah-**DREN**-ah-len), also respectively referred to as **epinephrine** (ep-ih-**NEF**-rin) and **norepinephrine** (**nor**-ep-ih-**NEF**-rin), and collectively as **catecholamines** (kat-eh-**KOHL**-ah-meenz). These are the so-called fight-and-flight hormones, because they prepare the body for physical exertion during times of stress.

Memory Key	• The adrenals sit on top of the kidneys.
	• Each adrenal cortex secretes mineralocorticoids, glucocorticoids, and sex hormones.
	• Each adrenal medulla secretes the fight-or-flight hormones adrenaline (epinephrine) and noradrenaline (norepinephrine).

PINEAL GLAND

The **pineal** (**PIN**-ee-al) **gland** is shown in Figure 11-2. It looks like a pine cone and is located deep within the brain. The pineal gland plays a role in the waking and sleeping cycle. It receives neural stimulation from the eye, which regulates its secretion of the hormone melatonin (**mel**-ah-**TOH**-nin). Light inhibits melatonin secretion; dark stimulates its production. This makes a person awake during the day and sleepy at night. Melatonin levels are also connected to mood.

> **Memory Key** | The pineal gland is located deep in the brain and secretes melatonin.

PANCREAS

The **pancreas** lies behind the stomach and secretes pancreatic juice, which travels along the pancreatic duct and into the duodenum. This is an exocrine function. The pancreas also secretes endocrine substances, the hormones **insulin** (**IN**-suh-lin) and **glucagon** (**GLOO**-kah-gon), which are important in the regulation of blood sugar. Insulin lowers blood sugar by stimulating the absorption of sugar by body cells. It also converts glucose into glycogen, which is the form in which sugar is stored in the liver. Glucagon increases blood sugar by converting glycogen back to glucose for use by the body when blood sugar is low.

> **Memory Key**
> - The pancreas lies near the stomach.
> - The pancreas has both exocrine and endocrine functions.
> - Its endocrine functions are to produce insulin and glucagon.
> - Insulin converts glucose into its storage form, glycogen, and stimulates the absorption of sugar by body cells.
> - Glucagon reconverts the glycogen into glucose when the body needs sugar.

Table 11-1 summarizes the endocrine glands, the hormones secreted, and their functions.

TABLE 11-1

SUMMARY OF ENDOCRINE GLANDS AND HORMONES

Gland	Hormone	Function
Anterior pituitary (adenohypophysis)	Growth hormone (GH); somatotropin	Stimulates growth in all body cells and release of somatomedin from the liver
	Thyroid-stimulating hormone (TSH); thyrotropin	Stimulates thyroid gland to produce T_3 and T_4
	Adrenocorticotropic hormone (ACTH)	Stimulates adrenal cortex to release cortisol aldosterone, estrogen, and progesterone
	Follicle-stimulating hormone (FSH); gonadotropin	Regulates development of ovaries and testes; promotes monthly growth of egg in females and sperm production in males
	Luteinizing hormone (LH) in females; interstitial cell-stimulating hormone (ICSH) in males; Gonadotropin	Triggers ovulation in females; regulates sex hormone secretion in males
	Prolactin (PRL)	Stimulates production of milk in mammary glands
	Melanocyte-stimulating hormone (MSH)	Produces melanin for skin pigmentation
Posterior pituitary (neurohypophysis)	Antidiuretic hormone (ADH); vasopressin	Regulates water retention in the body
	Oxytocin	Regulates flow of milk in mammary glands and stimulates uterine contractions during childbirth
Thyroid	Thyroxine (T_4) and triiodothyronine (T_3); thyroid-stimulating hormone	Increases metabolic rate; stimulates growth
	Calcitonin	Regulates blood calcium

continued on page 260

Table 11-1 *continued from page 259*

Gland	Hormone	Function
Parathyroids	Parathyroid hormone; parathormone (PTH)	Increases blood calcium; decreases blood phosphate
Adrenal cortex	Glucocorticoid hormones, including cortisol, also called hydrocortisone	Antibody production; response to stress; metabolism of carbohydrates, fats, and proteins
	Mineralocorticoid hormones including aldosterone	Regulates sodium and potassium levels
	Sex hormones estrogen and testosterone	Development of secondary female and male characteristics
Adrenal medulla	Catecholamines: epinephrine (adrenaline) and norepinephrine (noradrenaline)	Help body respond to stress
Pineal gland	Melatonin	Regulates waking and sleeping cycles
Pancreas	Insulin; glucagon	Insulin converts glucose to glycogen and stimulates the absorption of sugar. Glucagon converts glycogen to glucose.

Before you continue, review Sections 11.1 and 11.2. Then, complete Exercises 11–1 and 11–2 found at the end of the chapter.

11.3 Additional Word Parts

The following roots and suffixes will also be used in this chapter to build medical terms.

Root	Meaning
immun/o	safe
radi/o	radioactive

Suffix	Meaning
-genesis	production
-gen	producing

Prefix	Meaning
eu-	normal; good

11.4   Term Analysis and Definition

ROOTS

	acr/o	extremity; top
Term	**Term Analysis**	**Definition**
acromegaly (**ack**-roh-**MEG**-ah-lee)	-megaly = enlargement	enlargement of many skeletal structures, including the extremities, nose, forehead, and jaw (Figure 11-5)
	aden/o	**gland**
adenoma (**ad**-eh-**NO**-mah)	-oma = tumor; mass	benign tumor of a gland

FIGURE 11-5
Acromegaly; notice enlarged skeletal structures of nose and chin, and large lips

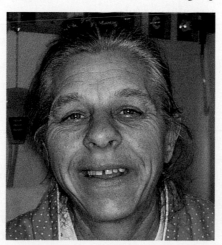

	adrenal/o; adren/o	adrenal
Term	**Term Analysis**	**Definition**
adrenalectomy (ah-**dree**-nal-**ECK**-toh-mee)	-ectomy = excision; surgical removal	excision of the adrenal gland
	andr/o	**male; man**
androgen (**AN**-droh-jen)	-gen = producing	substance producing male characteristics such as the hormone testosterone
	calc/o	**calcium**
hypercalcemia (**high**-per-kal-**SEE**-mee-ah)	-emia = blood condition hyper- = excessive; above normal	excessive amounts of calcium in the blood
	crin/o	**to secrete**
endocrinologist (**en**-doh-krih-**NOL**-oh-jist)	-logist = specialist endo- = within	specialist in the study of the diagnosis and treatment of disorders of the endrocrine glands and their hormones
endocrinology (**en**-doh-krih-**NOL**-oh-jee)	-logy = study of endo- = within	the study of the diagnosis and treatment of endocrine disorders
	estr/o	**female**
estrogen (**ES**-troh-jen)	-gen = producing	female sex hormones
	gluc/o (see also glyc/o)	**sugar**
glucogenesis (**gloo**-koh-**JEN**-eh-sis)	-genesis = production	production of sugar
gluconeogenesis (**gloo**-koh-**nee**-oh-**JEN**-eh-sis)	-genesis = production neo- = new	production of sugar from fats and proteins
	glyc/o	**sugar**
glycolysis (glye-**KOL**-ih-sis)	-lysis = breakdown; separation; destruction	breakdown of sugars
hyperglycemia (**high**-per-glye-**SEE**-mee-ah)	-emia = blood condition hyper- = excessive; above normal	excessive amounts of sugar in the blood

Term	Term Analysis	Definition
hypoglycemia (**high**-poh-glye-**SEE**-mee-ah)	-emia = blood condition hypo- = deficient; below normal	deficient amounts of sugar in the blood
	glycogen/o	**glycogen (storage form of sugar)**
glycogenolysis (**glye**-koh-jen-**OL**-ih-sis)	-lysis = breakdown; separation; destruction	breakdown of glycogen to form glucose
	gonad/o	**gonads; sex glands (testes and ovaries)**
hypergonadism (**high**-per-**GO**-nad-izm)	-ism = condition; process; state of hyper- = excessive; above normal	condition characterized by excessive secretion of gonadal hormones (resulting in early sexual development)
	gynec/o	**woman**
gynecomastia (**guy**-neh-koh-**MAS**-tee-ah)	-ia = condition **mast/o** = breast	abnormal enlargement of the male breast
	home/o	**same**
homeostasis (**hoh**-mee-oh-**STAY**-sis)	-stasis = standing; stable; stopping; controlling	a balanced, yet sometimes varying, state
	insulin/o	**insulin**
hypoinsulinism (**high**-poh-**IN**-suh-lin-izm)	-ism = condition; process; state of hypo- = deficient; below normal	condition characterized by decreased amounts of insulin secretion (resulting in hyperglycemia)
	kal/o	**potassium**
hyperkalemia (**high**-per-kah-**LEE**-mee-ah)	-emia = blood condition hyper- = excessive; above normal	excessive amounts of potassium in the blood
	natr/o	**sodium**
hyponatremia (**high**-poh-nah-**TREE**-mee-ah)	-emia = blood condition hypo- = deficient; below normal	deficient amounts of sodium in the blood

	pancreat/o	pancreas
Term	**Term Analysis**	**Definition**
pancreatogenic (**pan**-kree-ah-toh-**JEN**-ick)	-genic = produced by	produced by the pancreas
	parathyroid/o	**parathyroid gland**
hyperparathyroidism (**high**-per-**par**-ah-**THIGH**-roid-izm)	-ism = condition; process; state of hyper- = excessive; above normal	condition characterized by excessive secretion of parathormone (resulting in loss of calcium from the bone)
	pituitar/o	**pituitary gland**
panhypopituitarism (pan-**high**-poh-pih-**TOO**-ih-tar-izm)	-ism = condition; process; state of pan- = all hypo- = deficient; below normal	condition characterized by a deficiency of all pituitary hormones (resulting in dwarfism and a deterioration of secondary sex characteristics)
	thyr/o; thyroid/o	**thyroid gland; shield**
euthyroid (yoo-**THIGH**-roid)	-oid = resembling eu- = normal; good	normal thyroid gland
hyperthyroidism (**high**-per-**THIGH**-roid-izm)	-ism = condition; process; state of hyper- = excessive; above normal	condition characterized by excessive secretion of the thyroid hormones (resulting in **goiter**, an enlarged thyroid gland, and **exophthalmos**, an abnormal protrusion of the eyes as seen in Figure 11-6)
thyroiditis (thigh-roi-**DYE**-tis)	-itis = inflammation	inflammation of the thyroid gland
thyrotomy (thigh-**ROT**-oh-mee)	-tomy = process of cutting; incision	process of cutting into the thyroid gland
	ure/o	**urea (end product of protein breakdown, found in urine)**
antidiuretic hormone (**an**-tih-dye-yoo-**RET**-ick **HOR**-mohn)	-tic = pertaining to anti- = against dia- = through	a hormone that prevents the loss of excessive amounts of urine

Memory Key The *a* in dia- is dropped because the word element **ure/o** begins with a vowel.

FIGURE 11-6
Hyperthyroidism

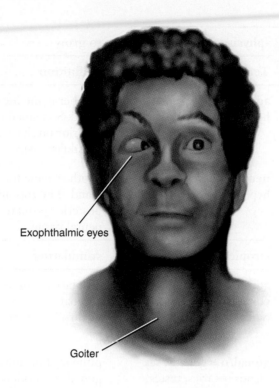

Exophthalmic eyes

Goiter

SUFFIXES

	-assay	analysis of a mixture to identify its contents
Term	**Term Analysis**	**Definition**
radioimmunoassay (RIA) (ray-dee-oh-**im**-yoo-no-**ASS**-ay)	**radi/o** = radioactive **immun/o** = safe	blood test used to identify hormonal levels in blood plasma. The hormones are labeled with a radioactive substance.
	-crine	**to secrete**
endocrine hormones (**EN**-doh-krin)	endo- = within	hormones secreted by the endocrine glands into the bloodstream
exocrine glands (**ECK**-soh-krin)	exo- = outside; outward	glands that secrete chemicals into ducts
	-dipsia	**thirst**
polydipsia (**pol**-ee-**DIP**-see-ah)	poly- = many	excessive thirst

	-physis	to grow
Term	**Term Analysis**	**Definition**
adenohypophysis (**ad**-eh-noh-high-**POF**-ih-sis)	**aden/o** = gland hypo- = below; under	another name for anterior pituitary gland. So named because the anterior pituitary is made up of glandular tissue
neurohypophysis (**noo**-roh-high-**POF**-ih-is)	**neur/o** = nerve hypo- = below; under	another name for posterior pituitary gland. The root indicates that the posterior pituitary is made up of neural tissue
	-tropic	stimulating
adrenocorticotropic hormone (ACTH) (ah-**dree**-noh-**kor**-tih-koh-**TROP**-ick)	**adren/o** = adrenal gland **cortic/o** = cortex; outer layer	pituitary hormone that stimulates the adrenal cortex to produce and secrete its own hormones
gonadotropic hormone (**gon**-ah-doh-**TROP**-ick)	**gonad/o** = gonads; sex glands (ovaries, testes)	pituitary hormone that stimulates the gonads to produce and secrete their own hormones
somatotropic hormone (**soh**-ma-toh-**TROP**-ick)	**somat/o** = body	pituitary hormone that stimulates growth of body tissues

PREFIXES

	oxy-	sharp; quick
Term	**Term Analysis**	**Definition**
oxytocin (**ock**-see-**TOH**-sin)	-tocin = labor	pituitary hormone that quickens childbirth by causing uterine contractions

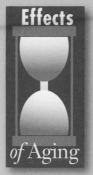

In Chapter 8, you learned that the decreased levels of testosterone, estrogen, and the growth hormone that occur with aging can cause muscle atrophy. These are not the only hormones that decrease. In fact, all hormones produced by the endocrine system decrease in production levels and activity as we age. However, because the body can produce far higher levels of hormones than we typically need, the loss of capacity is usually symptomless, or results in mild incapacity. For instance, the ability of the pancreas to produce insulin decreases, particularly in those over 65. In its mildest form, the result is higher than normal blood sugar levels for a longer period after a meal. However, this can lead to the development of diabetes in more severe cases.

11.5   Common Diseases

DIABETES MELLITUS

Diabetes mellitus (**dye**-ah-**BEE**-teez **MEL**-ih-tus) (**DM**) is a disease in which the body is unable to use sugar to produce energy. One cause is insufficient insulin secreted from the pancreas. Another cause is the production of ineffective insulin. When either of these occur, sugar is unable to move from the blood into body cells where it is normally used to produce energy. The result is abnormally high levels of blood glucose, known as hyperglycemia. It is a major symptom of diabetes. The normal blood glucose level is 70 to 100 mg/dL. Patients with blood glucose levels greater that 126 mg/dL are considered to be diabetic.

When the body doesn't have enough glucose, it breaks down fats and proteins for its energy. Over a long period of time, this results in a buildup of toxic wastes called **ketones** (**KEE**-tohnz). The condition is called **ketoacidosis** (**kee**-toh-**ass**-ih-**DOH**-sis). The excess sugars and ketones in the blood cause many diabetic complications such as blindness, arteriosclerosis, heart attacks, and gangrene of the lower extremities (loss of blood supply to the lower extremities causes decay of tissues).

There are two major types of diabetes.

Type 1 is an abrupt end to insulin production, often before the age of 25. This is thought to be due to an autoimmune reaction (the body's own antibodies destroy the pancreatic cells). Other factors such as genetics, viruses, and the environment might trigger the autoimmune reactions.

Type 2 is a reduction in insulin production, and often occurs after the age of 40. The pancreas continues to produce insulin, but one or two factors compromise that production: The pancreas produces reduced amounts of insulin; or body tissue fails to accept insulin into its cells for energy. Genetic factors and obesity play a role in the majority of cases. Obesity requires that the pancreas work harder to produce more insulin. Over time, the pancreatic cells wear out, and insulin production decreases.

Treatment for type 1 diabetes includes diet, exercise, and insulin injections. Type 2 diabetes is controlled by diet, exercise, and drugs that stimulate the pancreas to secrete insulin on its own. Some type 2 diabetics will also need insulin.

11.6 Abbreviations

Abbreviation	Meaning
ACTH	adrenocorticotropic hormone
ADH	antidiuretic hormone
Ca	calcium; cancer
FSH	follicle-stimulating hormone
GH	growth hormone
K	potassium
LH	luteinizing hormone
MSH	melanocyte-stimulating hormone
Na	sodium
OT	oxytocin
P	phosphorus
PRL	prolactin
PTH	parathyroid hormone (parathormone)
RIA	radioimmunoassay
T_3	triiodothyronine
T_4	thyroxine
TFT	thyroid function tests
TRH	thyrotropin-releasing hormone
TSH	thyroid-stimulating hormone

11.7   Putting It All Together

Exercise 11-1   IDENTIFICATION

Give alternative names for the following hormones.

1. growth hormone

2. thyroid-stimulating hormone

3. follicle-stimulating hormone

4. luteinizing hormone

5. hydrocortisone

6. adrenaline

Exercise 11-2   MATCHING

I. Match the gland in Column A with its hormonal secretion(s) in Column B.

Column A

_____ 1. anterior pituitary

_____ 2. posterior pituitary

_____ 3. thyroid gland

_____ 4. parathyroid

_____ 5. adrenal cortex

_____ 6. adrenal medulla

_____ 7. pineal gland

_____ 8. pancreas

Column B

A. growth hormone

B. calcitonin

C. luteinizing hormone

D. oxytocin

E. melatonin

F. cortisol

G. adrenocorticotropic

H. insulin

I. antidiuretic hormone

J. glucagon

K. prolactin

L. parathormone

M. aldosterone

N. adrenaline

II. Match the hormone in Column A with its function in Column B.

Column A	Column B
_____ 1. luteinizing hormone	A. stimulates milk production
_____ 2. prolactin	B. regulates calcium and phosphorus
_____ 3. thyroxine	C. antibody production
_____ 4. oxytocin	D. converts glucose to glycogen
_____ 5. parathormone	E. triggers ovulation in females
_____ 6. aldosterone	F. converts glycogen to glucose
_____ 7. cortisol	G. regulates metabolic rate
_____ 8. epinephrine	H. stimulates uterine contractions
_____ 9. insulin	I. regulates sodium and potassium
_____ 10. glucagon	J. prepares the body for physical exertion during times of stress

Exercise 11-3   BUILDING TERMS

I. Using -tropic, build terms for the following definitions.

1. pituitary hormone that stimulates the adrenal cortex to secrete their own hormones   _____

2. pituitary hormone that stimulates the gonads to secrete their own hormones   _____

3. pituitary hormone that stimulates growth of body tissues   _____

4. pituitary hormone that stimulates the thyroid to secrete its own hormones   _____

II. Using -emia, build terms for the following definitions.

5. excessive amounts of sugar in the blood   _____

6. deficient amounts of sugar in the blood   _____

7. excessive amounts of potassium in the blood   _____

8. deficient amounts of sodium in the blood   _____

9. excessive amounts of calcium in the blood   _____

III. Using -ism, build terms for the following definitions.

10. condition characterized by excessive secretions of gonadal hormones   _____

11. decreased amounts of insulin secretion   _____

12. condition characterized by excessive
    secretion of parathormone _____

13. condition characterized by a deficiency
    of all pituitary hormones _____

14. condition characterized by excessive
    secretion of the thyroid hormone _____

Exercise 11-4   WORD BUILDING

Build the medical terms from the following definitions.

1. production of sugar _____

   _____

2. breakdown of sugar _____

   _____

3. normal thyroid gland _____

   _____

4. balanced, yet varied, state _____

   _____

5. excessive thirst _____

6. abnormal enlargement of the male breast _____

   _____

7. tumor of a gland _____

   _____

Exercise 11-5   SPELLING

Circle any misspelled words in the following list and correctly spell them in the space provided.

1. pancrease _____

2. gynecomastia _____

3. epinephrine _____

4. endocrene _____

5. lutenizing _____

6. oxytocin _____

7. hypothalmus _____

8. euthyroid _____

9. adenohypophysis _____

10. hypercalcimia _____

Exercise 11-6   PATHOLOGY

Answer the following questions on diabetes mellitus.

1. Define diabetes mellitus: _____

2. Define the following terms relating to diabetes mellitus:

   a. ketoacidosis _____

   b. type I diabetes _____

   c. type II diabetes _____

   d. hyperglycemia _____

3. List and define three complications of diabetes mellitus:

   _____

   _____

   _____

4. What is the normal blood glucose level? _____

5. What is one cause of diabetes mellitus?

   _____

   _____

11.8   Review of Vocabulary

In the following tables, the medical terms found in this chapter are organized into these categories: anatomy, pathology, and diagnostic and surgical procedures. Define each term and decide into which category the word belongs. This will help you associate the term with its purpose and help you remember its meaning.

TABLE 11-2

REVIEW OF ANATOMICAL TERMS

1. adenohypophysis	2. adrenocorticotropic hormone	3. androgen
4. antidiuretic hormone	5. endocrine hormones	6. endocrinologist

continued on page 273

Table 11-2 *continued from page 272*

7. endocrinology	8. estrogen	9. exocrine glands
10. glucogenesis	11. gluconeogenesis	12. glycogenolysis
13. glycolysis	14. gonadotropic hormone	15. homeostasis
16. hypothalamus	17. neurohypophysis	18. oxytocin
19. pancreas	20. pancreatogenic	21. pineal gland
22. pituitary gland	23. somatotropic hormone	24. thyroid gland
25. tropic hormones		

TABLE 11-3

REVIEW OF PATHOLOGIC TERMS

1. acromegaly	2. adenoma	3. euthyroid
4. gynecomastia	5. hypercalcemia	6. hyperglycemia
7. hypergonadism	8 hyperkalemia	9. hyperparathyroidism
10. hyperthyroidism	11. hypoglycemia	12. hypoinsulinism

continued on page 274

Table 11-3 *continued from page 273*

13. hyponatremia	14. panhypopituitarism	15. polydipsia
16. thyroiditis		

TABLE 11-4

REVIEW OF DIAGNOSTIC TESTS AND SURGICAL PROCEDURES

1. adrenalectomy	2. radioimmunoassay	3. thyrotomy

. . . .

11.9 MEDICAL TERMS IN CONTEXT

After you read the following Discharge Summary, answer the questions that follow it. Use your text, medical dictionary, or other references if necessary.

DISCHARGE SUMMARY

DISCHARGE DIAGNOSIS: Type II diabetes with gangrene, cellulitis, and infection of bone and bone marrow of the left middle toe.

OPERATION: Proximal interphalangeal amputation, left middle toe.

HISTORY: This 65-year-old woman is extremely obese and has been most of her adult life. Her diabetes has been poorly controlled. Blood sugar levels are between 275 mg/dL to 425 mg/dL. She does not like taking her insulin and states, "I do not like giving myself needles." The toe and lower leg were erythematous, ulcerated, and bleeding. She has inflammation of the subcutaneous tissue of the skin, ulcer formation, and gangrene. The infection spread to the bone and bone marrow of her left middle toe. Antibiotics, prior to admission, did nothing to reduce the inflammation.

PHYSICAL EXAMINATION: Physical examination showed a patient with poorly controlled diabetes, along with neuropathy, retinopathy, and arteriosclerosis consistent with long-term type II diabetes. The patient is extremely obese with dyspnea on exertion. Pulses in her left foot could not be felt, nor could the patient feel pressure on deep palpation. No organomegaly. The left foot exhibited a gangrenous toe with ulceration and inflammation. There is also necrosis of the skin of the middle toe.

LABORATORY DATA: Showed blood sugar levels of 423 mg/dL on one occasion and 278 mg/dL on another. Her Hgb was 15.2. Urinalysis: normal. Culture of skin, left middle toe showed *Staphylococcus aureus*.

PROGRESS IN HOSPITAL: Patient was started on IV antibiotics and kept on bedrest. Her blood sugars were carefully controlled. Eventually, the swelling and redness due to the inflammation subsided, and after one week of drug therapy, the patient underwent an amputation at the proximal interphalangeal joint.

On the third postoperative day, the patient was discharged home accompanied by her daughter, who, as a nurse, will be able to care for her foot at home.

QUESTIONS ON THE DISCHARGE SUMMARY

Answer the following questions from information in the Discharge Summary.

1. The medical term for inflammation of the bone and bone marrow is:

    a. cellulitis

    b. osteoarthritis

    c. osteomyelitis

    d. myeloencephalitis

2. With blood sugars of 285 to 423 mg/dL, the patient has:

    a. hyperglycemia

    b. hypoglycemia

    c. hyperinsulinism

    d. both A and C

3. Antibiotics were given to the patient to resolve the:

    a. obesity

    b. dyspnea

    c. inflammation

    d. diabetes

4. Most likely, the gangrene of the middle toe would be due to:

    a. arteriosclerosis

    b. retinopathy

    c. neuropathy

    d. inflammation

5. Pulses in the patient's right foot could not be felt because of:

    a. arteriosclerosis

    b. retinopathy

    c. inflammation

    d. dyspnea on exertion

6. Erythematous means:

    a. hardening of the arteries

    b. red discoloration of the skin

    c. ulcer formation

    d. gangrenous

7. Obesity caused the patient to have difficulty:

    a. eating

    b. sleeping

    c. breathing

    e. walking

8. An ulcer is a(n):

    a. closed cavity or sac filled with fluid

    b. blister

    c. elevated area of skin filled with pus

    d. open sore

The Cardiovascular System

CHAPTER ORGANIZATION

This chapter will help you learn the cardiovascular system. It is divided into the following sections:

12.1	Structure of the Heart
12.2	Conduction System
12.3	Blood Pressure
12.4	Heart Sounds
12.5	Blood Vessels
12.6	Circulation
12.7	Additional Word Parts
12.8	Term Analysis and Definition
12.9	Common Diseases
12.10	Abbreviations
12.11	Putting It All Together
12.12	Review of Vocabulary
12.13	Medical Terms in Context

CHAPTER OBJECTIVES

On completion of this chapter, you will be able to do the following:

1. Name the major structures of the cardiovascular system
2. Define terms relating to the structure of the heart
3. Name and describe the walls of the heart
4. Identify the major structures of the heart on a diagram
5. Describe the pericardium
6. Describe the conduction system
7. Define common terminology used in an electrocardiogram
8. Describe blood pressure to include systole, diastole, systolic pressure, diastolic pressure, sphygmomanometer, hypertension, and hypotension
9. Differentiate between S_1 and S_2
10. Differentiate between the structure and function of arteries, veins, and capillaries
11. Describe the circulation of blood
12. Describe, in general, how arteries and veins are named
13. Analyze, define, pronounce, and spell terms relating to the cardiovascular system
14. Describe common diseases
15. Define abbreviations common to the cardiovascular system

277

INTRODUCTION

The 70 to 80 trillion cells in the human body require a continuous supply of oxygen and nutrients. At the same time, body cells must get rid of their accumulated waste products. The cardiovascular system (CVS) accomplishes these tasks. The CVS consists of the **heart** and **blood vessels**. Blood vessels are of three types: **arteries** (**AR**-ter-eez), **veins** (**VAYNZ**), and **capillaries** (ka-**PILL**-ah-reez). Arteries carry blood *away* from the heart. Veins carry blood *toward* the heart. Capillaries are tiny blood vessels that join the arterial and venous systems and carry blood to the organs.

As you study the cardiovascular system, keep in mind that the blood must travel to the lungs to become **oxygenated** (saturated with oxygen). Once oxygenated, the blood travels to the organs, where oxygen and nutrients are dropped off. **Deoxygenated blood** (blood released of oxygen) must travel through veins back to the heart, where that blood is pumped into the lungs to start the whole process over again. A more detailed discussion of blood circulation is in section 12.6.

Memory Key	• The cardiovascular system includes the:

Memory Key
- The cardiovascular system includes the:
  heart
  blood vessels (arteries, veins, and capillaries)
- It delivers oxygen and nutrients to all of the body's cells, and carries away carbon dioxide and waste products.

12.1   Structure of the Heart

Your heart is about the same size as your fist. It is surrounded by a fluid-filled sac called the **pericardium** (**per**-ih-**KAR**-dee-um), which lies within the thoracic cavity, posterior to the sternum and left of the midline. The heart is primarily composed of muscle tissue, which allows it to powerfully contract to pump blood throughout the body. As shown in Figure 12-1, the heart is connected to the aorta, the inferior and superior venae cavae, and the pulmonary veins and arteries.

Memory Key
- The heart is surrounded by the pericardium. It is located in the thoracic cavity.
- The heart is connected to the aorta, the inferior and superior venae cavae, and the pulmonary veins and arteries.

INTERIOR OF THE HEART

Figure 12-2 illustrates the interior of the heart. Note the four chambers: the right and left **atria** (**AY**-tree-ah) and the right and left **ventricles** (**VEN**-trick-ls). A structure called the **septum** (**SEP**-tum) separates the right and left sides of the heart.

The atria are separated from the ventricles by valves called **atrioventricular** (**ay**-tree-oh-ven-**TRICK**-you-lar) (**AV**) **valves**. They allow blood to flow only from the atrium into the ventricle. The right atrioventricular valve is also called the **tricuspid**

FIGURE 12-1
Structures of the heart

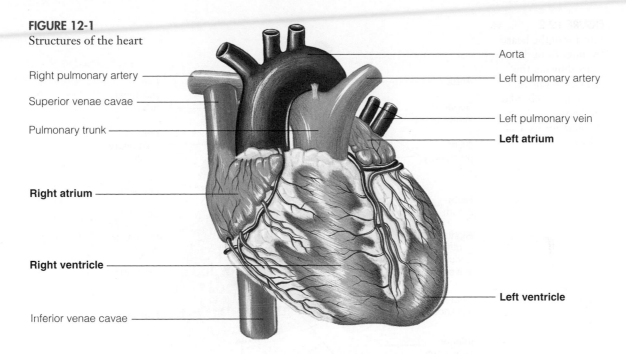

Right pulmonary artery

Superior venae cavae

Pulmonary trunk

Right atrium

Right ventricle

Inferior venae cavae

Aorta

Left pulmonary artery

Left pulmonary vein

Left atrium

Left ventricle

(trigh-**KUS**-pid) **valve**, because it consists of three triangular flaps called **cusps**. The left atrioventricular valve has only two cusps and is therefore called the **bicuspid valve**. Another common name for it is the **mitral** (**MY**-tral) **valve**. The cusps of each atrioventricular valve are attached to the walls of the heart by strong, fibrous cords called the **chordae tendineae** (**KOR**-dee **TEN**-din-ee), which ensure that the valves close tightly, preventing backflow of blood (see Figure 12-2B).

   Once blood has been pumped from the atria into the ventricles, it is pumped through half-moon-shaped valves called **semilunar valves**. The right ventricle pumps blood into the pulmonary artery through the **pulmonary semilunar valve**. The left ventricle pumps blood into the aorta through the **aortic semilunar valve**.

Memory Key

- The heart has four chambers: right and left atria and right and left ventricles.
- The septum separates the right and left sides of the heart.
- The atrioventricular valves allow blood to flow from atria to ventricles.
- The right atrioventricular valve is called the tricuspid valve. The left is called the bicuspid, or mitral, valve.
- The semilunar valves allow blood to flow from the ventricles to arteries.
- The pulmonary semilunar valve allows blood to flow from the right ventricle into the pulmonary artery.
- The aortic semilunar valve allows blood to flow from the left ventricle into the aorta.

FIGURE 12-2
Interior of the heart:
(A) interior of the
heart showing the
chambers, valves,
septum, and chordae
tendineae;
(B) superior view of
valves

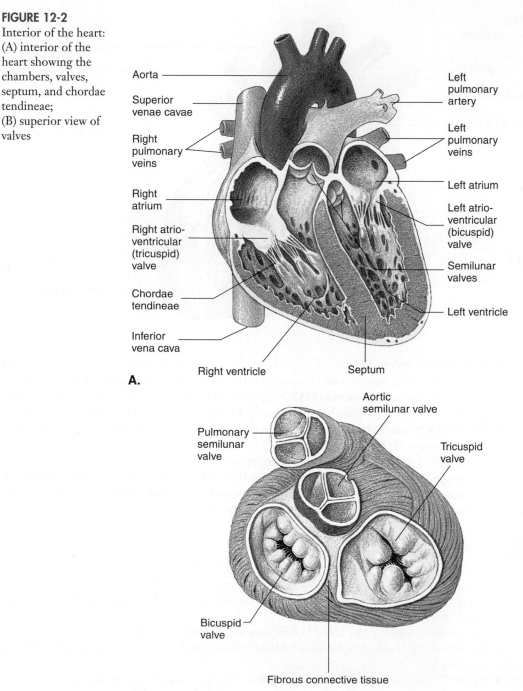

Aorta

Superior
venae cavae

Right
pulmonary
veins

Right
atrium

Right atrio-
ventricular
(tricuspid)
valve

Chordae
tendineae

Inferior
vena cava

Left
pulmonary
artery

Left
pulmonary
veins

Left atrium

Left atrio-
ventricular
(bicuspid)
valve

Semilunar
valves

Left ventricle

Right ventricle   Septum

A.

Aortic
semilunar valve

Pulmonary
semilunar
valve

Tricuspid
valve

Bicuspid
valve

Fibrous connective tissue

B.

WALLS OF THE HEART

The walls of the heart consist of three layers. The thick middle layer, the
myocardium (**my**-oh-**KAR**-dee-um), consists of cardiac muscle tissue. The thin inside
layer, the **endocardium** (**en**-do-**KAR**-dee-um), is epithelial tissue. The outer layer, the
epicardium (**ep**-ih-**KAR**-dee-um), is connective and epithelial tissue. Each layer is illustrated in Figure 12-3.

FIGURE 12-3
Heart walls

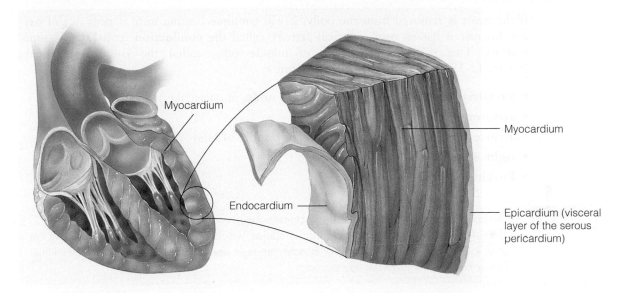

> **Memory Key**   From inside to out, the layers of the heart walls are endocardium, myocardium, and epicardium.

The heart is surrounded by the pericardium (Figure 12-4), which is a sac filled with **pericardial fluid**. Its outer covering is the **parietal** (pah-**RYE**-eh-tal) layer. The inner covering is the **visceral** (**VISS**-er-al) layer, which covers the heart and is another name for the epicardium referred to earlier.

> **Memory Key**   • The pericardium is a sac filled with pericardial fluid.
> • The outer covering of the pericardium is the parietal layer.
> • The inner lining of the pericardium is the visceral layer, also called the epicardium.

FIGURE 12-4
Pericardium

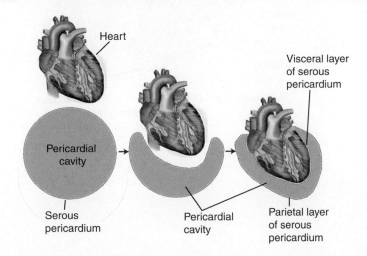

. . . .

12.2   Conduction System

If the heart is removed from the body, it will continue beating until it runs out of oxygen because it has its own electrical system, called the **conduction** (con-**DUCK**-shun) **system**. This specialized network of muscle cells, called the conduction system (Figure 12-5) includes the following structures:

- **sinoatrial** (**sigh**-no-**AY**-tree-al) **node** (**SA node**, or pacemaker)
- **atrioventricular node** (**AV node**)
- **atrioventricular bundle** (**AV bundle**, or **bundle of His**)
- **right** and **left bundle branches**
- **Purkinje** (per-**KIN**-jee) **fibers**

Memory Key	• The conduction system is the heart's electrical system.
	• The SA node (the pacemaker) initiates an impulse, which is sent to the AV node, causing the atria to contract, and then to the AV bundle, the right and left bundle branches and Purkinje fibers, causing the ventricles to contract.

FIGURE 12-5
Conduction system

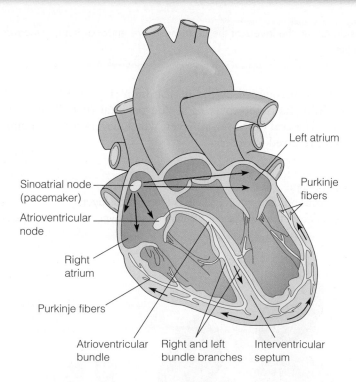

Left atrium

Purkinje fibers

Sinoatrial node (pacemaker)

Atrioventricular node

Right atrium

Purkinje fibers

Atrioventricular bundle

Right and left bundle branches

Interventricular septum

The SA node spontaneously initiates electrical impulses that cause the heart to contract at regular intervals (60 to 95 beats per minute is a normal range). Because the SA node sets the rhythm for the heart, it is referred to as the **pacemaker**. The impulses from the SA node are transmitted to the AV node, which, like the SA node, is situated in the wall of the right atrium. The AV node causes both the right and left atria to contract simultaneously. For the next beat, the AV node sends an impulse to the AV bundle of His, which in turn sends the signal down the right and left bundle branches to the Purkinje fibers. Because these fibers reach deep into the myocardium, they are able to stimulate the simultaneous contraction of the right and left ventricles.

An instrument called an **electrocardiograph** (ee-**leck**-troh-**KAR**-dee-oh-graff) can monitor and produce a written record of the electrical activity of the heart, called an electrocardiogram or ECG (EKG). This record consists of a series of waves, as illustrated in Figure 12-6. The P wave registers the atrial contraction, the QRS wave registers the ventricular contraction, and the T wave registers the recovery or repolarization of the ventricles. A measurement of the interval between P and R (the P–R interval) indicates how long it takes for impulses sent from the SA and AV nodes to reach the Purkinje fibers.

Memory Key	An ECG shows:	P waves (atrial contraction)
		QRS waves (ventricular contraction)
		T waves (ventricular recovery)

FIGURE 12-6

Electrocardiogram: (A) the heart's function is monitored during exercise; (B) normal electrocardiogram showing P waves, QRS wave, and T waves *(Courtesy of Space Labs Medical, Inc.)*

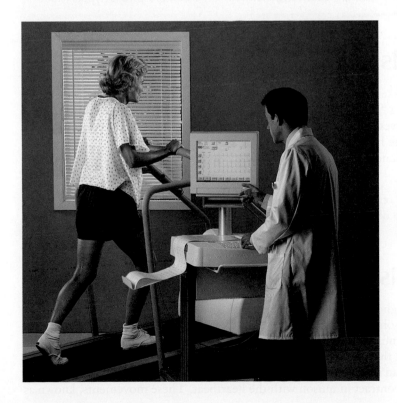

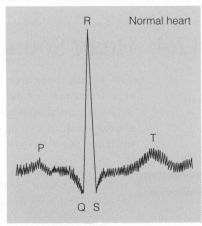

P = strength of atrial contraction

QRS = strength of ventricular contraction

T = resting state of ventricles

12.3 Blood Pressure

When the atria contract, the ventricles are at rest so that they can receive the blood pumped into them from the atria. Likewise, the atria are at rest when the ventricles contract. A heartbeat consists of one contraction phase of the ventricles, called the **systole** (**SIS**-toh-lee), and one resting phase, called the **diastole** (dye-**AS**-toh-lee). During the systole, blood is being forced under pressure out of the ventricles and into the arterial system. The arteries dilate, and this dilation is felt as a **pulse** at certain points in the body (Figure 12-7). The pressure of the blood against the arterial walls is called **blood pressure**. The pressure during systolic and diastolic phases is measured and expressed as two numbers by an instrument called a **sphygmomanometer** (**sfig**-moh-man-**OM**-eh-ter). **Systolic pressure** is the first number. It is higher because the ventricles contract during this phase. **Diastolic pressure**, the second number, is lower because it is a measure of pressure during the ventricular resting phase. A normal blood pressure measurement would range from 100/60 to 120/80 mm Hg. High blood pressure is called **hypertension**, and low blood pressure is called **hypotension**. Hypertension is defined as 140/90 mm Hg or greater. Hypotension is lower than 120/80 mm Hg. Many experts now suggest that 115/75 mm Hg is the optimum. Thus, a new category call **prehypertension** is defined as 120/80 to 139/89 mm Hg.

Memory Key	• A heartbeat consists of the systole (contraction phase) and diastole (resting phase).
	• The dilation of the arteries during the systolic phase is felt as a pulse.
	• Blood pressure is the pressure of blood against the arterial walls.
	• Systolic pressure is higher; diastolic pressure is lower.
	• Abnormally high blood pressure is called hypertension; low blood pressure is hypotension.

12.4 Heart Sounds

The sounds the heart makes as it beats come from the closing of the valves. When the atrioventricular valves close, a "lub" sound is heard. This is called the **first heart sound**, or S_1. When the semilunar valves close, a "dup" sound is heard. This is called the **second heart sound**, or S_2. A complete heartbeat, or a single cardiac cycle, consists of one "lub-dup." A **murmur** is a blowing sound indicative of abnormal blood flow.

Memory Key	• "Lub" (S_1) is the sound of the atrioventricular valves closing.
	• "Dup" (S_2) is the sound of the semilunar valves closing.

12.5 Blood Vessels

Blood is carried throughout the body by **blood vessels**, which consist of **arteries**, **arterioles** (ar-**TEE**-ree-ohlz), **veins**, **venules** (**VEN**-youlz), and **capillaries**.

Arteries are thick, muscular, and elastic, and capable of expanding to accommodate the surge of blood when the heart contracts. Arteries branch off into smaller vessels called arterioles, which then lead into the capillaries, which are discussed later (Figure 12-8). The arterial walls dilate and contract in unison with the heartbeat. These movements, known as a pulse, can be readily detected at certain sites. Pulses can be felt at the following arteries: temporal, carotid, brachial, radial, femoral, popliteal, and dorsalis pedis (see Figure 12-7).

Veins have the same composition as arteries, except that they are less elastic and muscular. Blood pressure in the veins is too low to push blood to the heart from areas such as the legs. Assistance is needed to overcome gravity. Skeletal muscle contraction helps, as does a system of tiny valves that prevent backflow of blood. If these valves are faulty, blood tends to pool in the veins of the legs, resulting in the condition known as varicose veins.

Capillaries are extremely tiny and have very thin walls, only one cell in thickness, composed of endothelium. They are embedded in the various organs of the body in **capillary beds**, which are large concentrations of capillaries. The capillary beds are the connection between the arterial and venous systems. The thin walls of the capillaries enable the transfer of oxygen to the organs and carbon dioxide from the organs. It is the capillaries that feed the walls of the arteries and veins. As discussed in the next section, blood from capillaries empties into small veins called venules, which then lead to the veins.

Figure 12-8 illustrates the capillary, arterial, and venous relationship.

FIGURE 12-7
Pulse points of
the body

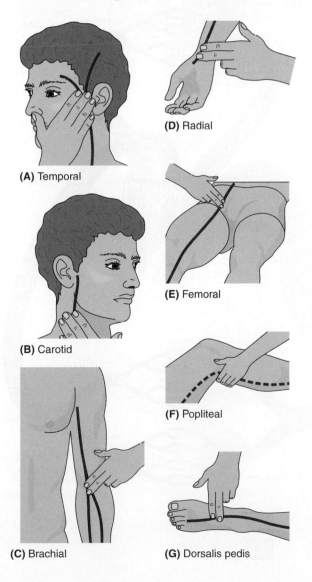

(A) Temporal

(B) Carotid

(C) Brachial

(D) Radial

(E) Femoral

(F) Popliteal

(G) Dorsalis pedis

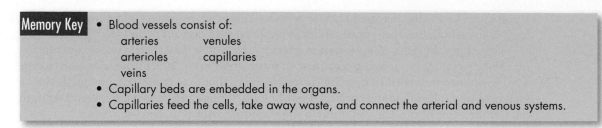

FIGURE 12-8
Schematic drawing of circulation through the lungs and body

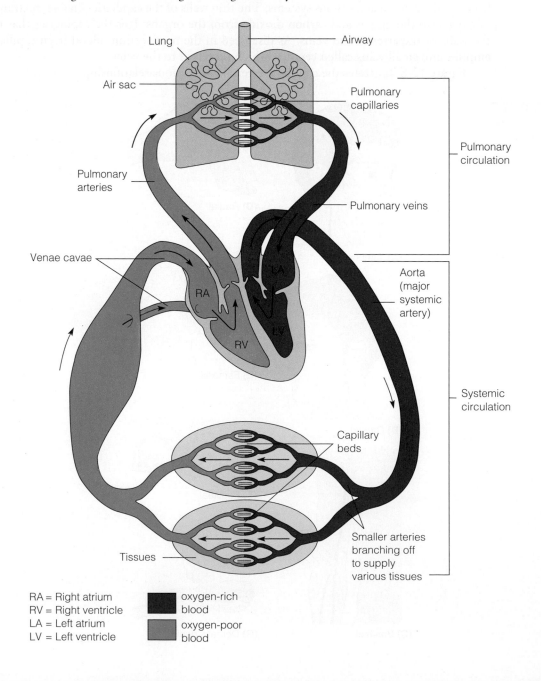

RA = Right atrium
RV = Right ventricle
LA = Left atrium
LV = Left ventricle

oxygen-rich blood

oxygen-poor blood

12.6   Circulation

Arteries (and arterioles) carry blood away from the heart, while veins (and venules) carry blood toward the heart. Although very tiny, capillaries are the most important vessels of all. Oxygenated blood is fed into them from the arterioles, and because capillaries are located within the organs and have very thin walls (only one cell in thickness), they give off the oxygen to the organs and then pick up carbon dioxide. The capillaries connect the arterial and venous systems, so that once oxygen is distributed to the organs and carbon dioxide is picked up, the blood enters the venous system to begin its journey back to the heart.

Veins in the head and arms drain into the **superior vena cava** (SVC). Veins in the rest of the body drain into the **inferior vena cava** (IVC). The SVC and IVC are the largest veins in the body. Each of these major veins returns blood to the **right atrium**, where it is pumped into the **right ventricle** through the **tricuspid valve**. From there, it is pumped into the **pulmonary trunk**, through the **pulmonary semilunar valve**, and through the **pulmonary arteries** to the **lungs**, where carbon dioxide in the blood is exchanged for oxygen, thus oxygenating the blood once again. The oxygenated blood returns through the **pulmonary veins** to the **left atrium** and is then pumped through the **bicuspid valve** into the **left ventricle**. Oxygenated blood is pumped out of the left ventricle, through the **aortic semilunar valve** into the **aorta**. It is then distributed to smaller arteries, branching out into the arterioles and ultimately reaching the capillaries, where oxygen and carbon dioxide transfer take place.

As you can see, all arteries except the pulmonary arteries carry oxygenated blood. Likewise, all veins except the pulmonary veins carry deoxygenated blood.

A simple illustration of the circulatory system appears in Figure 12-8.

Memory Key	• Circulation: superior and inferior venae cavae > right atrium > tricuspid valve > right ventricle > pulmonary semilunar valve > pulmonary arteries > lungs > pulmonary veins > left atrium > bicuspid valve > left ventricle > aortic semilunar valve > aorta > arteries > arterioles > capillaries > venules > veins. • All arteries except the pulmonaries carry oxygenated blood. • All veins except the pulmonaries carry deoxygenated blood.

The heart cannot feed itself from the blood that flows through it. Its walls are far too thick and muscular to absorb oxygen and give off carbon dioxide. It therefore requires its own system of capillaries to feed it, just as any other organ does; this system of capillaries needs a system of arteries and veins to furnish oxygenated blood and carry away deoxygenated blood. These are the **coronary** arteries and veins (Figure 12-9). A heart attack, or myocardial infarction (MI), is simply a blockage in one of the coronary arteries. Because oxygenated blood can no longer reach this part of the heart muscle, the muscle is damaged.

The risk of blockage in any of the arteries is minimized by the fact that the entire circulatory system has built-in parallel routes. Imagine it as a network of roads in a city. There is always more than one way to get somewhere. If one road is blocked off for repair, you just take another route. This is called **collateral** circulation.

Although there are some exceptions, arteries and veins are usually named after the organs through which they pass. For example, the kidneys have **renal** arteries and veins; the stomach has **gastric** arteries and veins. Capillaries are not named.

FIGURE 12-9
Major coronary arteries: right coronary artery, left coronary artery, circumflex artery, right marginal branch, and anterior and posterior interventricular arteries

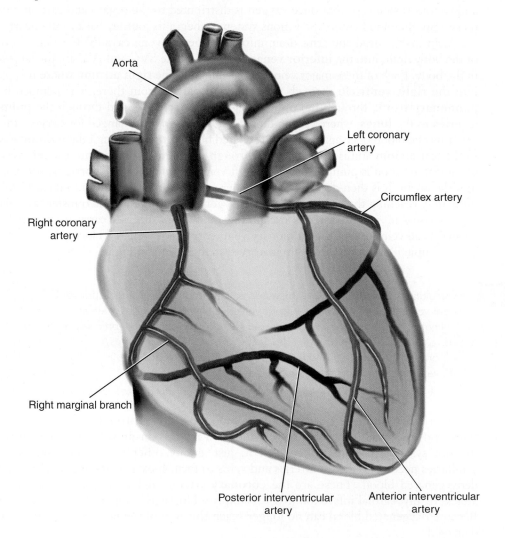

Before you continue, review Sections 12.1 to 12.6. Then, complete Exercises 12-1 and 12-2 found at the end of the chapter.

12.7   Additional Word Parts

The following roots will also be used in this chapter to build medical terms.

Root	Meaning
constrict/o	to draw together
dilat/o	to expand

12.8   Term Analysis and Definition

ROOTS

angi/o (see also vascul/o; vas/o)		**vessel**
Term	**Term Analysis**	**Definition**
angiography (**an**-jee-**OG**-rah-fee)	-graphy = process of recording	process of recording a blood vessel using x-rays following injection of a contrast medium (Figure 12-10). *NOTE:* A contrast medium highlights internal structures, which are otherwise difficult to observe on an x-ray film.

FIGURE 12-10
An angiogram showing
the femoral arteries

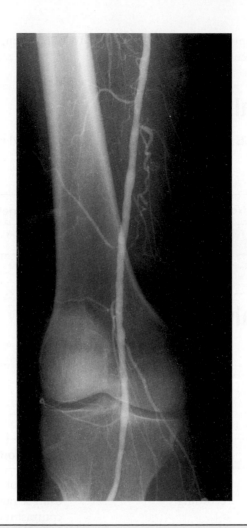

Term	Term Analysis	Definition
angioplasty (**AN**-jee-oh-**plas**-tee)	-plasty = surgical repair; surgical reconstruction	surgical repair of stenosed (narrowed) blood vessels. *NOTE:* Stenosis (narrowing) is caused by the accumulation of fatty debris on the artery wall. Balloon angioplasty flattens the fatty deposits against the walls of the artery, thereby increasing blood flow. One type of balloon angioplasty, percutaneous transluminal coronary angioplasty (PTCA), is shown in Figure 12-11. A balloon-tipped catheter flattens the fatty plaque. A tiny support structure called a **stent** might be placed inside the artery to keep the artery open. Cells quickly grow over the stent, providing a smooth inner lining.

FIGURE 12-11
Percutaneous transluminal coronary angioplasty (PTCA)

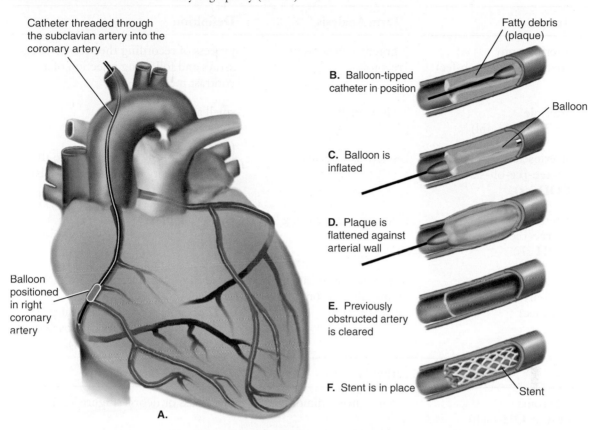

Catheter threaded through the subclavian artery into the coronary artery

Balloon positioned in right coronary artery

A.

Fatty debris (plaque)

B. Balloon-tipped catheter in position

Balloon

C. Balloon is inflated

D. Plaque is flattened against arterial wall

E. Previously obstructed artery is cleared

F. Stent is in place

Stent

Term	Term Analysis	Definition
angiospasm (**AN**-jee-oh-spazm)	-spasm = sudden, involuntary contraction	sudden, involuntary contraction of a blood vessel; vasospasm
	aort/o	**aorta**
aortostenosis (ay-**or**-toh-sten-**OH**-sis)	-stenosis = narrowing	narrowing of the aorta
aortotomy (**ay**-or-**TOT**-eh-mee)	-tomy = incision	incision into the aorta
transaortic (**tranz**-ay-**OR**-tick)	-ic = pertaining to trans- = across	pertaining to across the aorta

	arteri/o	artery
Term	**Term Analysis**	**Definition**
arteriography (**ar**-tee-ree-**OG**-rah-fee)	-graphy = process of recording	process of recording the arteries using x-rays and following injection of a contrast medium
arteriole (ar-**TEE**-ree-ohl)	-ole = small	small arteries
arteriosclerosis (ar-**tee**-ree-oh-skleh-**ROH**-sis)	-sclerosis = hardening	hardening of the arteries (due to the loss of elasticity of the arterial walls)
arteriostenosis (ar-**tee**-ree-oh-steh-**NOH**-sis)	-stenosis = narrowing	narrowing of an artery
endarterectomy (**end**-ar-ter-**ECK**-toh-mee)	-ectomy = surgical removal; excision endo- = within	removal of the inner lining of the arterial wall. *NOTE:* Endarterectomy is a surgical procedure used to treat atherosclerosis (see atherosclerosis below).
	ather/o	**fatty debris; fatty plaque**
atheroma (**ath**-er-**OH**-mah)	-oma = mass; tumor	fatty mass or debris (Figure 12-12)
atherosclerosis (**ath**-er-oh-skleh-**ROH**-sis)	-sclerosis = hardening	accumulation of fatty debris on the inner arterial wall; a type of arteriosclerosis
atherectomy (**ath**-er-**ECK**-toh-mee)	-ectomy = excision; removal	excision or removal of fatty debris (from an arterial wall)
	atri/o	**atrium (upper chamber of the heart)**
interatrial septum (**in**-ter-**AY**-tree-al)	-al = pertaining to inter- = between septum = wall	wall between the atria
	cardi/o	**heart**
cardiologist (**kar**-dee-**OL**-oh-jist)	-logist = specialist	specialist in the study of the diagnosis and treatment of heart disease and disorders

Term	Term Analysis	Definition
cardiology (**kar**-dee-**OL**-oh-jee)	-logy = study of	the study of the heart, including the diagnosis and treatment of heart disorders
cardiomegaly (**kar**-dee-oh-**MEG**-ah-lee)	-megaly = enlargement	enlarged heart
electrocardiogram (ee-**leck**-troh-**KAR**-dee-oh-**gram**)	-gram = record **electr/o** = electric	record of the electrical activity of the heart
myocardial (**my**-oh-**KAR**-dee-al)	-al = pertaining to **my/o** = muscle	pertaining to the heart muscle
cardiomyopathy (**kar**-dee-oh-**my-OP**-ah-thee)	-pathy = disease **my/o** = muscle	disease of the heart muscle
pancarditis (**pan**-kar-**DYE**-tis)	-itis = inflammation pan- = all	inflammation of all the walls of the heart
pericarditis (**per**-ih-kar-**DYE**-tis)	-itis = inflammation peri- = around	inflammation of the pericardium
pericardium (**per**-ih-**KAR**-dee-um)	-um = structure peri- = around	structure surrounding the heart
	coron/o	**crown**
coronary arteries (**KOR**-uh-**nerr**-ee)	-ary = pertaining to	the arteries that supply the heart with blood
	ech/o	**sound**
echocardiogram (**eck**-oh-**KAR**-dee-oh-**gram**)	-gram = record **cardi/o** = heart	record of the heart produced by high-frequency sound waves

Memory Key   The coronary arteries sit on top of the heart like a crown.

Term	Term Analysis	Definition
	embol/o	**plug**
embolus (**EM**-boh-lus)	-us = condition; thing	a plug of clotted blood that is transported through the bloodstream by the blood current. *NOTE:* An embolus can cause obstruction of blood flow, resulting in loss of blood to a part. It can be fatal.

Memory Key Embolus comes from Greek embolus, meaning "plug." An embolus was used as a cork in a liquor bottle.

	isch/o	**hold back**
myocardial ischemia (**my**-oh-**KAR**-dee-al iss-**KEE**-me-ah)	-emia = blood condition -al = pertaining to **my/o** = muscle **cardi/o** = heart	a hold back of blood to the heart muscle. *NOTE:* Myocardial ischemia leads to **myocardial infarction**, which is the area of tissue that has died due to a lack of blood supply to the heart (Figure 12-12). A common symptom of myocardial ischemia is **angina pectoris**, which is defined as severe chest pain.
	phleb/o (see also ven/o)	**vein**
phlebothrombosis (**fleb**-oh-throm-**BOH**-sis)	-osis = abnormal condition **thromb/o** = clot	abnormal condition of clots in a vein
thrombophlebitis (**throm**-boh-fleh-**BYE**-tis)	-itis = inflammation **thromb/o** = clot	inflammation of a vein with clot formation
	rhythm/o	**rhythm**
arrhythmia (ah-**RITH**-mee-ah)	-ia = state of; condition; process a(n)- = no; not	deviation from the normal heart rhythm

FIGURE 12-12
Ischemia

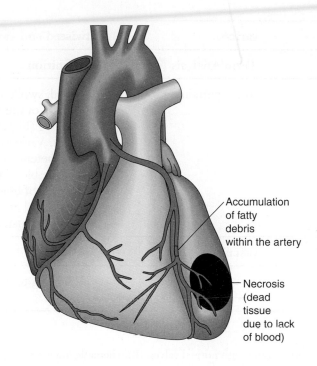

Accumulation
of fatty
debris
within the artery

Necrosis
(dead
tissue
due to lack
of blood)

	scler/o	hardening
Term	**Term Analysis**	**Definition**
sclerotherapy (**skleh**-roh-**THER**-ah-pee)	-therapy = treatment	injection of a solution into a vein for the purpose of destroying the vein's inner lining by hardening. *NOTE:* Sclerotherapy is very effective in treating varicose veins (term follows) and requires no hospitalization.
	thromb/o	**clot**
thrombus (**THROM**-bus)	-us = condition; thing	a blood clot that obstructs a blood vessel
	valvul/o	**valve**
valvuloplasty (**VAL**-vyoo-loh-**plas**-tee)	-plasty = surgical repair; surgical reconstruction	surgical repair of a valve

	varic/o	twisted and swollen
Term	**Term Analysis**	**Definition**
varicose veins (**VAR**-ih-kohs)	-ose = pertaining to	twisted, swollen superficial veins, typically of the **saphenous** vein of the lower leg (Figure 12-13). *NOTE:* Varicose veins occur when incompetent valves in the vein fail to push the blood forward, causing backflow of blood. Veins become dilated, and blood pools, creating unsightly clusters of protruding veins.
	vascul/o	**vessel**
avascular (a-**VAS**-kyoo-lar)	-ar = pertaining to a- = no; not; lack of	pertaining to no blood vessels

FIGURE 12-13
(A) Schematic drawing of normal veins with normal valves; (B) schematic drawing of varicose veins and abnormal valves; (C) photograph of varicose veins

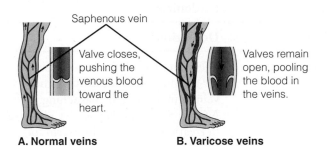

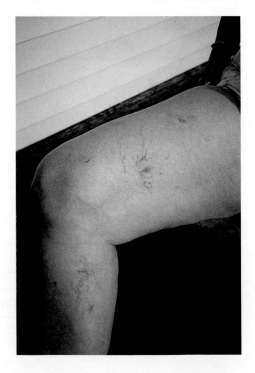

Term	Term Analysis	Definition
cerebrovascular accident (CVA) (**ser**-eh-broh-**VAS**-kyou-lar)	-ar = pertaining to **cerebr/o** = brain	disturbance in the flow of blood to one or more parts of the brain; commonly known as a stroke
	vas/o	**vessel**
extravasation (ecks-**trav**-ah-**SAY**-shun)	-ion = process extra- = outside	escape of fluid into the surrounding tissue; for example, the escape of blood from a blood vessel into the surrounding tissue
vasoconstriction (**vas**-oh-kon-**STRICK**-shun)	-ion = process **constrict/o** = to draw together; narrowing	narrowing of a vessel; vasospasm
vasodilation (**vas**-oh-dye-**LAY**-shun)	-ion = process **dilat/o** = to expand; widen	widening of the vessel; angiectasis
	ven/o	**vein**
venous (**VEE**-nus)	-ous = pertaining to	pertaining to a vein
venule (**VEN**-youl)	-ule = small	small vein
	ventricul/o	**ventricle (lower chamber of the heart)**
interventricular septum (**in**-ter-ven-**TRICK**-yoo-lar)	-ar = pertaining to inter- = between septum = wall	pertaining to the wall between the ventricles

SUFFIXES

Term	Term Analysis	Definition
	-ectasis	**dilation; dilatation; stretching**
angiectasis (**an**-jee-**ECK**-tah-sis)	**angi/o** = vessel	dilation of a blood vessel; vasodilation

PREFIXES

	-brady	slow
Term	**Term Analysis**	**Definition**
bradycardia (**brad**-ee-**KAR**-dee-uh)	-ia = condition; state of **cardi/o** = heart	slow heartbeat
	-tachy	**fast**
tachycardia (**tack**-ee-**KAR**-dee-ah)	-ia = condition; state of **cardi/o** = heart	fast heartbeat

Memory Key In *bradycardia* and *tachycardia*, both the *i* and the *o* are dropped from **cardi/o**; the suffix is -ia, meaning "condition" or "state of."

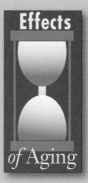

Effects *of Aging*

Aging heart muscle becomes stiffer because the muscle cells are gradually replaced with connective tissue. Therefore, the heart muscle cannot pump as effectively. An older heart cannot change its beat as quickly as a young one, and thus is less efficient in responding to the demands of exercise. Despite this, unless disease is present or the muscle has been damaged because of the lack of blood, an older heart functions perfectly well under normal stressors.

The walls of the arteries become thicker and less elastic as we age. Because the arteries can no longer expand and contract as quickly, elevated blood pressure is common in the elderly.

Avoidance of smoking and excessive alcohol as well as regular exercise can significantly reduce the effects of aging on the heart muscle and the arteries.

12.9   Common Diseases

ANEURYSM

An aneurysm (**AN**-yer-izm) is an abnormal bulge in the wall of an artery. It occurs most often in the aorta or in the brain. A ruptured aneurysm occurs when the wall of the artery bursts. This cause internal hemorrhaging, which might result in death.

CARDIAC ARREST

Cardiac arrest is when the heart suddenly stops pumping blood. The primary cause of cardiac arrest is dysfunction of the electrical activity through the heart. Other causes include airway obstruction and circulatory shock.

CEREBROVASCULAR ACCIDENT

Cerebrovascular accident (CVA), also known as a stroke, is a result of lack of blood to the brain, depriving it of oxygen and nutrients. CVA might be caused by a thrombus, an embolus, or a burst aneurysm.

Treatment of CVA involves restoring cerebral circulation by removing the thrombus or embolus by endarterectomy or angioplasty. Postoperatively, anticoagulant drugs are given to prevent blood clotting. When a stroke is caused by a burst aneurysm, surgery might be performed to remove the hematoma (clotted blood) from brain tissue, if it can be reached.

MYOCARDIAL INFARCTION

Myocardial infarction (MI), also called a heart attack, means death of the heart muscle. When one or more of the arteries that supply the heart with blood is blocked, blood flow to the heart muscle stops and the tissue dies. The heart is unable to function properly and not enough blood is pumped to the body's tissues.

Restoring blood supply to the heart muscle is a must to prevent further heart damage or death. Drugs such as nitroglycerin widen the arterial wall, thus improving blood flow to the heart muscle. Angioplasty and coronary artery bypass graft (CABG) are designed to improve circulation to one or more areas of the heart.

CABG or open-heart surgery is a procedure performed to re-establish adequate circulation to one or more segments of the heart when coronary artery disease diminishes blood flow. A section of vein is removed from the leg or breast and used as a graft to reroute the blood around the blockage.

12.10 Abbreviations

Abbreviation	Meaning
AV	atrioventricular
ASHD	arteriosclerotic heart disease (damage to the heart due to the obstruction of a coronary artery)
BP	blood pressure
CABG	coronary artery bypass graft
CAD	coronary artery disease
CCU	cardiac/coronary care unit

continued on page 300

continued from page 299

Abbreviation	Meaning
CHF	congestive heart failure (Myocardial disease results in the failure of the heart to pump blood effectively through the blood vessels, resulting in congestion or pooling of blood in the veins.)
CPR	cardiopulmonary resuscitation
CV	cardiovascular
CVA	cerebrovascular accident
ECG; EKG	electrocardiogram
HHD	hypertensive heart disease (With long-term high blood pressure, the heart needs to work harder to pump the blood through the blood vessels; over time this extra work damages the heart.)
IVC	inferior venae cavae
LA	left atrium
LV	left ventricle
MI	myocardial infarction
MVP	mitral valve prolapse (incomplete closure of the mitral valve resulting in the backflow of blood into the left atrium from the left ventricle)
PVC	premature ventricular contraction
RA	right atrium
RV	right ventricle
SA	sinoatrial
SVC	superior venae cavae

12.11 Putting It All Together

Exercise 12-1   SHORT ANSWER

1. List the structures through which blood passes as it circulates through the body. Start with the right atrium and end with the superior and inferior venae cavae.

_____

_____

_____

2. Differentiate between the pericardium, myocardium, endocardium, and epicardium. Which structure is the same as the visceral pericardium?

_____

_____

_____

3. What is the function of the conduction system? List five structures of the conduction system. Which structure is known as the pacemaker? Why?

_____

_____

_____

4. Define:

    a. systolic pressure   _____

    b. diastolic pressure   _____

    c. sphygmomanometer   _____

    d. P wave   _____

5. How are arteries and veins named?

_____

Exercise 12-2   OPPOSITES

Give the opposite of the following terms.

1. vasodilation   _____

2. hypertension   _____

3. bradycardia   _____

4. diastole   _____

Exercise 12-3   ROOTS AND DEFINITIONS

Underline the root(s), then give the definition of the following terms.

1. endarterectomy   _____

2. interatrial   _____

3. pancarditis   _____

4. echocardiogram   _____

5. phlebothrombosis   _____

6. cerebrovascular accident   _____

7. atheroma   _____

Exercise 12-4   BUILDING MEDICAL TERMS

Build the medical term for the following definitions.

1. dilation of a blood vessel   _____

2. process of recording a blood vessel   _____

3. surgical repair of a stenosed blood vessel   _____

4. sudden, involuntary contraction of
   blood vessels   _____

5. process of recording arteries   _____

6. small arteries   _____

7. hardening of the artery   _____

8. pertaining to a vein   _____

9. small vein   _____

10. specialist in the study of the heart   _____

Exercise 12-5   SPELLING

Circle any misspelled words in the following list and correctly spell them in the space provided.

1. paricardium   _____

2. ventrical   _____

3. atrium   _____

4. myocardeum   _____

5. capillaries   _____

6. Purkinje   _____

7. sfigmomanometer   _____

8. extravasashun _____

9. bicuspit _____

10. lumen _____

Exercise 12-6   ADJECTIVAL FORMS

Give the adjectival form for the following.

1. aorta _____

2. artery _____

3. atrium _____

4. valve _____

5. ventricle _____

Exercise 12-7   PATHOLOGY

I. Define the following:

a. cardiac arrest _____

_____

b. myocardial infarction _____

_____

c. cerebrovascular accident _____

_____

d. aneurysm _____

_____

II. Fill in the Blanks

a. Name three operative procedures that improve blood supply to an organ:

_____

_____

b. Write the name of the drug that is commonly given to widen the coronary arteries in myocardial ischemia: _____

c. Name the type of drug that prevents blood clotting:

_____

12.12 Review of Vocabulary

In the following tables, Tables 12-1 through 12-4, the medical terms found in this chapter are organized into these categories: anatomy, pathology, diagnostics, and surgical procedures. Define each term and decide into which category the word belongs. This will help you associate the term with its purpose, and help you remember it.

TABLE 12-1

REVIEW OF ANATOMICAL TERMS

1. aorta	2. arteriole	3. atria
4. cardiologist	5. cardiology	6. chordae tendinae
7. coronary arteries	8. interatrial septum	9. interventricular septum
10. mitral valve	11. myocardial	12. pericardium
13. semilunar valve	14. supreior venae cavae	15. venous
16. ventricles	17. venule	

TABLE 12-2

REVIEW OF PATHOLOGIC TERMS

1. angiectasis	2. angiospasm	3. aortostenosis
4. arrhythmia	5. arteriosclerosis	6. arteriostenosis

continued on page 305

Table 12-2 *continued from page 304*

7. atheroma	8. atherosclerosis	9. bradycardia
10. cardiomegaly	11. cerebrovascular accident	12. embolus
13. extravasation	14. myocardial ischemia	15. cardiomyopathy
16. pancarditis	17. pericarditis	18. phlebothrombosis
19. tachycardia	20. thrombophlebitis	21. thrombus
22. vasoconstriction	23. vasodilation	24. varicose veins

TABLE 12-3

REVIEW OF DIAGNOSTIC TERMS

1. angiography	2. arteriography	3. echocardiogram
4. electrocardiogram		

TABLE 12-4

REVIEW OF SURGICAL PROCEDURES

1. angioplasty	2. endarterectomy	3. sclerotherapy
4. valvuloplasty		

12.13 MEDICAL TERMS IN CONTEXT

After you read the following Personal History, answer the questions that follow. Use your text, medical dictionary, or other references if necessary.

PERSONAL HISTORY

HISTORY OF PRESENT ILLNESS: This patient was admitted through the emergency room from St. Edmund's Hospital with an acute onset of coldness and weakness in her lower extremities. She was found to have no pulse in her lower extremities.

PAST HISTORY: This patient had an aortofemoral bypass for chronic ischemia of her lower extremities five years ago. She also has a past history of hypertension, arrhythmia, and heart failure.

ALLERGIES: None known.

PHYSICAL EXAMINATION

General: A 75-year-old woman in severe distress with discomfort in her lower extremities.

Head and Neck: No audible abnormal sounds in the carotid or subclavian veins.

Cardiovascular System: Pulse was 72 per minute and irregular. BP 140/80. Heart sounds were unremarkable.

Abdomen: Healed midline abdominal incision. Normal palpable pulses in the aorta. No femoral pulses. No abdominal masses.

Periphery: Absent pulses in her lower extremities with ischemic lower extremities.

IMPRESSION

1. AORTOILIAC EMBOLUS
2. ATRIAL ARRHYTHMIA
3. HYPERTENSION

QUESTIONS ON THE PERSONAL HISTORY

1. Coldness in the lower extremities was likely due to:
   a. arrhythemia
   b. hypertension
   c. ischemia
   d. pallor

2. In the past, the patient had an aortofemoral bypass because of:
   a. an abnormal heart rhythm
   b. high blood pressure
   c. a holdback of blood
   d. necrotic tissue

3. Symptoms of coldness and weakness occurred in the:
   a. arms
   b. legs
   c. lower abdomen
   d. pelvis

4. Symptoms of coldness and weakness occurred:
   a. gradually
   b. consistently
   c. irregularly
   d. suddenly

5. Which of the following conditions is *not* included in the Past History?
   a. abnormal heart rate
   b. wandering blood clot
   c. high blood pressure
   d. holdback of blood to the legs

6. The carotid vein is in the:

    a. chest

    b. head

    c. lower extremities

    d. neck

7. Periphery means:

    a. away from the center

    b. away from the point of origin

    c. nearest the point of origin

    d. toward the center

8. The wandering blood clot was located in the:

    a. aortic and femoral arteries

    b. aortic and iliac arteries

    c. heart

    d. carotid and subclavian veins

Blood, Immune, and Lymphatic Systems

CHAPTER ORGANIZATION

This chapter will help you learn about blood and the immune and lymphatic systems. It is divided into the following sections:

13.1 Blood

13.2 Additional Word Parts

13.3 Term Analysis and Definition Pertaining to Blood

13.4 Common Diseases of Blood

13.5 Abbreviations Pertaining to Blood

13.6 Immune System

13.7 Lymphatic System

13.8 Term Analysis and Definition Pertaining to the Immune and Lymphatic Systems

13.9 Common Diseases of the Immune and Lymphatic Systems

13.10 Abbreviations Pertaining to the Immune and Lymphatic Systems

13.11 Putting It All Together

13.12 Review of Vocabulary Pertaining to Blood

13.13 Review of Anatomical Terms Pertaining to Immune and Lymphatic Systems

13.14 Medical Terms in Context

CHAPTER OBJECTIVES

On completion of this chapter, you will be able to do the following:

1. Name and describe the components of the blood

2. Define terms relating to the immune system

3. Locate and describe the organs of the lymphatic system

4. Analyze, define, pronounce, and spell terms related to blood, immune, and lymphatic systems

5. Describe common diseases

6. Define common abbreviations related to blood, immune, and lymphatic systems

INTRODUCTION

In the chapter on the skeletal system, you learned that blood cells are formed in the red bone marrow. When you studied the cardiovascular system, you learned about the veins and arteries that transport blood throughout the body and how blood functions to provide oxygen and nutrients to the organs and carry away wastes. In this chapter, you will learn about the makeup of blood, and the important role it plays in fighting disease. You will also learn about the body's other circulatory system, the lymphatic system, and how it functions together with the circulatory (blood) system to protect us from infection.

13.1   Blood

Whole blood is about 55% liquid and 45% solid, as illustrated in Figure 13-1. The liquid is called **plasma** (**PLAZ**-mah). The solid portion is referred to as **formed elements** and consists of three types of blood cells: **red blood cells** (**RBCs**), or **erythrocytes** (eh-**RITH**-roh-sights); **white blood cells** (**WBCs**), or **leukocytes** (**LOO**-koh-sights); and **platelets** (**PLAYT**-lets), or **thrombocytes** (**THROM**-boh-sights). Because plasma is more than 90% water, it is thin and almost colorless when it is separated from blood cells.

> **Memory Key**   Blood consists of plasma and the following formed elements: erythrocytes (RBCs), leukocytes (WBCs), and thrombocytes (platelets).

PLASMA

Plasma transports fats, proteins, gases, salts, and hormones to their various destinations throughout the body and picks up waste materials from organ cells. The fats, such as **triglyceride** (try-**GLIS**-er-eyed), **phospholipid** (fos-foh-**LIP**-id), and **cholesterol** (koh-**LES**-ter-ol), are transported to tissues by attaching to proteins. The plasma proteins are **albumin** (al-**BYOU**-min), **globulin** (**GLOB**-you-lin), and **fibrinogen** (figh-**BRIN**-oh-jen). Fibrinogen is the blood-clotting agent. When fibrinogen and other clotting factors are removed, the plasma is called **serum** (**SEER**-um).

> **Memory Key**   • Plasma carries fats (triglyceride, phospholipid, and cholesterol), proteins (albumin, globulin, and fibrinogen), gases, salts, and hormones.
> • Serum is plasma with fibrinogen and other clotting factors removed.

FORMED ELEMENTS

Erythrocytes (RBCs) are shaped like biconcave discs. They contain **hemoglobin** (Hgb) (**hee**-moh-**GLOH**-bin), a protein that contains iron and has the ability to bind with oxygen and carbon dioxide. This ability enables the blood to transport oxygen to the organ cells and carbon dioxide away from them. Erythropoiesis, the maturation process for red blood cells, involves several stages. In the second-to-last stage, the cell is called a **reticulocyte** (reh-**TICK**-you-loh-**sight**). After the reticulocyte becomes an erythrocyte, it leaves the red

FIGURE 13-1
Plasma, formed elements, erythrocytes, leukocytes, and thrombocytes

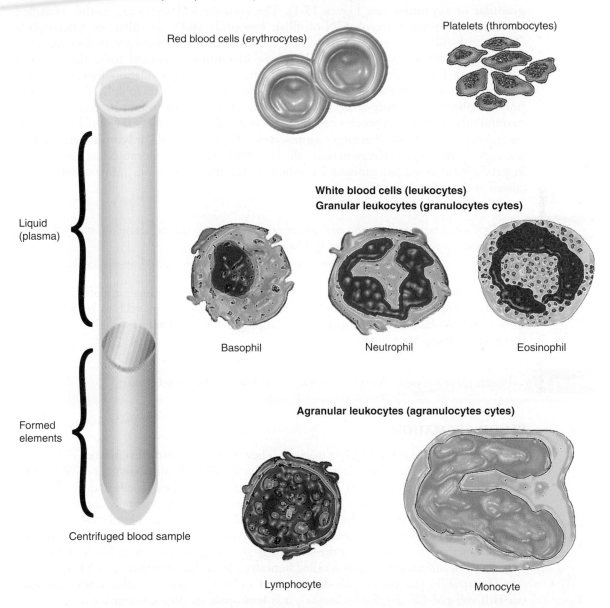

Red blood cells (erythrocytes)

Platelets (thrombocytes)

Liquid
(plasma)

Formed
elements

Centrifuged blood sample

White blood cells (leukocytes)
Granular leukocytes (granulocytes cytes)

Basophil

Neutrophil

Eosinophil

Agranular leukocytes (agranulocytes cytes)

Lymphocyte

Monocyte

bone marrow and enters the bloodstream, where it can be measured in a laboratory test called
a **reticulocyte count**. This test is a direct indication of the bone marrow's production of red
blood cells. After approximately 120 days, the erythrocyte ruptures and dies, releasing hemoglobin, which eventually finds its way back to the bone marrow to be recycled.

Memory Key	• RBCs (erythrocytes) contain hemoglobin, which transports oxygen and carbon dioxide.
	• Reticulocytes develop into RBCs.
	• RBCs live about 120 days, and then rupture.

Leukocytes (white blood cells) fight infections. They have the ability to migrate from the bloodstream into the tissues to the site of infection. They are classified as either **granular** or **agranular** (see Figure 13-1). The granular leukocytes are further classified as either **eosinophils** (ee-oh-**SIN**-oh-fills), **basophils** (**BAY**-soh-fills), or **neutrophils** (**NEW**-troh-fills). The eosinophils release chemicals into the bloodstream that can neutralize toxic substances. The basophils release **histamine**, a natural toxin that initiates the inflammatory process by dilating the blood vessels. This dilation increases blood flow into the site of the infection, thereby speeding recovery. Neutrophils, also known as **polymorphonuclear** (**poly**-more-foh-**NEW**-klee-ar) leukocytes, ingest bacteria and other harmful matter through a process called phagocytosis (**fag**-oh-sigh-**TOH**-sis). The agranular leukocytes are classified as either **monocytes** (**MON**-oh-sights) or **lymphocytes** (**LIM**-foh-sights). Monocytes change to cells called macrophages. They act much like neutrophils, ingesting harmful microorganisms. Lymphocytes are important in the immune system, discussed in the following section.

Memory Key   WBCs (leukocytes) fight infection and are either granular (eosinophils, basophils, and neutrophils) or agranular (monocytes and lymphocytes).

Thrombocytes (or platelets, because of their plate-like appearance) initiate blood clotting when bleeding occurs. Through the release of clotting agents such as **prothrombin** (pro-**THROM**-bin) and fibrinogen, a platelet plug is formed where a vessel wall has ruptured, thus halting bleeding.

Memory Key   Platelets (thrombocytes) release prothrombin and fibrinogen for blood clotting.

BLOOD FORMATION

Blood cells originate from the bone marrow. They start out as **undifferentiated** cells (nonspecialized cells) called **hemocytoblasts** (hee-moh-**SIGHT**-oh-blasts), or blood **stem cells**. Most stem cells are able to develop into many different types of cells in the body, such as muscle, skin, and nerve cells. However, blood stem cells can become only one of the three blood cell types: erythrocytes, leukocytes, or thrombocytes. As each blood stem cell develops into specific cells with different shapes and functions, they are said to be **differentiated**. This means that they cease being the same. The general process of their development into specialized or differentiated cells is called **hematopoiesis** (**hee**-mah-toh-poi-**EE**-sis).

The specific process for the development of erythrocytes is called **erythropoiesis** (eh-**rith**-roh-poi-**EE**-sis); for leukocytes, it is **leukopoiesis** (**loo**-koh-poi-**EE**-sis); and for thrombocytes, it is **thrombopoiesis** (**throm**-boh-poi-**EE**-sis).

Memory Key   • Hemocytoblasts develop into blood cells by hematopoiesis.
                 • The specific processes are erythropoiesis, leukopoiesis, and thrombopoiesis.

BLOOD TYPES

Any substance that stimulates the body's immune response (bacteria, viruses, and pollens, for example) is referred to as an **antigen** (**AN**-tih-jen), which is an abbreviation for the term "antibody generator." Specific to our discussion on blood cells, there are two types of proteins on the surface of red blood cells that are antigens. They are referred to as type A and type B antigens. Blood is classified as type **A**, **B**, **AB**, or **O**, depending on the presence or absence of these antigens. Type A blood has only type A antigens, type B has only type B antigens; AB has both, and O has neither. The type of blood a person receives in a transfusion depends on the presence or absence of the A, B, AB, and O antigens. If a person receives the wrong type of blood, blood that does not match his or her own blood type, **antibodies** will be formed against the specific antigen as they recognize the antigen to be foreign to the body. This is an antigen-antibody reaction. Persons with type A blood generate antibodies if type B blood is injected into them. Those with type B blood generate antibodies if type A blood is injected into them. Persons with AB blood can accept any type. Type O persons require type O blood but can donate to all others. The antigen-antibody reaction may cause a clumping of red blood cells, or agglutination. It is for this reason that blood must be cross-matched before it is transfused into a patient. In cross-matching, the donor's blood is mixed with the recipient's blood and analyzed for agglutination.

Memory Key	Type A blood has only type A antigens; type B blood has only type B antigens; type AB has both; and type O has neither.

There are several other blood antigens. The most important is the **Rh antigen**, which was first discovered by examining the blood of Rhesus monkeys. Most people are **Rh positive**, meaning they have the Rh antigen. Those who lack it are Rh negative.

Memory Key	Most people are Rh positive (have the Rh antigen).

Before you continue, review Section 13.1. Then, complete Exercise 13-1, questions 1 and 2 found at the end of the chapter.

13.2   Additional Word Parts

The following roots, suffixes and prefix will aslo be used in this chapter to build medical terms.

Root	Meaning
anis/o	unequal
bilirubin/o	bilirubin (a bile pigment)
cholesterol/o	cholesterol

Root	Meaning
granul/o	granules
lipid/o	fat
norm/o	normal
poikil/o	variation; irregular

Suffix	Meaning
-edema	accumulation of fluid
-plastic	pertaining to formation

Prefix	Meaning
mono-	one

13.3   Term Analysis and Definition Pertaining to Blood

ROOTS

	chrom/o	color
Term	**Term Analysis**	**Definition**
hyperchromia (**high**-per-**KROH**-mee-ah)	-ia = condition; state of hyper- = excessive;	excessively pigmented red blood cells above normal
hypochromia (**high**-poh-**KROH**-mee-ah)	-ia = condition; state of hypo- = below; deficient	under-pigmented red blood cells
normochromia (**nor**-moh-**KROH**-mee-ah)	-ia = condition; state of **norm/o** = normal	normally pigmented red blood cells

	erythr/o	red
Term	**Term Analysis**	**Definition**
erythrocyte (eh-**RITH**-roh-sight)	-cyte = cell	red blood cell
	hemat/o; hem/o	**blood**
hemolysis (hee-**MOL**-ih-sis)	-lysis = breakdown separation; destruction	breakdown of blood
hematologist (**hee**-mah-**TOL**-oh-jist)	-logist = specialist	specialist in the study of blood and blood disorders
hematology (**hee**-mah-**TOL**-oh-jee)	-logy = study of	study of blood and blood disorders
	leuk/o	**white**
leukocyte (**LOO**-koh-sight)	-cyte = cell	white blood cell
	myel/o	**bone marrow**
myelogenous (**my**-eh-**LOJ**-en-us)	-genous = produced by	produced by the bone marrow
myeloid (**MY**-eh-loid)	-oid = resembling	resembling bone marrow
	reticul/o	**network**
reticulocyte (reh-**TICK**-yoo-loh-sight)	-cyte = cell	a young red blood cell characterized by a network of granules within the cell membrane
	thromb/o	**clot**
thrombocyte (**THROM**-boh-sight)	-cyte = cell	clotting cell; platelet
thrombolysis (throm-**BOL**-ih-sis)	-lysis = destruction; breakdown; separation	breakdown of a clot that has formed in the blood
thrombosis (throm-**BOH**-sis)	-osis = abnormal condition	blood clot; abnormal condition of clot formation

SUFFIXES

Term	Term Analysis	Definition
	-blast	**immature, growing thing**
hemocytoblast (**hee**-moh-**SIGHT**-oh-blast)	**hem/o** = blood **cyt/o** = cell	immature blood cell
lymphoblast (**LIM**-foh-blast)	**lymph/o** = lymph	immature lymphocyte, type of white blood cell
monoblast (**MON**-oh-blast)	**mono-** = one	immature monocyte, type of white blood cell
	-crit	**separate**
hematocrit (HCT) (hee-**MAT**-oh-krit)	**hemat/o** = blood	a laboratory test that determines the percentage of erythrocytes in a blood sample
	-cytosis	**increase in the number of cells**
anisocytosis (an-**eye**-soh-sigh-**TOH**-sis)	**anis/o** = unequal	increased variation in the size of cells, particularly red blood cells
leukocytosis (**loo**-koh-sigh-**TOH**-sis)	**leuk/o** = white	marked increase in the number of white blood cells. NOTE: The increase in the number of white blood cells is not permanent. They are temporarily increased to fight an infection. After the infection has subsided, the number of white blood cells returns to normal.
poikilocytosis (**poi**-kil-oh-sigh-**TOH**-sis)	**poikil/o** = variation; irregular	increased variation in the shape of cells, particularly red blood cells
	-emia	**blood condition**
anemia (ah-**NEE**-mee-ah)	**an-** = no; not; lack of	lack of red blood cells or hemoglobin content in the blood
erythremia (**er**-ih-**THREE**-mee-ah)	**erythr/o** = red	abnormal increase in the number of red blood cells

Term	Term Analysis	Definition
hyperbilirubinemia (high-per-bil-ih-roo-bih-NEE-mee-ah)	hyper- = excessive; above normal bilirubin/o = bilirubin (a bile pigment)	above normal levels of bilirubin in the blood *NOTE*: Bilirubin comes from the breakdown of hemoglobin.
hypercholesterolemia (**high**-per-koh-**les**-ter-ol-**EE**-mee-ah)	hyper- = excessive; above normal **cholesterol/o** = cholesterol	above normal levels of cholesterol in the blood
hyperlipidemia (**high**-per-**lip**-ih-**DEE**-mee-ah)	hyper- = excessive; above normal **lipid/o** = fat	above normal levels of fats in the blood
leukemia (loo-**KEE**-mee-ah)	**leuk/o** = white	malignant increase in the number of white blood cells in the blood; considered a form of cancer
	-penia	**deficient; decrease**
erythrocytopenia (eh-**rith**-roh-**sigh**-toh-**PEE**-nee-ah)	**erythr/o** = red **cyt/o** = cell	decrease in the number of red blood cells; erythropenia
leukocytopenia (**loo**-koh-**sigh**-toh-**PEE**-nee-ah)	**leuk/o** = white **cyt/o** = cell	decrease in the number of white blood cells; leukopenia
pancytopenia (**pan**-sigh-toh-**PEE**-nee-ah)	pan- = all **cyt/o** = cell	decrease in the number of all blood cells
thrombocytopenia (**throm**-boh-**sigh**-toh-**PEE**-nee-ah)	**thromb/o** = clot **cyt/o** = cell	decrease in the number of clotting cells; thrombopenia
	-phoresis	**transmission; carry**
electrophoresis (ee-**leck**-troh-for-**EE**-sis)	**electr/o** = electric	a laboratory test in which substances in a mixture, usually proteins, are separated by an electrical current
	-poiesis	**production; manufacture; formation**
erythropoiesis (eh-**rith**-roh-poi-**EE**-sis)	**erythr/o** = red	production of red blood cells

Term	Term Analysis	Definition
hematopoiesis (**hee**-mah-toh-poi-**EE**-sis)	**hemat/o** = blood	production of blood cells
	-poietin	**hormones regulating the production of various cell types**
erythropoietin (eh-**rith**-roh-**POI**-eh-tin)	**erythr/o** = red	a hormone in the kidneys that stimulates the production of red blood cells
	-stasis	**stopping; controlling**
hemostasis (**hee**-moh-**STAY**-sis)	**hem/o** = blood	stoppage of blood

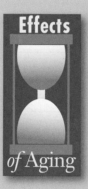

Effects of Aging on Blood

Red blood cells are produced in the red bone marrow. Because the aging process is accompanied by a decrease in red bone marrow, the body's ability to produce red blood cells decreases with age. Under normal conditions, this is not significant. However, under stress, such as a hemorrhage, the body might not be able to produce red blood cells quickly enough.

Hemoglobin levels in males and females are significantly different after age 30. Levels in males slowly decrease, while females produce higher levels until about age 60, after which their production declines to the level of males.

13.4   Common Diseases of Blood

LEUKEMIA

Leukemia is a form of cancer of the bone marrow that results in a malignant increase in the number of white blood cells in the blood. The vast numbers of white blood cells eventually replace red blood cells, platelets, and normal-functioning white blood cells. Oxygen delivery to tissues, blood clotting, and immunity become impaired. Leukemic cells might spread to other organs, including the spleen, lymph nodes, and the central nervous system.

Chemotherapy is the prominent form of treatment. **Radiation therapy** is also used to damage leukemia cells and prevent their growth. **Bone marrow transplantation** is sometimes used. It involves the replacement of diseased bone marrow with leukemia-free bone marrow from a closely related donor. Before a transplant can be successful, the patient must undergo chemotherapy and radiation therapy to kill all the diseased bone marrow that causes leukemia.

Stem cell transplantation can be used to treat acute forms of leukemia. The stem cells can be taken from the patient's healthy cells or from a compatible donor. After the stem cells are placed into the patient's body, they develop and grow into mature, healthy blood cells. As in the bone marrow transplant, the patient first receives chemotherapy and radiation therapy to kill the diseased bone marrow before the stem cells are transplanted.

13.5   Abbreviations Pertaining to Blood

Abbreviation	Meaning
ABO	three main blood groups
CBC	complete blood count
diff	differential count (laboratory test to determine the number of different types of white blood cells)
eos	eosinophil
ESR	erythrocyte sedimentation rate
Hb; Hgb	hemoglobin
HCT; HcT	hematocrit
lymphs	lymphocytes
mono	monocyte
PMN	polymorphonuclear
polys	polymorphonuclear leukocytes
RBC; rbc	red blood cell
segs	segmented polymorphonuclear leukocytes
WBC; wbc	white blood cell

13.6   Immune System

As mentioned earlier, lymphocytes are one of the two types of agranular (or nongranular) leukocytes and are responsible for initiating the immune response. Two types of lymphocytes are involved: **T lymphocytes (T cells)**, which are produced in the red bone marrow but mature in the thymus, and **B lymphocytes (B cells)**, which develop and mature in the red bone marrow.

> **Memory Key**   Lymphocytes are agranular leukocytes. They are of two types: T lymphocytes (T cells) and B lymphocytes (B cells).

T cells protect us through a process called **cellular immunity**. These cells have the ability to recognize viral invasion of the body's cells. The T cell attacks and kills the infected cell, and the virus is unable to replicate itself. When enough infected cells have been killed, the viral infection abates. T cells also recognize and kill cancerous cells. Because T cells will detect and kill foreign cells, their activity will lead to rejection of transplanted organs unless drugs are administered to prev ent their doing so.

> **Memory Key**   T cells provide cellular immunity by killing virus-infected cells. They also kill cancerous cells and foreign cells.

B cells utilize a different process called **humoral** (**YOO**-moh-ral) **immunity**. They produce **antibodies** called immunoglobulins (Ig). **Immunoglobulins** (im-yoo-no-**GLOB**-yoo-lins) are proteins that travel through the circulatory system and have the ability to attach to foreign cells, labeling them for destruction by bacteria-eating white blood cells called **phagocytes** (**FAG**-oh-sights). B cells are particularly effective against bacterial infections. **Humoral** refers to body fluids or substances contained in them. Antibodies, which play a significant part in humoral immunity, are substances found in blood.

> **Memory Key**   B cells provide humoral immunity by producing antibodies that attach to foreign cells, such as bacteria, labeling them for destruction by phagocytes.

T cells and B cells create memory cells that remember how a particular invader was killed. These memory cells are permanently stored in the **lymphoid** (**LIM**-foid) tissue. When the same invader comes along again, the memory cells know precisely how to deal with it and dispatch it much more quickly than the first time, so quickly in fact, that we are usually unaware of these subsequent infections.

> **Memory Key**   T cells and B cells create memory cells that remember how an invader was killed, thus allowing the body to readily deal with a new infection of that type.

13.7   Lymphatic System

The **lymphatic** (lim-**FAH**-tick) **system** consists of a vascular system, fluid called **lymph** (**LIMF**), the lymph nodes, the **thymus** (**THIGH**-mus) **gland**, the **spleen**, the **tonsils**, and **Peyer's** (**PIE**-erz) **patches**. It is illustrated in Figure 13-2. The lymphatic system serves several important functions in the body. Of primary importance is the task of draining excess fluids away from body tissues into the bloodstream. The system also carries nutrients, hormones, and oxygen to body tissues and transports lipids (fat) from the digestive system. Because of the presence of lymphocytes and monocytes, this system also plays an important role in the body's defense against infection.

Memory Key	• The lymphatic system consists of:

• The lymphatic system consists of:

a vascular system	thymus gland	Peyer's patches
lymph	spleen	
lymph nodes	tonsils	

• This system drains fluids; carries nutrients, hormones, oxygen, and fats; and fights infection.

The vascular system consists of three types of vessels. The smallest are the **lymphatic capillaries**, which are present in all body tissue and originate in capillary beds with those of the circulatory system (see Figure 13-3). Plasma routinely seeps out of arterial capillaries into body tissues. This fluid, called interstitial fluid, picks up bacteria and cellular wastes and seeps back into the circulatory system or into the lymphatic capillaries. Once the fluid enters the lymphatic capillaries, it is called lymph. Lymph drains from the lymphatic capillaries into larger vessels called **lymphatics**, which ultimately drain into the largest vessels of the lymphatic system, the **right** and **left lymph ducts**. The right lymph duct receives lymph from the right side of the head, neck, and chest and the right arm. Lymph from the rest of the body drains into the left duct, also known as the thoracic duct. Both of the lymph ducts drain into the bloodstream (see Figure 13-4).

Memory Key

• The vascular system consists of:
  lymphatic capillaries
  lymphatics
  two lymph ducts
• The right lymph duct drains the right side of the head, neck, and chest and the right arm.
• The left thoracic lymph duct drains the rest of the body.

As illustrated in Figures 13-3 and 13-4, some lymphatics drain into **lymph nodes**. They are concentrated at various sites in the body. The lymph nodes act as filtration devices for lymph and contain great concentrations of phagocytes, which consume bacteria. This process is called **phagocytosis** (**fag**-oh-sigh-**TOH**-sis). With bacterial infections, the lymph nodes can become swollen and tender because of the huge concentration of bacteria in them. This condition is referred to as **lymphadenopathy** (lim-**fad**-eh-**NOP**-ah-thee). The principal clusters of nodes are the **cervical**, **submandibular**, **axillary**, and **inguinal**, as illustrated in Figure 13-4.

Memory Key

• Lymph nodes contain phagocytes, which consume bacteria (phagocytosis).
• The nodes are clustered as follows: cervical, submandibular, axillary, and inguinal.
• Lymphadenopathy is swollen lymph nodes.

FIGURE 13-2
Lymphatic system

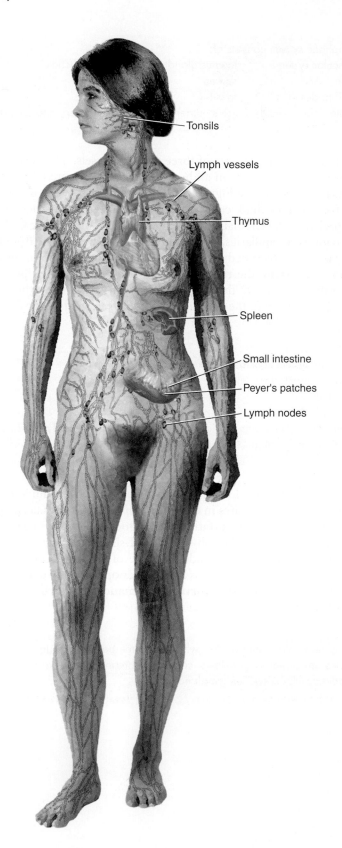

Tonsils

Lymph vessels

Thymus

Spleen

Small intestine

Peyer's patches

Lymph nodes

FIGURE 13-3
Lymph vessels

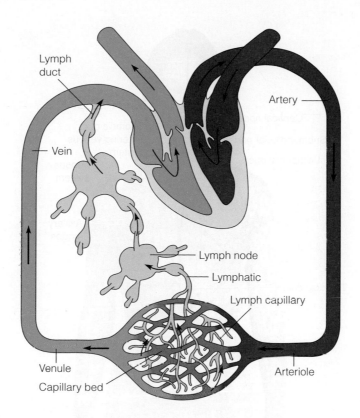

The **thymus gland**, located near the heart in the thoracic cavity, is both a lymph organ and an endocrine gland. It secretes a hormone called **thymosin** (thigh-**MOH**-sin), which stimulates red bone marrow to produce T cells. The T cells mature in the thymus.

Memory Key The thymus gland secretes thymosin, which stimulates red bone marrow to produce T cells.

The **spleen** is located in the left side of the abdominal cavity. It is a storehouse for red blood cells, releasing them when the body requires them. It also contains a great many phagocytes and thus plays a role in ridding the body of cellular debris, old red blood cells, and bacteria. In adults, if the bone marrow is damaged, the spleen can function to produce red blood cells.

Memory Key The spleen stores blood and contains many phagocytes.

FIGURE 13-4
Body areas served by
the two lymph ducts

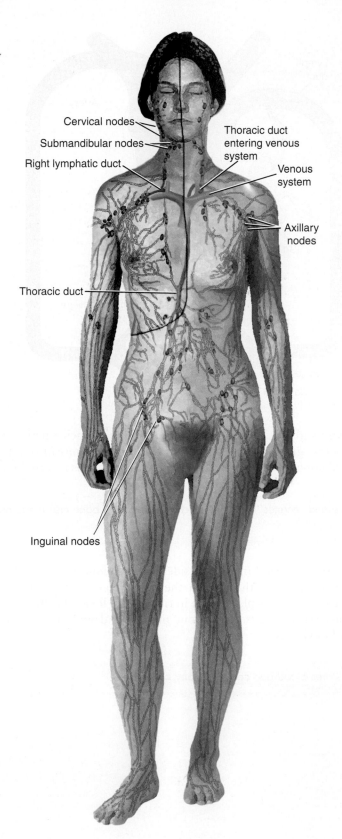

Cervical nodes

Submandibular nodes

Right lymphatic duct

Thoracic duct entering venous system

Venous system

Axillary nodes

Thoracic duct

Inguinal nodes

Tonsils are filters for bacteria and are made of lymphatic tissue. Three pairs are located in the throat. The **palatine** (**PAL**-ah-tine) tonsils, normally referred to simply as tonsils, are at the back of the oropharynx. The **pharyngeal** (far-**IN**-jee-al) tonsils, also called the **adenoids** (**AD**-eh-noids), are in the nasopharynx. The **lingual** (**LING**-gwal) tonsils are near the base of the tongue.

Peyer's patches are lymphatic filters located in the small intestine.

Memory Key	• Tonsils are made of lymphatic tissue.
	• Tonsils filter bacteria and consist of the palatine, pharyngeal (adenoids), and lingual tonsils.
	• Peyer's patches are lymphatic filters located in the small intestine.

Before you continue, review Sections 13.6 and 13.7. Then, complete questions 3, 4, and 5 of Exercise 13-1 found at the end of the chapter.

13.8   Term Analysis and Definition Pertaining to the Immune and Lymphatic Systems

ROOTS

	immun/o	immunity; safe
Term	**Term Analysis**	**Definition**
immunodeficiency (**im**-yoo-no-dee-**FISH**-en-see)	deficiency = lacking	inadequate immune response
immunology (**im**-yoo-**NOL**-oh-jee)	-logy = study of	study of the immune system; study of how the body responds to foreign substances
	lymphaden/o	**lymph node**
lymphadenitis (lim-**fad**-eh-**NIGH**-tis)	-itis = inflammation	inflammation of the lymph nodes
lymphadenopathy (lim-**fad**-eh-**NOP**-ah-thee)	-pathy = disease	disease (particularly enlargement) of the lymph nodes
	lymphangi/o	**lymph vessels**
lymphangiography (lim-**fan**-jee-**OG**-rah-fee)	-graphy = process of recording; producing images	process of recording the lymph vessels by the use of x-rays, following injection of a contrast medium

Term	Term Analysis	Definition
lymphangitis (**lim**-fan-**JIGH**-tis)	-itis = inflammation	inflammation of the lymph vessels
	lymph/o	**lymph**
lymphedema (lim-feh-**DEE**-mah)	-edema = accumulation of fluid	accumulation of interstitial fluid due to obstruction of lymphatic structures
lymphoma (lim-**FOH**-mah)	-oma = tumor; mass	tumor of the lymphatic structures
	splen/o	**spleen**
splenomegaly (**splee**-noh-**MEG**-ah-lee)	-megaly = enlargement	enlargement of the spleen
splenorrhagia (**splee**-noh-**RAY**-jee-ah)	-rrhagia = bursting forth	hemorrhage from the spleen
splenorrhaphy (splee-**NOR**-ah-fee)	-rrhaphy = suture	suture of the spleen
	thym/o	**thymus gland**
hemithymectomy (**HEM**-ee-thigh-**MECK**-toh-mee)	-ectomy = excision; surgical removal hemi- = half	excision of half the thymus gland

SUFFIXES

Term	Term Analysis	Definition
	-immune	**immunity; safe**
autoimmune disease (**aw**-toh-ih-**MYOON**)	auto- = self	an immune response to one's own body tissue; destruction of one's own cells by the immune system
	-stitial	**pertaining to a place**
interstitial fluid	-al = pertaining to inter- = between	fluid placed or lying between the tissue spaces

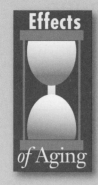

Effects of Aging on the Immune System

The immune system decreases in effectiveness as we age. Infections last longer and are more intense. Recovery times are increased. In addition, because it is the immune system that kills cancer cells, cancer rates in the elderly are much higher than for any other sector of the population.

13.9   Common Diseases of the Lymphatic and Immune Systems

HUMAN IMMUNODEFICIENCY VIRUS (HIV)/AUTOIMMUNODEFICIENCY SYNDROME (AIDS)

HIV/AIDS is an infection with the **human immunodeficiency virus (HIV)**. This virus obstructs the body's ability to fight off bacteria, viruses, parasites, and fungi.

With the appropriate treatment, a person can live with HIV for many years, and function normally without major problems. As the disease progresses, however, the immune system becomes weakened and incapacitated. A diagnosis of **AIDS** is given at that time. HIV infection and AIDS are the same disease. The label HIV is used when the disease is in its early stages. The label AIDS is used in the late stages of the disease.

Human immunodeficiency virus (HIV) causes AIDS. HIV is transmitted by contact with infected body fluids. The most common forms of transmission are sexual contact with an infected partner, sharing of hypodermic needles among IV drug users infected with HIV, and blood transfusions using HIV-infected blood. HIV can also be transmitted from an infected mother to her baby in the uterus or at the time of birth.

There is no cure for AIDS. Treatment is aimed at reducing the symptoms and preventing infectious complications to maintain a reasonable quality of life. A combination of drugs is given to stop viral replication and prevent advancement of the disease. This regimen is known as HAART (highly active antiretroviral therapy).

13.10 Abbreviations Pertaining to the Immune and Lymphatic Systems

Abbreviation	Meaning
Ab	antibody (a protein substance, formed by lymphocytes, that is stimulated by the presence of antigens in the body. An antibody then helps neutralize or inactivate the antigen that stimulated its formation.)
Ag	antigen (a foreign substance that stimulates the production of an antibody)
AIDS	acquired immune deficiency syndrome
HIV	human immunodeficiency virus (the agent attacking the immune system and causing AIDS)
Ig	immunoglobulin (antibody occurring naturally in the body)

13.11 Putting It All Together

Exercise 13-1   SHORT ANSWER

1. Name three plasma proteins found in the blood.

   _____

2. Differentiate between:

   (a) plasma and serum

   _____

   _____

   (b) eosinophils, basophils, and neutrophils

   _____

   _____

(c) A, B, AB, and O type blood

_____

_____

(d) How do the functions of erythrocytes, leukocytes, and thrombocytes differ?

_____

_____

(e) Differentiate between an antigen and an antibody, and describe how they relate to each other.

_____

_____

3. List three functions of the lymphatic system.

_____

_____

4. Define:

(a) phagocytes

_____

_____

(b) thymosin

_____

_____

(c) pharyngeal tonsils

_____

_____

(d) T lymphocytes

_____

_____

(e) B lymphocytes

_____

_____

5. Name four groups of lymph nodes.

_____

_____

Exercise 13-2 IDENTIFICATION

Give the meaning for the following component parts.

1. chrom/o _____

2. reticul/o _____

3. -poietin _____

4. -penia _____

5. leuk/o _____

6. thromb/o _____

7. -crit _____

8. -phoresis _____

9. -poiesis _____

10. -stasis _____

Exercise 13-3 BUILDING MEDICAL TERMS

I. Use -penia to build terms for the following definitions.

1. decrease in the number of red blood cells _____

2. decrease in the number of white blood cells _____

3. decrease in the number of clotting cells _____

4. decrease in the number of all blood cells _____

II. Use -cytosis to build terms for the following definitions.

5. increased variation in the size of cells _____

6. marked increase in the number of white blood cells _____

7. increased variation in the shape of cells _____

III. Use -emia to build terms for the following definitions.

8. lack of red blood cells or hemoglobin _____

9. abnormal increase in the number of red blood cells _____

10. excessive amounts of bilirubin in the blood _____

11. excessive amounts of cholesterol in the blood _____

12. excessive amounts of fats in the blood _____

Exercise 13-4   BUILDING MEDICAL TERMS

Build the medical term for each of the following definitions.

1. excessively pigmented red blood cells _____

2. process of recording the lymph vessels _____

3. accumulation of fluid due to obstruction
   of lymphatic structures _____

4. resembling bone marrow _____

5. suturing of the spleen _____

6. abnormal condition of clot formation _____

7. production of red blood cells _____

8. stoppage of blood _____

9. immunity against one's own body tissue _____

10. produced by the bone marrow _____

Exercise 13-5   DEFINITIONS

Define the following terms.

1. hypochromia _____

2. hematology _____

3. immunodeficiency _____

4. lymphadenopathy _____

5. hematocrit _____

6. hemoglobin _____

7. electrophoresis _____

8. erythropoietin _____

Exercise 13-6   PATHOLOGY

Answer the following questions

1. Describe how leukemia affects the body.

   _____

   _____

2. Name the microorganism that causes AIDS:

   _____

   _____

3. How is AIDS treated? How does this treatment work?

_____

_____

4. List four possible treatments for leukemia:

_____

_____

13.12 Review of Vocabulary Pertaining to Blood

In the following tables, the medical terms are organized into these categories: anatomy, pathology, diagnostics, and surgical procedures. Define each term and decide into which category the word belongs. This will help you associate the term with its purpose, and help you remember its meaning.

TABLE 13-1		
REVIEW OF ANATOMICAL TERMS PERTAINING TO BLOOD		
1. antibody	2. antigen	3. erythrocyte
4. erythropoiesis	5. erythropoietin	6. formed elements
7. globulin	8. hematologist	9. hematology
10. hematopoiesis	11. hemocytoblast	12. leukocyte
13. lymphoblast	14. monoblast	15. myelogenous
16. myeloid	17. neutrophils	18. normochromia

continued on page 333

Table 13-1 *continued from page 332*

19. plasma	20. reticulocyte	21. serum
22. thrombocyte		

TABLE 13-2

REVIEW OF PATHOLOGIC TERMS PERTAINING TO BLOOD

1. anemia	2. anisocytosis	3. erythremia
4. erythrocytopenia	5. hemolysis	6. hyperbilirubinemia
7. hypercholesterolemia	8. hyperchromia	9. hyperlipidemia
10. hypochromia	11. leukemia	12. leukocytopenia
13. leukocytosis	14. pancytopenia	15. poikilocytosis
16. thrombocytopenia	17. thrombolysis	18. thrombosis

TABLE 13-3

REVIEW OF DIAGNOSTIC TESTS AND CLINICAL PROCEDURES PERTAINING TO BLOOD

1. electrophoresis	2. hematocrit	3. hemostasis

13-13 Review Of Anatomical Terms Pertaining To The Immune And Lymphatic Systems

TABLE 13-4		
REVIEW OF ANATOMICAL TERMS PERTAINING TO THE IMMUNE AND LYMPHATIC SYSTEMS		
1. B lymphocytes	2. cellular immunity	3. immunoglobulins
4. lymph node	5. phagocytes	6. spleen
7. thymus gland	8. tonsils	

TABLE 13-5		
REVIEW OF PATHOLOGIC TERMS PERTAINING TO THE IMMUNE AND LYMPHATIC SYSTEMS		
1. autoimmune disease	2. HIV	3. immunodeficiency
4. lymphadenitis	5. lymphadenopathy	6. lymphangitis
7. lymphedema	8. lymphoma	9. splenorrhagia

TABLE 13-6
REVIEW OF DIAGNOSTIC TERMS PERTAINING TO THE IMMUNE AND LYMPHATIC SYSTEMS
1. lymphangiography

TABLE 13-7

REVIEW OF SURGICAL PROCEDURES PERTAINING TO THE IMMUNE AND LYMPHATIC SYSTEMS

1. splenomegaly	2. splenorrhaphy	3. thymectomy

13.14 Medical Terms in Context

After you read the following Morphology Report, answer the questions that follow it. Use your text, medical dictionary, or other references if necessary.

MORPHOLOGY REPORT—PERIPHERAL BLOOD

The red cells are normochromic with moderate anisocytosis. Occasional microcytes are seen. There is reduction in platelets.

The white cell count is markedly elevated with many blast forms present and showing scanty cytoplasm. An occasional blast shows folded nuclei. Occasional nucleated red cells also are noted. Occasional neutrophils are present.

IMPRESSION: This is a marked leukocytosis with many blast forms present that morphologically appear lymphoblastic.

QUESTIONS ON MORPHOLOGY REPORTS

1. Peripheral blood would most likely be obtained from the:

    a. aorta

    b. arm

    c. neck

    d. pulmonary arteries

2. The white blood cell count indicated _____, with many _____.

    a. anisocytosis; microcytes

    b. erythrocytosis; nucleated cells

    c. increased lymphoblasts; platelets

    d. leukocytosis; immature white blood cells

3. Morphology means the study of:

   a. blood

   b. color

   c. disease

   d. shape

4. On examining the blood, there was a decrease in the number of:

   a. red blood cells

   b. thrombocytes

   c. white blood cells

5. The red blood cells were of _____ size and _____ color.

   a. equal size; normal

   b. equal size; over-pigmented

   c. unequal size; normal

   d. unequal size; under-pigmented

6. Lymphoblasts are:

   a. platelets

   b. red blood cells

   c. white blood cells

7. Leukocytosis is:

   a. a form of cancer characterized by a malignant increase in the number of white blood cells

   b. also known as leukopenia

   c. marked decrease in the number of white blood cells

   d. marked increase in the number of white blood cells

The Respiratory System

CHAPTER ORGANIZATION

This chapter will help you learn the respiratory system. It is divided into the following sections:

14.1   Nose, Nasal Cavities, and Paranasal Sinuses

14.2   Pharynx, Larynx, and Trachea

14.3   Bronchi and Lungs

14.4   Additional Word Parts

14.5   Term Analysis and Definition

14.6   Common Diseases

14.7   Abbreviations

14.8   Putting It All Together

14.9   Review of Vocabulary

14.10   Medical Terms in Context

CHAPTER OBJECTIVES

On completion of this chapter, you will be able to do the following:

1. State the difference between inhalation and expiration

2. Name, locate, and describe the functions of the respiratory structures

3. Define Adam's apple, epiglottis, cilia, bronchial tree, and paranasal sinuses

4. Define the terms that describe the structures of the lung

5. Analyze, define, pronounce, and spell terms relating to the respiratory system

6. Describe common diseases

7. Define abbreviations common to the respiratory system

INTRODUCTION

In the chapter on the cardiovascular system, you learned that the body's trillions of cells need to take in oxygen and eliminate carbon dioxide on a continuous basis. This interchange of gases, called **respiration**, or **breathing**, occurs when oxygen is inhaled into the lungs from the air and passes into the blood, and when carbon dioxide moves from the blood to the lungs and is exhaled into the air. Breathing in is called **inhalation** or **inspiration**. Breathing out is called **exhalation** or **expiration**.

Figure 14-1 illustrates all of the structures of the respiratory system: the **nose**, **nasal cavity**, **pharynx** (**FAR**-inks), **larynx** (**LAR**-inks), **trachea** (**TRAY**-kee-ah), **bronchi** (**BRONG**-kye), and **lungs**. Each of these structures is described in the following sections.

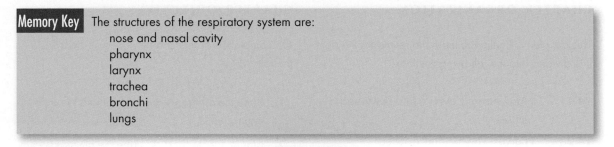

Memory Key | The structures of the respiratory system are:
nose and nasal cavity
pharynx
larynx
trachea
bronchi
lungs

FIGURE 14-1
Structures of the
respiratory system

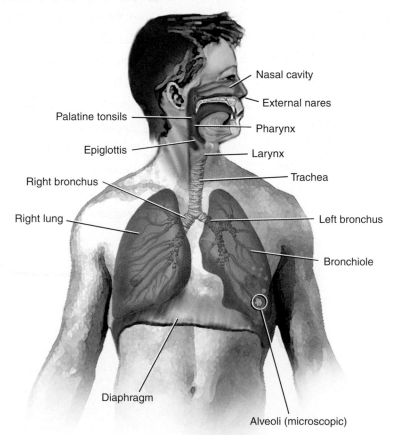

Nasal cavity

External nares

Palatine tonsils

Pharynx

Epiglottis

Larynx

Right bronchus

Trachea

Right lung

Left bronchus

Bronchiole

Diaphragm

Alveoli (microscopic)

14.1   Nose, Nasal Cavities, and Paranasal Sinuses

The **external nares** (**NAH**-reez), or nostrils, allow both inspiration and expiration of air. The hairs, or **cilia** (**SIL**-ee-ah), in the nares filter out dust particles in the air. The **nasal cavity** extends from the external nares to the pharynx. It is divided into right and left cavities by the **nasal septum** (**SEP**-tum). The nasal cavity warms and moistens air and provides us with our sense of smell through **olfactory** (ol-**FACK**-toh-ree) **neurons** in the lining of the nasal tract. Hollow spaces within the skull called **paranasal sinuses** lighten the skull. Because they are lined with mucous membrane, the paranasal sinuses also play a role in respiration by moistening air. They lie above, between, and under the eyes in pairs and are called the frontal, ethmoid, sphenoid, and maxillary sinuses (see Figure 14-2).

Memory Key	• The nostrils are called external nares.
	• The nasal cavity extends from the external nares to the pharynx.
	• The nasal cavity is divided by the nasal septum.
	• The paranasal sinuses are the frontal, ethmoid, sphenoid, and maxillary.

FIGURE 14-2
Paranasal sinuses

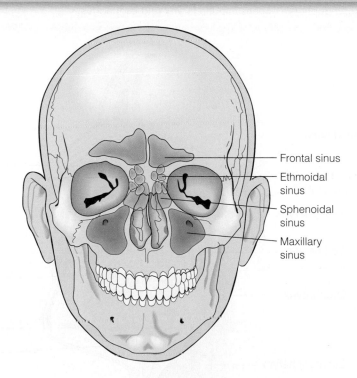

Frontal sinus

Ethmoidal sinus

Sphenoidal sinus

Maxillary sinus

14.2 Pharynx, Larynx, and Trachea

PHARYNX

The pharynx is the throat. It consists of the **nasopharynx** (**nay**-zoh-**FAR**-inks), the **oropharynx** (**or**-oh-**FAR**-inks), and the **laryngopharynx** (lar-**ING**-oh-**FAR**-inks). The nasopharynx lies posterior to the nasal cavity (Figure 14-3). Two openings called **internal nares** lead from the nasopharynx to the nasal cavity and are separated by the nasal septum. Two other openings lead from the nasopharynx into the **eustachian** (yoo-**STAY**-shun) tubes and through them to the ears. The nasopharynx also contains the adenoids, or pharyngeal tonsils. The oropharynx is posterior to the oral cavity and contains the **palatine** (**PAL**-ah-tine) **tonsils** and the **lingual** (**LING**-gwal) **tonsils**. The laryngopharynx opens into the larynx and esophagus.

> **Memory Key**
> - The nasopharynx contains internal nares opening into the nasal cavity and openings into the eustachian tube.
> - The oropharynx contains the tonsils.
> - The laryngopharynx opens into the larynx and esophagus.

FIGURE 14-3
Nasal cavity, nasopharynx, oropharynx, and largngopharynx

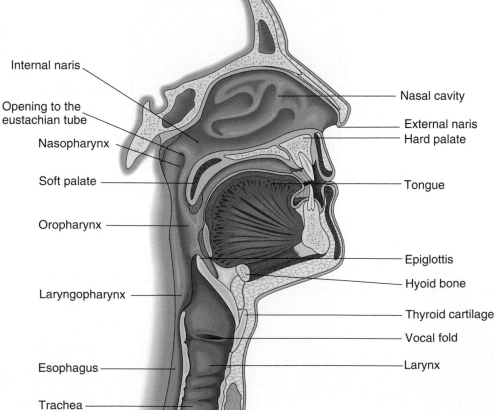

Internal naris

Opening to the eustachian tube

Nasopharynx

Soft palate

Oropharynx

Laryngopharynx

Esophagus

Trachea

Nasal cavity

External naris

Hard palate

Tongue

Epiglottis

Hyoid bone

Thyroid cartilage

Vocal fold

Larynx

LARYNX

The larynx (Figure 14-4) is the voice box. A portion of the larynx is the **Adam's apple**, a large shield of cartilage protecting inner structures. Another structure of the larynx is the **epiglottis** (**ep**-ih-**GLOT**-is), which swings up and down like a lid, covering the opening of the larynx during swallowing so that the air passage is sealed. The **vocal cords**, responsible for sound, are folds of mucous membrane. The slit between them is the **glottis**. Sound is produced as air moves out of the lungs through the glottis, causing vibrations in the vocal cords. Voice pitch is determined by the length and tension of the vocal cords.

> **Memory Key**
> - The larynx is the voice box.
> - The Adam's apple is a shield of cartilage.
> - The epiglottis is a flap that swings up and down to close off air passage during swallowing.
> - The vocal cords are mucous membrane containing a slit called the glottis.
> - Vibration of vocal cords produces sound.

TRACHEA

The trachea (see Figure 14-4) is the windpipe. It extends from the larynx to the bronchi. It is lined with mucous membrane and cilia, which filter the air. The trachea is composed mostly of muscle fibers. It also contains C-shaped cartilage, which prevents the trachea from collapsing.

> **Memory Key**
> The trachea is the windpipe, connecting to the bronchi. It consists of muscle and C-shaped cartilage, lined with mucous membrane and cilia.

FIGURE 14-4

Larynx, trachea, and bronchioles: (A) anatomy of larynx, trachea, and bronchial tree; (B) end of bronchial tree showing terminal bronchioles, alveolar duct, and alveoli

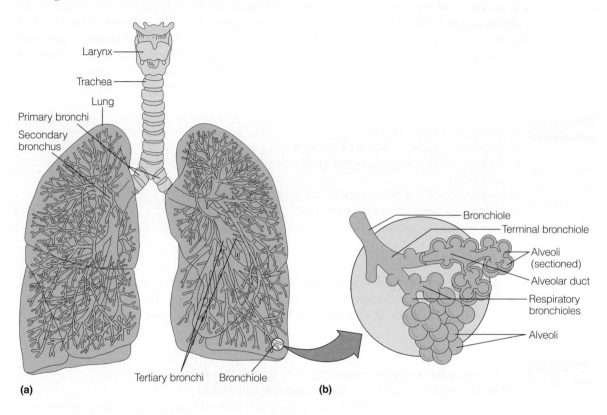

Larynx

Trachea

Lung

Primary bronchi

Secondary bronchus

Tertiary bronchi   Bronchiole

(a)

Bronchiole

Terminal bronchiole

Alveoli (sectioned)

Alveolar duct

Respiratory bronchioles

Alveoli

(b)

14.3   Bronchi and Lungs

THE BRONCHI

The trachea divides into two **primary bronchi**, each of which leads to a lung. The primary bronchi split off into smaller bronchi, the **secondary** and **tertiary bronchi**, within the lungs. The tertiary bronchi connect to even smaller tubes called **bronchioles** (**BRONG**-kee-ohlz). Because of its resemblance to an inverted tree, the bronchial system is referred to as the **bronchial tree** (Figure 14-4).

A common condition of the bronchial tubes is **bronchial asthma**, in which the bronchi spasm, cutting off the patient's air supply. The patient then experiences **paroxysmal dyspnea** (**par**-ox-**SYS**-mal **DISP**-nee-ah), which is difficulty in breathing of an off-and-on nature. These attacks are recurrent and often allergic in nature.

Memory Key   In the lungs, the two primary bronchi divide into secondary and tertiary bronchi, which connect to bronchioles.

LUNGS

The lungs lie in the thoracic cavity. The top of each lung is called the **apex**, and the bottom is the **base**.

The right lung is divided into three **lobes**: the **superior**, **middle**, and **inferior**. The left has only superior and inferior lobes. Inside each lung are approximately 300 million microscopic **alveoli** (al-**VEE**-oh-lye), which are connected to the bronchioles by **alveolar ducts** (Figure 14-4). The alveoli are like tiny balloons, expanding and contracting with inspiration and expiration. The alveoli are surrounded by **pulmonary capillaries**, which deliver carbon dioxide to the alveoli and absorb oxygen from them. The carbon dioxide is then expelled from the lungs. The oxygenated blood flows from the pulmonary capillaries, into the pulmonary vein, and then on to the heart, to be pumped to the cells of the body (see Figure 14-5).

FIGURE 14-5

Lungs: (A) anatomical structures of the lung; (B) capillary network surrounding the alveoli

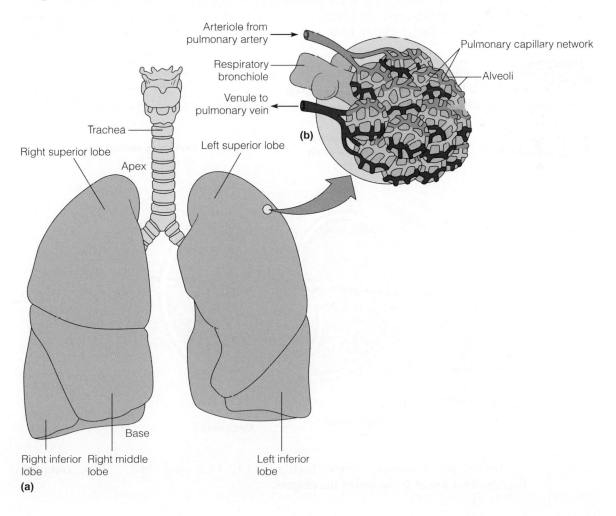

Memory Key
- The lungs lie in the thoracic cavity.
- The top of the lung is the apex; the bottom, the base.
- The right lung has superior, middle, and inferior lobes; the left, superior and inferior.
- The respiratory bronchioles connect by alveolar ducts with the alveoli, which are tiny balloons responsible for gas exchange with the pulmonary capillaries.
- Carbon dioxide moves from the pulmonary capillaries to the alveoli and then is expelled from the lungs.
- Oxygen moves from the alveoli to the pulmonary capillaries, into the pulmonary vein, and then into the heart.

PLEURAL AND MEDIASTINAL CAVITIES

The thoracic cavity contains two smaller cavities: the **pleural** (**PLOOR**-al) and **mediastinal** (**me**-dee-as-**TYE**-nal) cavities. The pleural cavity surrounds the lungs (Figure 14-6). Its outer layer is the parietal pleura. The inner layer is the visceral pleura. Between these two layers is the pleural cavity, filled with pleural fluid. The mediastinal cavity lies between the lungs (Figure 14-6) and contains the heart, aorta, trachea, and esophagus.

Memory Key
- The pleural cavity surrounds the lungs.
- The mediastinal cavity is between the lungs.

FIGURE 14-6
Pleural cavities and mediastinal cavity

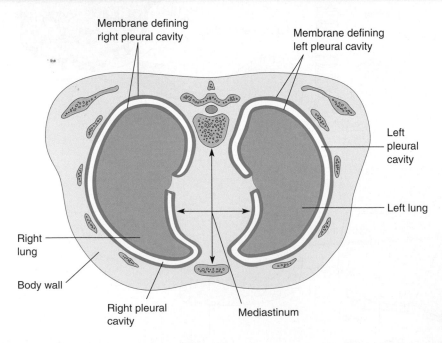

Membrane defining right pleural cavity

Membrane defining left pleural cavity

Left pleural cavity

Left lung

Right lung

Body wall

Right pleural cavity

Mediastinum

Before you continue, review Sections 14.1, 14.2, and 14.3. Then, complete Exercise 14-1 found at the end of the chapter.

14.4   Additional Word Parts

The following roots and prefix will also be used in this chapter to build medical terms.

Root	Meaning
coni/o	dust
dilat/o	widening; dilation

Prefix	Meaning
oligo-	scanty; few

14.5   Term Analysis and Definition

ROOTS

	adenoid/o	adenoids
Term	**Term Analysis**	**Definition**
adenoidectomy (**ad**-eh-noid-**ECK**-toh-mee)	-ectomy = excision	excision of the adenoids *NOTE:* If the adenoids become enlarged, airflow is obstructed, necessitating adenoidectomy.
	alveol/o	**alveoli; air sacs**
alveolar (al-**VEE**-oh-lar)	-ar = pertaining to	pertaining to the alveoli
alveolitis (**al**-vee-oh-**LYE**-tis)	-itis = inflammation	inflammation of the alveoli
	bronchi/o; bronch/o	**bronchus**
bronchiectasis (**brong**-kee-**ECK**-tah-sis)	-ectasis = dilation; stretching	dilation of the bronchus
bronchitis (brong-**KYE**-tis)	-itis = inflammation	inflammation of the bronchus

Term	Term Analysis	Definition
bronchodilator (**brong**-koh-**DYE**-lay-tor)	-or = person or thing that does something **dilat/o** = dilation; widening	drugs that dilate the bronchus to relieve bronchospasm
bronchoscopy (brong-**KOS**-koh-pee)	-scopy = process of visual examination	process of visually examining the bronchus
bronchospasm (**BRONG**-koh-spazm)	-spasm = sudden, involuntary contraction	sudden, involuntary contraction of the bronchus
bronchogenic carcinoma (**BRONG**-koh-jen-ic)	-genic = produced by carcinoma = malignant tumor of epithelial tissue	a malignant tumor of the lung that originates in the bronchi *NOTE*: Bronchogenic carcinoma is the most common form of lung cancer. It metastasizes (spreads) rapidly to other body parts such as the liver, kidney, and bones. Smoking is the leading cause of lung cancer.
	bronchiol/o	**bronchioles; small bronchi**
bronchiolitis (**brong**-kee-oh-**LYE**-tis)	-itis = inflammation	inflammation of the bronchioles
	laryng/o	**larynx; voice box**
laryngeal (lar-**INN**-jee-al)	-eal = pertaining to	pertaining to the voice box
laryngospasm (lar-**ING**-oh-spazm)	-spasm = sudden, involuntary contraction	sudden, involuntary contraction of the voice box
	lob/o	**lobe**
lobar (**LOH**-bar)	-ar = pertaining to	pertaining to the lobe of the lung
lobectomy (loh-**BECK**-toh-mee)	-ectomy = excision; surgical removal	excision of a lobe of the lung

Term	Term Analysis	Definition
	mediastin/o	**mediastinum (cavity between the lungs)**
mediastinoscopy (**mee**-dee-**as**-tih-**NOS**-kah-pee)	-scopy = process of visually examining a body cavity or organ	process of visually examining the mediastinum (cavity between the lungs) *NOTE:* An endoscope is placed through an incision above the sternum. The area is examined and tissue samples excised.
	muc/o	**mucus (a sticky, thick secretion of mucous membrane)**
mucolytic (**myoo**-koh-**LIH**-tick)	-lytic = breakdown; destruction; separate	drugs used to break down thick mucus so it can be coughed up

Memory Key
- Mucus is the noun.
- Mucous is the adjective, as in mucous membrane.

Term	Term Analysis	Definition
	nas/o	nose
nasolacrimal (**nay**-zoh-**LACK**-rih-mal)	-al = pertaining to **lacrim/o** = lacrimal apparatus; tears	pertaining to the nose and lacrimal apparatus
nasopharyngeal (**nay**-zoh-far-**INN**-jee-al)	-eal = pertaining to **pharyng/o** = pharynx; throat	pertaining to the nasopharynx (the portion of the pharynx located behind the nose)
	ox/o; ox/i	**oxygen**
anoxia (ah-**NOCK**-see-ah)	-ia = state of; condition a(n)- = no; not; lack of	lack of oxygen *NOTE: Anoxia* is often used interchangeably with *hypoxia.*

Memory Key   An- is used instead of a- before word parts beginning with a vowel.

Term	Term Analysis	Definition
hypoxia (high-**POCK**-see-ah)	-ia = state of; condition hypo- = deficient; abnormal decrease	deficiency of oxygen
oximeter (ock-**SIM**-ih-ter)	-meter = instrument used to measure	the instrument used to measure the percentage of hemoglobin in arterial blood saturated with oxygen
	pector/o (see also steth/o; thorac/o)	**chest**
pectoral (**PECK**-toh-rahl)	-al = pertaining to	pertaining to the chest
expectoration (ex-**peck**-tor-**AY**-shun)	ex- = out -ation = process (noun ending)	process of coughing out materials from the lungs
	pharyng/o	**pharynx; throat**
pharyngoglossal (feh-**ring**-goh-**GLOS**-al)	-al = pertaining to **gloss/o** = tongue	pertaining to the pharynx and tongue
oropharyngeal (**or**-oh-far-**IN**-jee-al)	-eal = pertaining to **or/o** = mouth	pertaining to the mouth and pharynx
	phren/o	**diaphragm**
phrenic (**FREN**-ick)	-ic = pertaining to	pertaining to the diaphragm
phrenotomy (fren-**OT**-oh-mee)	-tomy = process of cutting	process of cutting into the diaphragm
	pleur/a; pleur/o	**pleura; pleural cavity**
pleuralgia (ploor-**AL**-jee-ah)	-algia = pain	pain in the pleura
	pneumat/o	**air; respiration**
pneumatic (new-**MAT**-ick)	-ic = pertaining to	pertaining to air or respiration

	pneumon/o	lungs
Term	**Term Analysis**	**Definition**
pneumoconiosis (**new**-moh-**koh**-nee-**OH**-sis)	-osis = abnormal condition **coni/o** = dust	abnormal condition of dust in the lung; black lung. *NOTE:* Dust particles are inhaled into the lungs, and over time, they will coat the alveoli. This fine coat of dust prevents the exchange of oxygen and carbon dioxide. Lung tissue deteriorates, breathing becomes difficult, and the patient dies because of the lack of oxygen.
pneumopleuritis (**new**-moh-ploo-**RYE**-tis)	-itis = inflammation **pleur/o** = pleura	inflammation of the lungs and pleura
	pneum/o;	**lungs**
pneumonia (new-**MOH**-nee-ah)	-ia = condition; state of	inflammation of the lung; also known as pneumonitis (Figure 14-7)
pulmonary edema (**PUL**-moh-ner-ee eh-**DEE**-mah)	-ary = pertaining to edema = accumulation of fluid in body tissues	accumulation of excess fluid in the lungs

FIGURE 14-7
Types of pneumonia

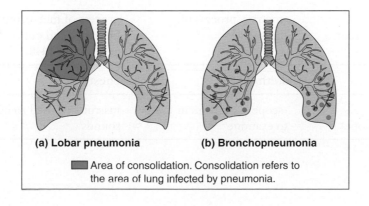

(a) Lobar pneumonia   (b) Bronchopneumonia

Area of consolidation. Consolidation refers to the area of lung infected by pneumonia.

	rhin/o	nose
Term	**Term Analysis**	**Definition**
otorhinolaryngology (**oh**-toh-**rye**-noh-**lar**-in-**GOL**-oh-jee)	-logy = study of **ot/o** = ear **laryng/o** = voice box; larynx	the study of the ear, nose, and throat (ENT)
rhinitis (rye-**NIGH**-tis)	-itis = inflammation	inflammation of the mucous membrane of the nose
rhinorrhea (**rih**-noh-**REE**-ah)	-rrhea = discharge	discharge from the nose
rhinoplasty (**RYE**-noh-**plas**-tee)	-plasty = surgical recon-struction; surgical repair	surgical repair of the nose; plastic surgery on the nose for cosmetic or reconstructive purposes; a nose job
	sinus/o	**sinuses**
pansinusitis (**pan**-sigh-nuhs-**EYE**-tis)	-itis = inflammation pan- = all	inflammation of all the paranasal sinuses
sinusotomy (**sigh**-nuhs-**OT**-oh-mee)	-tomy = process of cutting	process of cutting into the sinus
	spir/o	**breathing**
spirometer (spye-**ROM**-et-er)	-meter = instrument used to measure	instrument used to measure airflow and volume into and out of the lungs
spirometry (spye-**ROM**-eh-tree)	-metry = process of measuring	process of measuring airflow and vol-ume into and out of the lungs (see Figure 14-8)
	steth/o	**chest**
stethoscope (**STETH**-oh-skope)	-scope = instrument used to examine	instrument used to listen to chest sounds

FIGURE 14-8
Spirometry

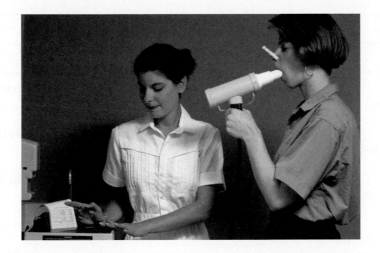

	thorac/o	**chest**
Term	**Term Analysis**	**Definition**
thoracocentesis (**thoh**-rah-koh-sen-**TEE**-sis)	-centesis = surgical puncture	surgical puncture to remove fluid from the pleural cavity; also known as thoracentesis, pleurocentesis, and pleuracentesis (Figure 14-9)
thoracodynia (**thor**-ack-oh-**DIN**-ee-ah)	-dynia = pain	chest pain
thoracoplasty (**thor**-ah-koh-**PLAS**-tee)	-plasty = surgical reconstruction; surgical repair	surgical reconstruction of the thorax
thoracotomy (**thor**-ah-**KOT**-toh-mee)	-tomy = process of cutting	process of cutting into the chest

FIGURE 14-9
Thoracocentesis

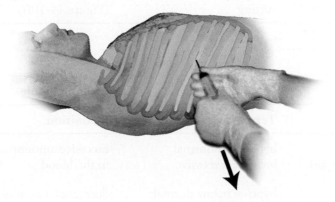

	tonsill/o	tonsils
Term	**Term Analysis**	**Definition**
tonsillar (**TON**-sih-lar)	-ar = pertaining to	pertaining to the tonsils
tonsillectomy (**ton**-sih-**LECK**-toh-mee)	-ectomy = surgical excision; removal	excision of the tonsils
tonsillitis (**ton**-sih-**LYE**-tis)	-itis = inflammation	inflammation of the tonsils
tonsillotome (ton-**SIL**-oh-tohm)	-tome = instrument used to cut	instrument used to cut the tonsils
	trache/o	**trachea; windpipe**
endotracheal (**en**-doh-**TRAY**-kee-al)	-eal = pertaining to endo- = within	pertaining to within the trachea
laryngotracheobronchitis (lah-**ring**-goh-**tray**-kee-oh-brong-**KYE**-tis)	-itis = inflammation **laryng/o** = larynx; voice box **bronch/o** = bronchus	inflammation of the larynx, trachea, and bronchus; also known as **croup**
tracheoesophageal (**tray**-kee-oh-ee-**sof**-ah-**JEE**-al)	-eal = pertaining to **esophag/o** = esophagus	pertaining to the trachea and esophagus
tracheostomy (**tray**-kee-**OS**-toh-mee)	-stomy = new opening	new opening into the trachea is created through the neck and a tube is inserted to assist breathing. The tracheostomy tube may be temporary or permanent (Figure 14-10A)
tracheotomy (**tray**-kee-**OT**-oh-mee)	-tomy = process of cutting	process of cutting into the trachea (Figure 14-10B)

SUFFIXES

	-capnia	carbon dioxide
Term	**Term Analysis**	**Definition**
hypercapnia (**high**-per-**KAP**-nee-ah)	hyper- = abnormal increase; excessive	excessive amounts of carbon dioxide in the blood
hypocapnia (**high**-poh-**KAP**-nee-ah)	hypo- = below normal; decrease	decreased amounts of carbon dioxide in the blood

FIGURE 14-10
(A) Tracheostomy; (B) Tracheotomy

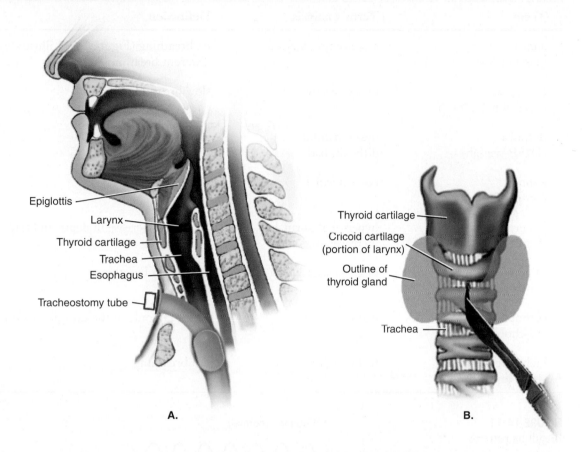

Epiglottis

Larynx

Thyroid cartilage

Trachea

Esophagus

Tracheostomy tube

A.

Thyroid cartilage

Cricoid cartilage
(portion of larynx)

Outline of
thyroid gland

Trachea

B.

	-graphy	**process of recording; producing images**
Term	**Term Analysis**	**Definition**
bronchography (brong-**KOG**-rah-fee)	**bronch/o** = bronchus	process of producing an image of the bronchi, following injection of contrast medium
pulmonary angiography (**PUL**-moh-**nar**-ee an-jee-**OG**-rah-**fee**)	**angi/o** = vessel -ary = pertaining to **pulmon/o** = lungs	process of producing an image of the blood vessels of the lung, following injection of contrast medium
	-phonia	**voice**
aphonia (ah-**FOH**-nee-ah)	a- = no; not; lack of	loss of voice
dysphonia (dis-**FOH**-nee-ah)	dys- = difficult bad; painful	difficulty in speaking

	-pnea	breathing
Term	**Term Analysis**	**Definition**
apnea (**AP**-nee-ah)	a- = no; not; lack of	no breathing (Figure 14-11 illustrates different breathing pattern)
bradypnea (**brad**-ihp-**NEE**-ah)	brady- = slow	slow breathing
dyspnea (**DISP**-nee-ah)	dys- = painful; difficult; bad	painful breathing
eupnea (yoop-**NEE**-ah)	eu- = normal	normal breathing
hyperpnea (**high**-perp-**NEE**-ah)	hyper- = abnormal increase; excessive	abnormal increase in depth and rate of breathing
oligopnea (**ol**-ih-gop-**NEE**-ah)	oligo- = scanty; few	infrequent breathing
orthopnea (**or**-thop-**NEE**-ah)	ortho- = straight	breathing only in the upright position
tachypnea (**tack**-ihp-**NEE**-ah)	tachy- = fast	fast breathing

FIGURE 14-11
Breathing patterns

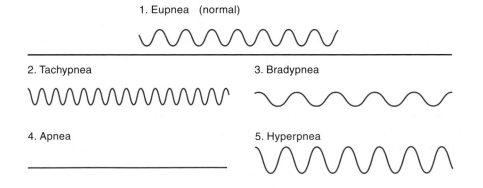

1. Eupnea   (normal)

2. Tachypnea

3. Bradypnea

4. Apnea

5. Hyperpnea

	-ptysis	**spitting**
hemoptysis (he-**MOP**-tih-sis)	**hem/o** = blood	spitting up of blood
	-thorax	**chest**
hemothorax (**he**-moh-**THOR**-acks)	**hem/o** = blood	blood in the pleural cavity
hydrothorax (**high**-droh-**THOR**-acks)	**hydr/o** = water	watery fluid in the pleural cavity
pneumothorax (**new**-moh-**THOR**-acks)	**pneum/o** = air	collection of air in the pleural cavity (Figure 14-12)
pyothorax (**pye**-oh-**THOR**-acks)	**py/o** = pus	pus in the pleural cavity; also known as **empyema** (Figure 14-12)
	-sphyxia	**pulse**
asphyxia (as-**FICK**-see-ah)	a- = no; not; lack of	lack of oxygen to body tissues; can interfere with respiration and eventually lead to a loss of pulse

FIGURE 14-12
Pneumothorax and pyothorax

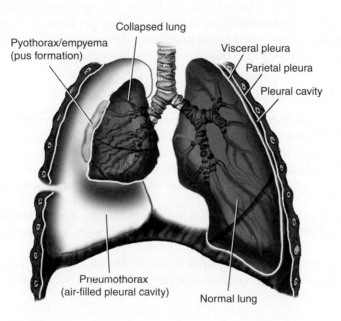

Collapsed lung

Pyothorax/empyema (pus formation)

Visceral pleura

Parietal pleura

Pleural cavity

Pneumothorax (air-filled pleural cavity)

Normal lung

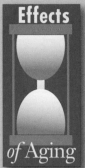

Physical changes associated with aging make it more difficult for air to flow into and out of the lungs. The costal cartilage hardens and the thoracic cage becomes rigid, which prevents the lungs from expanding fully. The elasticity of the lungs diminishes, allowing air to be trapped in the alveoli. The respiratory muscles weaken, making breathing more difficult.

Other factors impair the efficiency of the respiratory system even more. Because the cilia, tiny hairs in the respiratory tract, become less active, they therefore have diminished ability to move foreign particles and mucus out of the respiratory tract. The coughing reflex becomes less powerful, which also impairs our ability to eject foreign material.

All of these factors increase the chance of respiratory infections and complicate recovery from such infections.

14.6   Common Diseases

ASTHMA

Asthmatic attacks stemming from asthma (**AZ**-mah) involve severe constriction of the bronchi, which blocks airflow to the lungs. This is called a bronchospasm. Bronchospasms can usually be reversed with proper treatment, but sometimes can be fatal.

Asthma is thought to be an inherited disease, but environmental factors also play a part. Foreign particles, such as airborne chemicals, pollen, pet hairs, and dust, are common triggers of attacks. Drugs called **bronchodilators** (bron-koh-**DYE**-lay-torz) improve airflow to the lungs by relieving the constriction of the bronchial muscles.

EMPHYSEMA

Emphysema (**em**-fih-**SEE**-mah) is a disease of unknown cause, although it is strongly associated with long-term smoking. The alveoli become overexpanded (dilated) due to loss of elasticity. Because they do not return to their normal size, air is not expelled and becomes trapped. This obstructs the passage of oxygen from the lungs into the bloodstream, and to body tissues. Eventually, this leads to loss of pulmonary function and the breakdown of the alveoli walls.

Destruction of the alveoli makes breathing difficult. The patient compensates by force breathing, which over time reshapes the thoracic cavity into what is known as a **barrel chest**.

There is no cure for emphysema. Once the alveoli are destroyed, they do not regenerate. The patient must use supplemental oxygen to improve ventilation.

LUNG CANCER

Lung cancer is the leading cause of cancer deaths in North America. It is classified as **primary** if the cancer starts in the lungs, and **secondary** if it has metastasized to the lungs. The following discussion is concerned with primary lung cancer.

Primary lung cancers are classified as either **small cell** or **non-small cell**. As the name suggests, small cell cancer cells are small, mainly consisting of the nucleus. About 20% of cancers diagnosed are of this type. Smoking is almost always the cause. Another name for small cell cancer is oat cell carcinoma.

Non-small cell lung cancer is divided into three types: adenocarcinoma, squamous cell carcinoma, and large cell carcinoma. Treatment is identical for each type, and different from that used in small cell cancer.

Cigarette smoking causes most but not all lung cancers. The risk of cancer in smokers is decreased when smoking is stopped. Other factors may be radiation exposure, secondhand smoke, and inhalation of carcinogenic agents such as asbestos.

Lung cancer rarely occurs in people younger than 40 years of age. Genetic studies have proposed a predisposition to cancer.

MRI (magnetic resonance imaging) and CT scans (computed tomography) are common methods of diagnosing lung cancer. SPECT (single-photon emission computed tomography) provides visualization of how a patient's organ or body system functions. This diagnostic technique utilizes radiation tagged with a pharmaceutical: a radiopharmaceutical. It is placed into the body by injection, ingestion, or inhalation. As the radioactive substance decays, gamma rays are emitted (single-photon emission). The gamma rays (rather than x-rays as in CT scans, or a magnetic field as in MRIs) provide a picture of what is happening inside the body. Biopsies are performed to confirm the diagnosis.

Chemotherapy, radiation therapy, and surgical removal of the tumor are common forms of treatment. There is no cure. Metastases to the brain and bone are common in all lung cancers.

PNEUMONIA

Pneumonia involves infection and inflamation of the lung. As the condition progresses, the effects of the inflammatory process (redness, swelling, heat, and pain) deteriorate lung function, hindering the exchange of oxygen and carbon dioxide between blood vessels. The lung or a portion of it, can become a solid mass due to the infection. This solid mass is called an area of consolidation (Figure 14-7).

Pneumonia can be caused by viruses, bacteria, fungi or foreign substances being inhaled. A pneumonia commonly seen in AIDS patients is *Pneumocystis carinii* pneumonia (PCP), caused by the fungus *Pneumocystis carinii* now renamed *Pneumocystis jiroveci*.

Pneumonias are sometimes named in accordance with the location of the consolidation: **lobar pneumonia**, affecting a lobe of the lung; **basal pneumonia** the base of the lung; **interstitial pneumonia**, the tissue spaces within the lung; and **bronchopneumonia**, along the bronchus. **Aspiration pneumonia** is caused by the inhalation (aspiration) of foreign matter such as liquids or bits of food into the respiratory tract causing inflammation of the lung.

Pneumonia is treated differently depending upon the cause. Antibiotics are used to treat bacterial and aspiration pneumonia, rest and fluids are recommended for viral pneumonia, and anti-infective drugs for PCP.

14.7 Abbreviations

Abbreviation	Meaning
AP	anteroposterior
CO_2	carbon dioxide
CXR	chest x-ray
ERV	expiratory reserve volume (test of pulmonary function)
IRV	inspiratory reserve volume (test of pulmonary function)
O_2	oxygen
PA	posteroanterior
PCP	pneumocystis carinii
PFT	pulmonary function tests (various tests of lung performance using a spirometer) *NOTE:* Pulmonary function tests include tidal volume (TV), inspiratory reserve volume (IRV), expiratory reserve volume (ERV), and residual volume (RV).
R	respiration
RV	residual volume (test of pulmonary function)
SOA	shortness of air
SOB	shortness of breath
T&A	tonsillectomy and adenoidectomy
TV	tidal volume (test of pulmonary function)
URI	upper respiratory infection
URT	upper respiratory tract

14.8   Putting It All Together

1. Differentiate between inhalation and expiration.

   _____

   _____

2. Name the respiratory structures. Describe their functions.

   _____

   _____

   _____

   _____

   _____

   _____

   _____

3. Define: a. Adam's apple   _____

   b. epiglottis   _____

   c. cilia   _____

   d. bronchial tree   _____

   e. paranasal sinuses   _____

4. Define the following terms describing the structures of the lung: apex, base, lobes, alveoli.

   _____

   _____

   _____

   _____

   _____

   _____

5. Complete the following short answer exercises.

   a. Name the organs surrounded by the pleural cavity: _____

   b. The pleural cavity is filled with   _____

   c. Name the two layers of the pleura: _____

Exercise 14-2   ADJECTIVAL FORMS

Give the adjectival form for each of the following.

1. alveolus _____   6. larynx _____

2. bronchus _____   7. diaphragm _____

3. lobe _____   8. pleura _____

4. nose _____   9. lungs _____

5. pharynx _____   10. chest _____

Exercise 14-3   IDENTIFICATION

Place an **X** beside the terms that indicate treatment.

1. bronchodilator _____   8. rhinorrhea _____

2. bronchiectasis _____   9. thoracocentesis _____

3. laryngospasm _____   10. thoracodynia _____

4. lobectomy _____   11. thoracoplasty _____

5. mucolytic _____   12. tracheoesophageal _____

6. pneumoconiosis _____   13. dysphonia _____

7. phrenotomy _____   14. hemoptysis _____

Exercise 14-4   BUILDING MEDICAL TERMS

Build the medical terms for the following definitions.

1. no breathing _____

2. slow breathing _____

3. painful breathing _____

4. normal breathing _____

5. abnormal increase in depth and rate
   of breathing _____

6. infrequent breathing _____

7. breathing in only the upright position _____

8. fast breathing _____

9. excessive amounts of carbon dioxide
   in the blood _____

10. decreased amounts of carbon dioxide
    in the blood _____

11. blood in the pleural cavity _____

12. watery fluid in the pleural cavity _____

13. collection of air in the pleural cavity _____

14. pus in the pleural cavity _____

15. instrument used to listen to chest sounds _____

Exercise 14-5 DEFINITIONS

Define the following word elements.

1. -ectasis _____

2. lacrim/o _____

3. ox/o _____

4. pector/o _____

5. phren/o _____

6. pleur/o _____

7. -rrhagia _____

8. pan- _____

9. -tome _____

10. pneum/o _____

11. trache/o _____

12. rhin/o _____

13. ot/o _____

14. spir/o _____

15. –metry _____

16. steth/o _____

17. –ar _____

18. thorac/o _____

19. -capnia _____

20. -phonia _____

21. dys- _____

22. angi/o _____

23. eu- _____

24. -pnea _____

25. olig/o _____

26. ortho- _____

27. -tachy _____

28. -ptysis _____

29. hydr/o- _____

30. pyo- _____

Exercise 14-6 ALTERNATIVE TERMS

I. Write alternative term(s) for the following conditions.

   a. pleuracentesis _____

   b. laryngotracheobronchitis _____

II. a. Write three combining forms meaning chest: _____, _____, and
_____

   b. Write one combining form and one suffix meaning breathing: _____

Exercise 14-7 PLURALS

Give the plural of the following terms. Use your medical dictionary if necessary.

1. alveolus _____

2. bronchus _____

3. larynx _____

4. tonsil _____

5. trachea _____

Exercise 14-8 SPELLING

Circle any misspelled words in the following list and correctly spell them in the space provided.

1. alveolor _____

2. pulmonary _____

3. bronchiolitis _____

4. mucolytic _____

5. diaphram _____

6. pneumoconioses _____

7. pneumopluritis _____

8. sperometer _____

9. rhinorrhea _____

10. dispnea _____

11. oligopnea _____

12. bronchography   _____

13. bronhectasis   _____

14. tonsilar   _____

15. adenoidectomy   _____

14.9   Review of Vocabulary

In the following tables, the medical terms found in this chapter are organized into these categories: anatomy, pathology, diagnostics, clinical and surgical procedures, and treatment. Define each term and decide into which category the word belongs. This will help you associate the term with its purpose and help you remember its meaning.

TABLE 14-1

REVIEW OF ANATOMICAL TERMS

1. alveolar	2. endotracheal	3. laryngeal
4. lobar	5. nasolacrimal	6. nasopharyngeal
7. otorhinolaryngology	8. pectoral	9. pharyngoglossal
10. phrenic	11. pneumatic	12. pulmonary
13. tonsillar	14. tracheoesophageal	15. inhalation
16. exhalation	17. cilia	18. nasal septum
19. olfactory neurons	20. paranasal sinuses	21. laryngopharynx
22. glottis	23. mediastinal cavity	24. pleural cavity

TABLE 14-2

REVIEW OF PATHOLOGIC TERMS

1. alveolitis	2. anoxia	3. aphonia
4. apnea	5. bradypnea	6. bronchiectasis
7. bronchiolitis	8. bronchitis	9. bronchogenic carcinoma
10. bronchospasm	11. dysphonia	12. dyspnea
13. eupnea	14. hemoptysis	15. hemothorax
16. hydrothorax	17. hypercapnia	18. hyperpnea
19. hypocapnia	20. hypoxia	21. laryngospasm
22. laryngotracheobronchitis	23. oliopnea	24. orthopnea
25. pansinusitis	26. pleuralgia	27. pneumoconiosis
28. pneumonia	29. pneumopleuritis	30. pneumothorax
31. pyothorax	32. rhinitis	33. rhinorrhea
34. tachypnea	35. thoracodynia	36. tonsillitis

TABLE 14-3

REVIEW OF DIAGNOSTIC TERMS

1. bronchography	2. bronchoscopy	3. pulmonary angiography
4. spirometer	5. spirometry	6. stethoscope

TABLE 14-4

REVIEW CLINICAL PROCEDURES, SURGICAL PROCEDURES, AND SURGICAL INSTRUMENTS

1. adenoidectomy	2. lobectomy	3. phrenotomy
4. pneumonectomy	5. rhinoplasty	6. sinusotomy
7. thoracocentesis	8. thoracoplasty	9. thoracotomy
10. tonsillectomy	11. tonsillotome	12. tracheostomy
13. tracheotomy		

TABLE 14-5

REVIEW OF TERMS USED IN TREATMENT

1. bronchodilator	2. mucolytic

14.10 Medical Terms in Context

After you read the following Medical Note, answer the questions that follow it. Use your text, medical dictionary, or other references if necessary.

MEDICAL NOTE

This 57-year-old white male presented to the hospital approximately three weeks ago with a respiratory infection, an eight-month history of anorexia, a 40-pound weight loss, and dyspnea, especially on exertion. An initial chest x-ray showed a large mass at the top of the right lung, a smaller right hilar mass, and right hydrothorax. A CT of the chest showed metastases in the mediastinum and right adrenal gland. A 5-cm abdominal mass was also noted, and biopsy revealed the mass to be cancerous. Bronchoscopy showed an endobronchial mass on the right side where the primary bronchus splits off into the secondary bronchi. There was no hemoptysis or hemothorax.

QUESTIONS ON THE MEDICAL NOTE

1. The 40-pound weight loss was most likely due to:

    a. dyspnea

    b. anorexia

    c. hydrothorax

2. On doing physical exercise, the patient experienced:

    a. dyspnea

    b. anorexia

    c. hydrothorax

3. Name the area of the lung where a large mass was found on the chest x-ray:

    a. apex

    b. base

    c. right middle lobe

4. Name the structure that passes through the hilar area:

    a. trachea

    b. bronchus

    c. alveolar duct

5. Name the material found in the pleural cavity on the chest x-ray:

   a. air

   b. blood

   c. water

   d. none of the above

6. Following several diagnostic tests, it was determined that the cancer had spread to the:

   a. hilum

   b. kidney

   c. mediastinum

   d. lung

7. Name the organ within the mediastinum:

   a. heart

   b. lung

   c. adrenal gland

8. Where are the adrenal glands located?

   a. pharynx

   b. on top of the kidneys

   c. lungs

   d. kidneys

9. Name the procedure that diagnosed the spread of cancer to the adrenal gland.

   a. biopsy

   b. bronchoscopy

   c. computed tomography

   d. none of the above

10. A symptom of this cancer was the spitting up of blood.

   a. true

   b. false

15 CHAPTER

The Digestive System

CHAPTER ORGANIZATION

This chapter will help you understand the digestive system. It is divided into the following sections:

15.1	Oral Cavity
15.2	Pharynx
15.3	Esophagus
15.4	Stomach
15.5	Small Intestine
15.6	Large Intestine
15.7	Accessory Organs
15.8	Peritoneum
15.9	Additional Word Parts
15.10	Term Analysis and Definition
15.11	Common Diseases
15.12	Abbreviations
15.13	Putting It All Together
15.14	Review of Vocabulary
15.15	Medical terms in Context

CHAPTER OBJECTIVES

On completion of this chapter, you will be able to do the following:

1. Name, locate, and describe the functions of the six major organs of the digestive system
2. Name, locate, and describe the functions of the accessory organs of the digestive system
3. Name the three portions of the small intestine
4. Name the three regions of the large intestine
5. Describe the peritoneum
6. State the major functions of the digestive system
7. Analyze, define, pronounce, and spell terms relating to the digestive system
8. Describe common diseases
9. Define abbreviations common to the digestive system

INTRODUCTION

Figure 15-1 is an overview of the digestive system. You can see that it is essentially a long tube, plus four accessory organs described in the following. The tube is called the **digestive tract** or **gastrointestinal tract** (GIT). It extends from the mouth to the anus. Its functions are to take in food, break it down into simpler molecules that may be utilized by the body, and eliminate wastes. The process of breaking food down is called **digestion**. Once the food is broken down, the molecules move through the wall of the digestive tract into the blood and lymph for distribution throughout the body. This process is called **absorption**.

Six regions along the digestive tract perform specialized functions. They are the **oral cavity**, or mouth; the **pharynx** (**FAR**-inks), or throat; the **esophagus** (eh-**SOF**-ah-gus); the **stomach**; the **small intestine**; and the **large intestine**.

The accessory organs are the **salivary glands**, **pancreas** (**PAN**-kree-as), **liver**, and **gallbladder**. They are connected to the digestive tract by ducts and secrete substances into the tract that aid the processes of digestion and absorption.

FIGURE 15-1
Structures of the
digestive tract

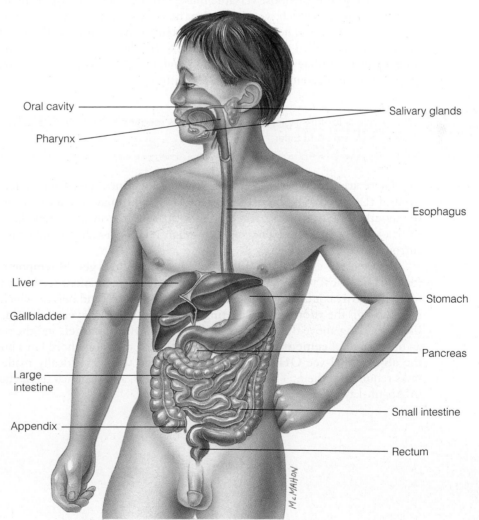

Oral cavity

Pharynx

Salivary glands

Esophagus

Liver

Stomach

Gallbladder

Pancreas

Large
intestine

Small intestine

Appendix

Rectum

. . . .

15.1   Oral Cavity

All the structures of the mouth are considered to be part of the oral cavity. The only external structure is the lips, which are muscular folds. The inside lining of the cheeks (bucca) is mucous membrane called **buccal mucosa** (**BUK**-ahl myoo-**KOH**-sa). The **palate** (**PAL**-at), the roof of the mouth, separates the mouth from the nasal cavity. Its anterior portion (the **hard palate**) is bony; the posterior portion (the **soft palate**) consists of muscle and connective tissue. At the back of the palate is the **uvula** (**YOO**-vyoo-lah), a saclike structure that hangs into the throat and closes off the nasal passage during swallowing.

Memory Key	• Cheeks are lined with buccal mucosa. • The hard and soft palates separate the mouth from the nasal cavity. • The uvula closes off the nasal passage during swallowing.

The **tongue** is the most versatile muscle in the body. It is tremendously important in the production of speech; yet its primary functions are to provide a sense of taste and to assist in swallowing. The tongue is connected to the bottom of the mouth by a mucous membrane cord called the **frenulum** (**FREN**-yoo-lum). Projections on the surface of the tongue called **papillae** (pah-**PIL**-ee) add roughness to aid licking and contain taste buds for sensing sweetness, sourness, saltiness, and bitterness.

Memory Key	The tongue is for talk, taste, and swallowing. Its roughness comes from papillae, which sense sweet, sour, salt, and bitter.

There are four types of teeth. **Incisors** and **canines** (**cuspids**) are located toward the front of the mouth, and **bicuspids** (premolars) and **molars** are located toward the back of the mouth. The two main parts of the tooth are the crown, located above the gums, and the root, below the gums. The gums, or gingiva (**JIN**-jih-vah), are mucous membranes that surround the tooth socket.

Between the ages of 6 months and 2 years, children get 20 temporary or **deciduous** (deh-**SID**-yoo-us) teeth, which are replaced with 32 permanent teeth. At the core of each tooth is a cavity containing **pulp** made up of blood vessels and nerves, which extend into the root through the **root canal**. Covering the pulp cavity is a layer of **dentin**. The portion of the tooth lying above the gum is covered by hard, white **enamel**, and the root is covered by an outer layer of **cementum** (seh-**MEN**-tum). The root is anchored in a bony socket called the **alveolus** (al-vee-**OH**-lus) (Figure 15-2). The teeth are ideally made for the simple tasks required of them. The front teeth slice or tear, and the back teeth chew or **masticate** (**MAS**-tih-kayt) food.

FIGURE 15-2
Structures of a tooth

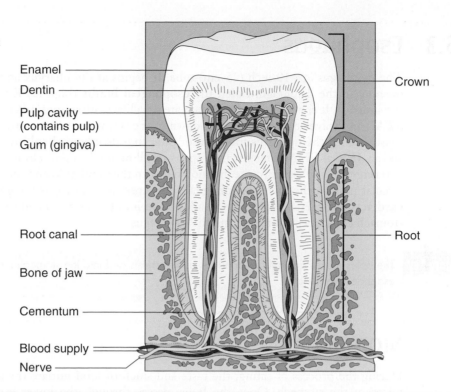

Enamel

Dentin

Pulp cavity
(contains pulp)

Gum (gingiva)

Crown

Root canal

Bone of jaw

Cementum

Blood supply

Nerve

Root

Memory Key
- Temporary teeth are called deciduous.
- Types of teeth are:

  incisors   bicuspids
  canines   molars

- The crown is located above the gums; the root, below the gums.
- From inside out, teeth consist of pulp, dentin, cementum, enamel.
- Front teeth tear food, and back teeth masticate it.

15.2   Pharnyx

During mastication, the food is mixed with saliva, producing a softened ball of food called a **bolus** (**BO**-lus), which is pushed by the tongue into the throat, or **pharynx**. This pushing commences the process of swallowing, also called **deglutition** (**deg**-loo-**TISH**-un). Because the pharynx opens to both the respiratory system via the larynx and to the digestive system via the **esophagus**, swallowing must be precisely coordinated to avoid aspirating food (taking it into the lungs). A small flap of tissue on the voice box called the **epiglottis** (**ep**-ih-**GLOT** -is) performs this function by reflexively covering the larynx during swallowing.

Memory Key   Swallowing is deglutition. The food (bolus) passes through the pharynx to the esophagus.

15.3   Esophagus

The esophagus is a 10-inch (25-cm) tube. It begins at the pharynx and passes through an opening in the diaphragm called the **esophageal hiatus** (high-**AYE**-tus) before reaching the stomach. It contains muscles that create wavelike contractions called **peristaltic** (**per**-ih-**STAL**-tik) **waves** to push the bolus down to the stomach. At the proximal end is a circular muscle called the **upper esophageal** or **pharyngoesophageal sphincter** (**far**-ing-goh-ee-**sof**-ah-**JEE**-al **SFINK**-ter), which opens to allow food in and closes to prevent air from entering the esophagus. At the junction between the esophagus and the stomach is a second circular muscle, the **lower esophageal sphincter**, also known as the **gastroesophageal** or **cardiac sphincter**, which opens to allow food into the stomach and then closes to prevent stomach contents from reentering the esophagus.

Memory Key The bolus moves down the esophagus by peristalsis and into the stomach through the lower esophageal sphincter.

15.4   Stomach

During the process of eating, the taste and smell of food initiate the secretion of gastric juices in the stomach. Once the bolus passes through the lower esophageal sphincter into the stomach, muscle action causes churning, mixing the bolus with the gastric juices (mucus, hydrochloric acid, enzymes, and other chemicals) into a semiliquid called **chyme** (**KYM**).

Figure 15-3 is a cutaway illustration of the stomach. Note the inner lining of the stomach. It consists of a series of folds called **rugae** (**ROO**-jee), which stretch to accommodate food. Structurally, the stomach is J-shaped, with four regions: the **cardia** (**KAR**-dee-ah), **fundus** (**FUN**-dus), **body**, and **antrum**. The medial curve is called the **lesser curvature**, and the lateral curve is called the **greater curvature**. Food leaves the stomach for the small intestine through another circular muscle called the **pyloric** (pye-**LOR**-ik) **sphincter**.

Memory Key
- Food enters the stomach through the lower esophageal sphincter and leaves through the pyloric sphincter.
- The bolus is mixed with gastric juices to form chyme.
- The folds of the stomach walls are rugae.
- The regions are cardia, fundus, body, and antrum.
- The curves are called lesser and greater.

FIGURE 15-3
Stomach

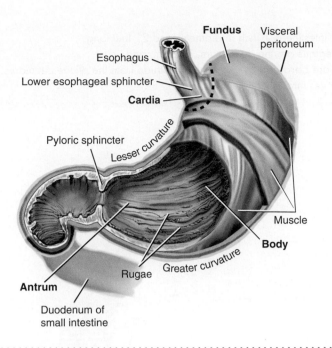

15.5   Small Intestine

Figure 15-4 illustrates the small intestine. Coiled within the abdominopelvic cavity, the 21-foot-long (7-m) small intestine has three regions: the **duodenum** (**dew**-oh-**DEE**-num), the **jejunum** (jeh-**JOO**-num), and the **ileum** (**ILL**-ce-um). Although the diameter is only about 1 inch (2.54 cm), the inner surface area is greatly increased by folds called **plicae circulares** (**PLYE**-kee **sir**-kyoo-**LAR**-eez), illustrated in Figure 15-5. Many fingerlike projections called **villi** (**VIL**-eye) protrude from the plicae circulares. Each villus has a network of capillaries that permit the absorption of nutrients from digested food into the bloodstream. The remaining waste product enters the large intestine through a valve at the end of the ileum called the **ileocecal** (**ill**-ee-oh-**SEE**-kal) **valve**.

FIGURE 15-4
Small intestine

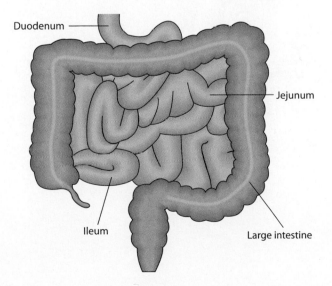

Memory Key
- The small intestine is 1 inch in diameter and 21 feet long.
- Its three regions are the duodenum, jejunum, and ileum.
- Nutrients are absorbed by villi, which protrude from the plicae circulares.
- Waste leaves through the ileocecal valve.

FIGURE 15-5
Structures of absorption in the small intestine: (A) plicae circulares; (B) villi; (C) capillaries

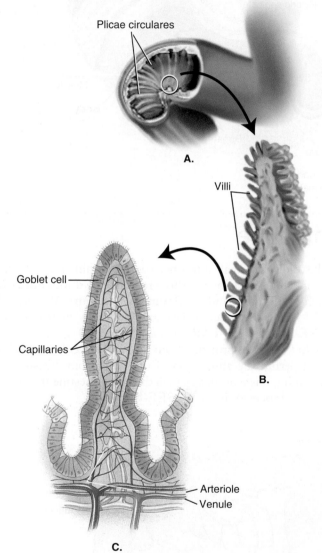

Plicae circulares

A.

Villi

Goblet cell

Capillaries

Arteriole
Venule

B.

C.

15.6   Large Intestine

The large intestine is about 5 feet (1.8 m) long and 2.4 inches (6 cm) in diameter. Its functions are to absorb water, vitamin K, and some B vitamins and to eliminate waste by **defecation** (def-eh-**KAY**-shun). It has three regions, as illustrated in Figure 15-6: a pouch called the **cecum** (**SEE**-kum), the **colon**, and the **rectum**. The colon forms a long, square arch consisting of the **ascending colon**, **transverse colon**, **descending colon**, and **sigmoid colon**. The rectum is about 8 inches long and is lined with mucous folds. The final segment of the rectum is the **anal canal**. It is surrounded by the **internal** and **external sphincters**, circular muscles that regulate the evacuation of feces through the anus. The **appendix**, which has no known function, hangs down from the cecum.

Memory Key	• The large intestine is 5 feet long and 2.4 inches in diameter.

- The large intestine is 5 feet long and 2.4 inches in diameter.
- It absorbs water, vitamin K, and some B vitamins and eliminates waste.
- The regions of the large intestine are:
  - cecum   rectum
  - colon
- The regions of the colon are:
  - ascending   descending
  - transverse   sigmoid
- The rectum includes:
  - anal canal   external and internal sphincters
  - anus

FIGURE 15-6
Large intestine

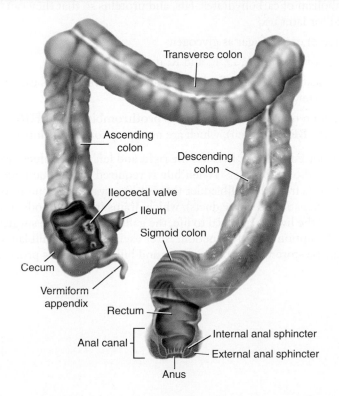

Transverse colon

Ascending colon

Descending colon

Ileocecal valve

Ileum

Sigmoid colon

Cecum

Vermiform appendix

Rectum

Anal canal

Internal anal sphincter

External anal sphincter

Anus

15.7 Accessory Organs

SALIVARY GLANDS

There are three pairs of **salivary glands**: the **parotid** (pah-**ROT**-id), the **submandibular** (sub-man-**DIB**-yoo-lar), and **sublingual** (sub-**LING**-gwal). They drain saliva into the oral cavity via salivary ducts. Saliva contains an important enzyme, **salivary amylase** (**AM**-ih-lays), which begins the digestion of carbohydrates.

Memory Key	• The salivary glands are the:
	  parotid
	  submandibular
	  sublingual
	• Saliva contains salivary amylase, which begins the digestion of carbohydrates.

LIVER AND BILIARY TRACT

The **biliary tract** includes the **liver**, **gallbladder** (**GB**), the **hepatic ducts**, the **cystic duct**, and the **common bile duct** (**CBD**). The liver weighs about 4 pounds (1.75 kg). It is located below the diaphragm, in the right upper quadrant (RUQ) of the abdomen. As illustrated in Figure 15-7, the liver is divided into right and left lobes, which in turn divide into smaller lobes. The liver performs the following functions:

1. Production of bile for the breakdown of fat in the duodenum
2. Metabolism of carbohydrates, fats, and proteins so that they can be absorbed or stored for later use
3. Storage of excess sugar as glycogen
4. Storage of vitamins A, D, E, and K; iron; and copper
5. Detoxification of harmful substances by the action of cells called **Kupffer's** (**KOOP**-ferz) cells
6. Production of blood proteins such as **prothrombin** (pro-**THROM**-bin) and **fibrinogen** (figh-**BRIN**-oh-jen), which are necessary for blood clotting

Bile is transported from the liver via the right and left hepatic ducts and into the cystic duct for storage in the gallbladder. When bile is required in the duodenum for the breakdown of fats, it travels from the gallbladder through the cystic duct and into the CBD (the union between the hepatic and cystic ducts), which drains into the duodenum.

Whereas the liver is essential to life, the gallbladder may be surgically removed without too much disruption to body function. After excision of the gallbladder (cholecystectomy), the bile may be stored in the biliary ducts and biliary processes proceed normally.

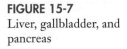

FIGURE 15-7
Liver, gallbladder, and pancreas

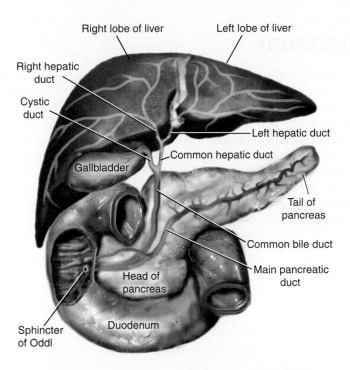

Right lobe of liver

Left lobe of liver

Right hepatic duct

Cystic duct

Left hepatic duct

Common hepatic duct

Gallbladder

Tail of pancreas

Common bile duct

Main pancreatic duct

Head of pancreas

Sphincter of Oddi

Duodenum

Memory Key

- The liver:
  produces bile
  breaks down carbohydrates, fats, and proteins
  stores sugar; vitamins A, D, E, and K; iron; and copper
  detoxifies harmful substances
  synthesizes blood-clotting factors prothrombin and fibrinogen
- The gallbladder stores bile.
- The biliary system consists of the gallbladder, hepatic ducts, cystic ducts, and common bile duct.

PANCREAS

The pancreas, illustrated in Figure 15-7, is a long, fish-shaped organ lying behind the stomach. It secretes **pancreatic juice** (enzymes and sodium bicarbonate). The enzymes break down food in the duodenum. The sodium bicarbonate provides the proper environment for the action of enzymes because it neutralizes the acid in chyme. The juice travels along the **pancreatic duct** running the length of the pancreas. The pancreatic duct fuses with the common bile duct and then empties into the duodenum, where the pancreatic juice is deposited. The **sphincter of Oddi** at the entrance to the duodenum regulates the flow of pancreatic juice and bile into the duodenum. The pancreas also secretes the hormones **insulin** (**IN**-suh-lin) and **glucagon** (**GLOO**-kah-gon), which together regulate the amount of sugar in the bloodstream. See Chapter 11, under pancreas, for details of sugar regulation.

Memory Key   The pancreas secretes pancreatic juice, which runs through the pancreatic duct to the duodenum. The pancreas also secretes the hormones insulin and glucagon, which regulate blood sugar.

15.8   Peritoneum

The peritoneum is a membrane lining the abdominopelvic cavity and covering the abdomino-pelvic organs. The abdominopelvic cavity lies below the diaphragm. The membrane lining its walls is called the **parietal peritoneum** (pah-**RYE**-eh-tal **per**-ih-toh-**NEE**-um) (pariet/o = wall). The covering of the organs is referred to as **visceral** (**VIS**-er-al) **peritoneum** (viscer/o = organ). The space between the parietal and visceral peritoneum is called the **peritoneal** (**per**-ih-toh-**NEE**-al) **cavity**. It is filled with **peritoneal fluid**, a watery fluid that prevents friction between the parietal and visceral layers. Organs such as the kidneys that lie near the posterior abdominal wall but behind the peritoneal cavity are in a **retroperitoneal** (**ret**-roh-**per**-ih-toh-**NEE**-al) position. Figure 15-8 illustrates the preceding terms regarding the peritoneum.

FIGURE 15-8
Abdominal cavity and peritoneal membranes

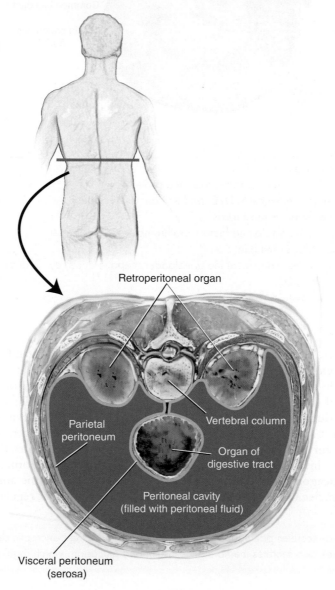

Retroperitoneal organ

Vertebral column

Parietal peritoneum

Organ of digestive tract

Peritoneal cavity (filled with peritoneal fluid)

Visceral peritoneum (serosa)

| Memory Key | Peritoneum lining the abdominopelvic cavity is called parietal peritoneum. Peritoneum covering the organs in the abdominopelvic cavity is called visceral peritoneum. |

Before you continue, review Sections 15.1 to 15.8. Then, complete Exercises 15-1 and 15-2 found at the end of the chapter.

15.9   Additional Word Parts

The following roots, suffixes, and prefixes will also be used in this chapter to build medical terms.

Root	Meaning
chol/e	bile; gall
hiat/o	gape; opening
intestin/o	intestine
umbilic/o	navel

Suffix	Meaning
-clysis	washing; irrigation
-flux	flow
-lytic	pertaining to destruction, separation, or breakdown
-tresia	opening
-tripsy	crushing

Prefix	Meaning
re-	back
retro-	backward; back

15.10 Term Analysis and Definition

ROOTS

	abdomin/o (see also lapar/o)	abdomen
Term	**Term Analysis**	**Definition**
abdominal (ab-**DOM**-ih-nal)	-al = pertaining to	pertaining to the abdomen
	an/o	**anus**
anorectal (**ay**-noh-**RECK**-tal)	-al = pertaining to **rect/o** = rectum	pertaining to the anus and rectum
perianal (**peh**-ree-**AY**-nal)	-al = pertaining to peri- = around	pertaining to around the anus
	append/o; appendic/o	**appendix**
appendectomy (**ap**-en-**DECK**-toh-mee)	-ectomy = excision; surgical removal	surgical removal of the appendix
appendicitis (ah-**pen**-dih-**SIGH**-tis)	-itis = inflammation	inflammation of the appendix
	bil/i	**bile**
biliary (**BILL**-ee-ayr-ee)	-ary = pertaining to	pertaining to bile
	bucc/o	**cheek**
buccal mucosa (**BUK**-ahl myoo-**KOH**-sa)	-al = pertaining to mucosa = mucous membrane	pertaining to the mucous membrane of the cheek
	cec/o	**cecum**
cecopexy (**SEE**-koh-**peck**-see)	-pexy = surgical fixation	surgical fixation of the cecum

	cheil/o (see also labi/o)	lips
Term	**Term Analysis**	**Definition**
cheiloplasty (**KYE**-loh-**plas**-tee)	-plasty = surgical recon- struction; surgical repair	surgical repair of the lips
cheilorrhaphy (kye-**LOR**-ah-fee)	-rrhaphy = suture (to sew)	suturing of the lips
cheilosis (kye-**LOH**-sis)	-osis = abnormal condition	abnormal condition of the lips characterized by deep, cracklike sores
	cholangi/o	**bile duct; bile vessel**
cholangiogram (koh-**LAN**-jee-oh-gram)	-gram = record; writing	a record of the bile ducts
cholangiopancreatography (koh-**lan**-jee-oh-**pan**- kree-ah-**TOG**-rah-fee)	-graphy = process of recording **pancreat/o** = pancreas	process of recording the bile ducts and pancreas *NOTE:* In endoscopic retrograde cholangiopancreatography (ERCP), an endoscope is inserted through the mouth and into the duodenum. A contrast medium is introduced through the endoscope and flows backward (retrograde), highlighting the biliary ducts and pancreas. X-rays are then taken.
	cholecyst/o	**gallbladder**
cholecystectomy (**koh**-lee-sis-**TECK**- toh-mee)	-ectomy = excision; surgical removal	excision of the gallbladder
cholecystitis (**koh**-lee-sis-**TYE**-tis)	-itis = inflammation	inflammation of the gallbladder
	choledoch/o	**common bile duct (CBD)**
choledochotomy (**koh**-led-uh-**KOT**- oh-mee)	-tomy = to cut; to cut into; incision	incision into the common bile duct

	col/o; colon/o	colon
Term	**Term Analysis**	**Definition**
colitis (koh-**LYE**-tis)	-itis = inflammation	inflammation of the colon
colocolostomy (**koh**-loh-koh-**LAHS**-toh-mee)	-stomy = new opening	creation of a new opening between two segments of the colon *NOTE:* The surgical joining of two structures that are normally separate is called **anastomosis**. An anastomosis of the colon might be performed after excision of a cancerous portion of colon.
colostomy (koh-**LAHS**-toh-mee)	-stomy = new opening	creation of a new opening between the colon and the abdominal wall (Figure 15-9)

Memory Key Be aware when spelling words using **chol/e** and **col/o**. The first syllable is pronounced the same, but is spelled differently.

FIGURE 15-9
Colostomies. The type of colostomy depends on which part of the intestine is removed. The part of the intestine remaining after the colostomy is shown in blue.

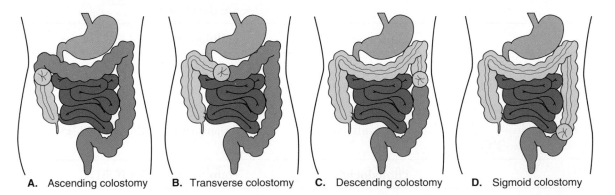

A. Ascending colostomy   **B.** Transverse colostomy   **C.** Descending colostomy   **D.** Sigmoid colostomy

	dent/o (see also odont/o)	tooth
Term	**Term Analysis**	**Definition**
edentulous (ee-**DEN**-tyoo-lus)	-ous = pertaining to e- = without	without teeth; having had teeth but lost them
dental caries (**DEN**-tal **KAYR**-eez)	-al = pertaining to caries = decay; cavities	tooth decay
	duoden/o	**duodenum (proximal portion of small intestine)**
duodenal (**doo**-oh-**DEE**-nal)	-al = pertaining to	pertaining to the duodenum
	enter/o	**small intestine; intestine**
gastroenteritis (**gas**-troh-en-ter-**EYE**- tis)	-itis = inflammation **gastr/o** = stomach	inflammation of the stomach and intestines
gastroenterologist (**gas**-troh-**en**-ter-**OL**-oh-jist)	-ist = specialist **gastr/o** = stomach	specialist in the study and treatment of diseases of the digestive tract
	esophag/o	**esophagus**
esophageal atresia (eh-**sof**-ah-**JEE**-al ah-**TREE**-zha)	-eal = pertaining to -tresia = opening a- = no; not	closure of the esophagus
gastroesophageal reflux (GER) (**gas**-troh-eh-**sof**-ah-**JEE**-al **REE**-flucks)	-eal = pertaining to **gastr/o** = stomach -flux = flow re- = back	backward flow of gastric contents into the esophagus
	gastr/o	**stomach**
gastrectomy (gas-**TRECK**-toh-mee)	-ectomy = excision; surgical removal	excision of the stomach
gastrointestinal (**gas**-troh-in-**TES**-tih-nal)	-al = pertaining to **intestin/o** = intestine	pertaining to the stomach and intestine
gastrotomy (gas-**TROT**-oh-mee)	-tomy = to cut; incise process of cutting	to cut into the stomach

Term	Term Analysis	Definition
nasogastric tube (**nay**-zoh-**GAS**-trick)	-ic = pertaining to **nas/o** = nose	a tube placed into the nose and extending into the stomach for the insertion or withdrawal of substances
	gingiv/o (see also lingulo)	**gums**
gingivobuccal (**jin**-jih-voh-**BUK**-ahl)	-al = pertaining to **bucc/o** = cheek	pertaining to the gums and cheeks
gingivitis (**jin**-jih-**VYE**-tis)	-itis = inflammation	inflamed gums
	gloss/o (see also lingu/o)	**tongue**
glossectomy (glos-**ECK**-toh-mee)	-ectomy = excision; surgical removal	excision of the tongue
	hepat/o	**liver**
hepatocellular (**hep**-ah-toh-**SEL**-you-lar)	-ar = pertaining to **cellul/o** = cell	pertaining to liver cells
hepatitis (**hep**-ah-**TYE**-tis)	-itis = inflammation	inflammation of the liver
hepatoma (**hep**-ah-**TOH**-mah)	-oma = tumor; mass	tumor of the liver
	herni/o	**hernia; protrusion or displacement of an organ through a structure that normally contains it**
femoral hernia (**FEM**-or-al **HER**-nee-ah)	-al = pertaining to **femor/o** = thigh	displacement of intestines through the femoral canal; more common in females than males *NOTE:* The femoral canal is a small tubular channel for the passage of blood vessels and nerves to the thigh.
herniorrhaphy (**her**-nee-**OR**-ah-fee)	-rrhaphy = suture	hernia repair *NOTE:* This surgical procedure is performed by making an incision over the hernial site. The organ, usually the intestine, is returned to its normal position and the area secured.
hiatal hernia (high-**AY**-tal **HER**-nee-ah)	-al = pertaining to **hiat/o** = gape; opening	displacement of the stomach above the diaphragm into the thoracic cavity (Figure 15-10A)

FIGURE 15-10
(A) hiatal hernia;
(B) inguinal hernia

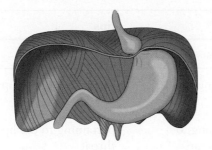

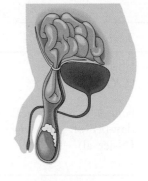

(A) **(B)**

Term	Term Analysis	Definition
inguinal hernia (**ING**-gwih-nal **HER**-nee-ah)	-al = pertaining to **inguin/o** = groin	displacement of intestines through the inguinal canal; more common in males than females (Figure 15-10B) *NOTE:* The inguinal canal is a 1-inch long channel in the lower abdominal wall. In the male it serves for the passage of the spermatic cord (blood vessels, nerves, and other vessels). In the female it serves for the passage of the round ligament.
umbilical hernia (um-**BILL**-ih-kuhl **HER**-nee-ah)	-al = pertaining to **umbilic/o** = navel	displacement of intestines through a weak spot in the abdominal wall near the umbilicus (navel)
	ile/o	**ileum (distal portion of small intestine)**
ileostomy (**ill**-ee-**OS**-toh-mee)	-stomy = new opening	creation of a new opening between the ileum and the abdominal wall
ileotomy (**ill**-ee-**OT**-oh-mee)	-tomy = to cut; incise, process of cutting	to cut into the ileum
	jejun/o	**jejunum (middle portion of small instestine)**
gastrojejunostomy (**gas**-troh-**jeh**-joo-**NOS**-toh-me)	-stomy = new opening **gastr/o** = stomach	new opening between the stomach and jejunum; anastomosis between the stomach and jejunum
jejunal (jeh-**JOO**-nal)	-al = pertaining to	pertaining to the jejunum

	labi/o	**lips**
Term	**Term Analysis**	**Definition**
labial (**LAY**-bee-al)	-al = pertaining to	pertaining to the lips
labioglossopharyngeal (**lay**-bee-oh-**glos**-oh-far-**IN**-jee-al)	-eal = pertaining to **gloss/o** = tongue **pharyng/o** = throat; pharynx	pertaining to the lips, tongue, and throat
	lapar/o	**abdomen**
laparoscope (**LAP**-ah-roh-skohp)	-scope = instrument used to visually examine	instrument used to visually examine the inside of the abdomen
laparoscopy (lap-ah-**ROS**-koh-pee)	-scopy = process of visually examining (a body cavity or organ)	process of visually examining the inside of the abdomen (Figure 4-1)
laparotomy (lap-ah-**ROT**-oh-mee)	-tomy = to cut; incise	incision into the abdominal wall
	lingu/o	**tongue**
sublingual (sub-**LING**-gwal)	-al = pertaining to sub- = under	pertaining to under the tongue
	lith/o	**stone**
cholecystolithiasis (**koh**-lee-**sis**-toh-lih-**THIGH**-ah-sis)	-iasis = abnormal condition **cholecyst/o** = gallbladder	condition of stones in the gallbladder (Figure 15-11)
choledocholithiasis (koh-**led**-uh-koh-lih-**THIGH**-ah-sis)	-iasis = abnormal condition **choledoch/o** = common bile duct	abnormal condition of stones in the common bile duct (Figure 15-11)
litholytic agent (lith-oh-**LIT**-ick)	-lytic = pertaining to destruction, separation, or breakdown	oral drugs used to break down gallstones, thereby eliminating the need for surgery
lithotripsy (**LITH**-oh-**trip**-see)	-tripsy = crushing	crushing of gallstones into pebbles tiny enough to be eliminated without surgical removal
choledocholithotripsy (koh-**led**-uh-koh-**LITH**-oh-**trip**-see)	-tripsy = crushing **choledoch/o** = common bile duct	crushing of stones in the common bile duct

FIGURE 15-11
Cholelithiasis and
choledocholithiasis

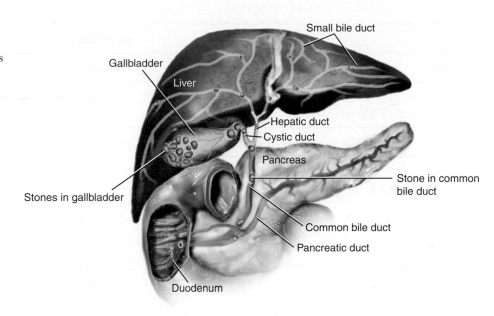

	odont/o	tooth
Term	**Term Analysis**	**Definition**
endodontist (**en**-doh-**DON**-tist)	-ist = specialist endo- = within	dentist who specializes in the diagnosis and treatment of diseases within the tooth such as in the pulp
orthodontist (**or**-thoh-**DON**-tist)	-ist = specialist ortho- = straight	dentist who specializes in the correction of deformed or maloccluded teeth
periodontist (**per**-ee-oh-**DON**-tist)	-ist = specialist peri- = around	specialist in diseases of tissues around the tooth such as the gums and cementum *NOTE:* The structures around the tooth are collectively known as the periodontium.
	orex/i	**appetite**
anorexia (**an**-oh-**RECK**-see-ah)	-ia = condition an- = no; not; lack of	loss of appetite *NOTE:* Do not confuse **anorexia**, which is often caused by a disorder of the digestive system, with **anorexia nervosa**, a psychiatric condition.
	or/o (see also stomat/o)	**mouth**
oral (**OR**-al)	-al = pertaining to	pertaining to the mouth

	pancreat/o	pancreas
Term	**Term Analysis**	**Definition**
pancreatitis (**pan**-kree-ah-**TYE**-tis)	-itis = inflammation	inflammation of the pancreas
	peritone/o	**peritoneum**
peritonitis (**per**-ih-toh-**NYE**-tis)	-itis = inflammation	inflammation of the peritoneum *NOTE:* A life-threatening condition, often due to a ruptured appendix, which releases intestinal bacteria resulting in an inflamed peritoneum.
retroperitoneal (**ret**-roh-**per**-ih-toh-**NEE**-al)	-al = pertaining to	behind the peritoneum retro- = behind
ventriculoperitoneal shunt (ven-**trick**-yoo-loh-**per**-ih-toh-**NEE**-al)	-al = pertaining to **ventricul/o** = ventricles of the brain	the use of a shunt to divert cerebro-spinal fluid from the ventricles to the peritoneum shunt = a device used to divert the flow of fluid
	pharyng/o	**throat; pharynx**
pharyngeal (**far**-in-**JEE**-al)	-eal = pertaining to	pertaining to the pharynx
	proct/o (see also rect/o)	**rectum**
proctologist (prock-**TOL**-oh-jist)	-ist = specialist	specialist in the study of the rectum
proctoclysis (prock-**TOCK**-lih-sis)	-clysis = washing;	irrigation of the rectum irrigation
	pylor/o	**pylorus (distal portion of the stomach); pyloric sphincter**
pyloric stenosis (pie-**LOR**-ick steh-**NOH**-sis)	-ic = pertaining to stenosis = narrowing; stricture	narrowing of the pylorus
pylorospasm (pie-**LOR**-oh-spasm)	-spasm = sudden, invol-untary contraction	sudden, involuntary contraction of the pylorus
pyloromyotomy (pye-**lor**-oh-my-**OT**-oh-mee)	-tomy = to cut; incise; process of cutting **my/o** = muscle	incision into the pyloric sphincter *NOTE:* Pyloromyotomy widens the stricture caused by pyloric stenosis.

	rect/o	rectum
rectostenosis (**reck**-toh-sten-**OH**-sis)	-stenosis = narrowing; stricture	narrowing or stricture of the rectum *NOTE:* -stenosis can be used as a suffix as evident in this example, or it can be a stand-alone medical word as in *pyloric stenosis*.
	sial/o	saliva
Term	**Term Analysis**	**Definition**
salivary (**SAL**-ih-ver-ee)	-ary = pertaining to	pertaining to the saliva
	sialaden/o	salivary gland
sialadenitis (**sigh**-al-**ad**-eh-**NYE**-tis)	-itis = inflammation	inflammation of the salivary gland
	sigmoid/o	sigmoid colon
sigmoidoscopy (**sig**-moi-**DOS**-koh-pee)	-scopy = process of visually examining (a body organ or cavity)	process of visually examining the sigmoid colon
	steat/o	fat
steatorrhea (**stee**-ah-toh-**REE**-ah)	-rrhea = discharge; flow	discharge of fat in the feces
	stomat/o	mouth
stomatitis (**sto**-mah-**TYE**-tis)	-itis = inflammation	inflammation of the mouth

Memory Key **Stomat/o**, rather than **or/o**, is commonly used in reference to pathology of the mouth.

	viscer/o	internal organs
visceroptosis (**vis**-er-op-**TOH**-sis)	-ptosis = drooping; sagging; prolapse	drooping of the internal organs

SUFFIXES

	-chalasia	relaxation
Term	**Term Analysis**	**Definition**
achalasia (**ack**-ah-**LAY**-zee-ah)	a- = no; not; lack of	inability of the muscles of the digestive tract to relax
	-grade	**to step; to go**
retrograde (**RET**-roh-grayd)	retro- = backward; back	backward flow, especially of fluid
	-emesis	**vomiting**
hyperemesis (**high**-per-**EM**-eh-sis)	hyper- = excessive; above normal	excessive vomiting
hematemesis (**hem**-ah-**TEM**-eh-sis)	**hemat/o** = blood	vomiting of blood
melanemesis (**mel**-ah-**NEM**-eh-sis)	**melan/o** = black	black vomit caused by the mixing of blood with intestinal contents *NOTE:* Melanemesis might be an indication of bleeding ulcers.
	-lith	**stone**
cholelith (**KOH**-lee-lith)	**chol/e** = bile; gall	gallstones
sialolith (sigh-**AL**-oh-lith)	**sial/o** = saliva	stone in the salivary gland or duct
	-phagia	**eating; swallowing**
aphagia (ah-**FAY**-jee-ah)	a- = no; not; lack of	no eating
dysphagia (dis-**FAY**-jee-ah)	dys- = difficult; painful; bad	difficulty in eating
polyphagia (**pol**-ee-**FAY**-jee-ah)	poly- = many; much	excessive eating

	-plakia	patches
Term	**Term Analysis**	**Definition**
leukoplakia (**loo**-koh-**PLAY**-kee-ah)	**leuk/o** = white	white patches on the mucous membrane
	-pepsia	**digestion**
dyspepsia (dis-**PEP**-see-ah)	dys- = difficult; painful; bad	indigestion
	-prandial	**meal**
postprandial (pohst-**PRAN**-dee-al)	post- = after	after a meal

PREFIXES

	endo-	within
Term	**Term Analysis**	**Definition**
endoscopy (en-**DOS**-koh-pee)	-scopy = process of visually examining (a body cavity or organ)	process of visually examining the internal body cavities by inserting a tube equipped with a light and lens system; examples are gastroscopy, laparoscopy, and colonoscopy (Figure 4-1)

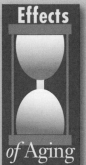

The entire digestive tract incurs subtle changes with age. Saliva production decreases, affecting taste and swallowing, and contributing to the development of periodontal disease, which leads to tooth loss. The esophageal muscles contract with less force, and the lower esophageal sphincter might not relax as readily, making swallowing more difficult. Alternatively, the sphincter might become lax, allowing stomach acid into the esophagus, which might cause heartburn.

The stomach cannot hold as much food because of loss of elasticity, and the secretion of gastric juices might decrease. In some people, a reduced production of lactase might lead to lactose intolerance, and cause digestive disturbances when dairy products are consumed.

Constipation is common among the elderly for several reasons. Fluid intake and exercise might be reduced. Overuse of laxatives earlier in life might have a rebound effect. The inner linings of the intestine might develop weaknesses that cause the formation of small pouches in the lining, leading to pain and constipation.

The liver becomes smaller and enzyme production might decrease, making the liver less able to detoxify substances. Thus, older people tend to feel the effects of drugs for longer periods of time.

15.11 Common Diseases

CROHN'S DISEASE

Crohn's (**KROHNZ**) is a form of inflammatory bowel disease that can involve any part of the digestive tract, but is most often found in the ileum. The inflammation causes obstruction of intestinal contents.

In severe cases, an **ostomy** is done to remove the diseased bowel and create an artifical opening between the intestine and abdominal wall. If this is done at the colon, the operation is called a **colostomy**. If it is done at the ileum, it is called an **ileostomy**.

ULCERS

An ulcer occurs when the mucous membrane lining the digestive tract wears away, creating an open sore (Figure 15-12). Ulcers of the duodenum, stomach, and esophagus are often referred to by the general term **peptic ulcers** (peptic = digestion). Ulcers might be caused by the bacterium *Helicobacter pylori (H. pylori)*. Another cause is the extended use of nonsteroidal anti-inflammatory drugs (NSAID) such as aspirin. Sometimes, the cause is idiopathic (unknown). Factors that contribute to the disease include hyperacidity, stress, smoking, and alcohol.

Ulcers are treated with drug therapy that includes antibiotics to kill *H. pylori* and drugs to reduce acid secretions.

FIGURE 15-12
Ulcer of the stomach

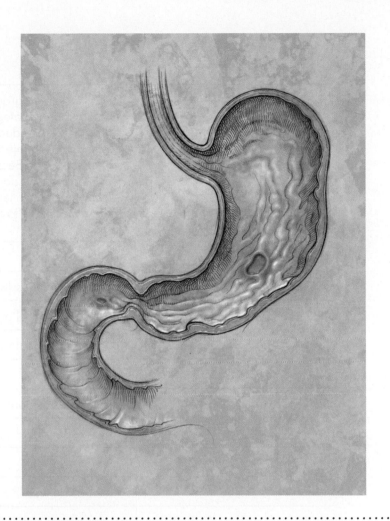

15.12 Abbreviations

Abbreviation	Meaning
BE	barium enema (X-ray of the large bowel following the placement of barium into the rectum. Barium is a contrast medium used to highlight the large bowel.)
CBD	common bile duct

continued on page 394

continued from page 393

Abbreviation	Meaning
ERCP	endoscopic retrograde cholangiopancreatography (X-ray of the bile ducts and pancreas following injection of a contrasting dye. Because the dye flows against the normal flow of substances, the term *retrograde*, meaning "to flow back," is used.)
GB	gallbladder
GBS	gallbladder series (type of x-ray)
GER	gastroesophageal reflux
GERD	gastroesophageal reflux disorder
GI	gastrointestinal
IVC	intravenous cholangiogram
LES	lower esophageal sphincter
NG	nasogastric
NGT	nasogastric tube
NPO	nothing by mouth
PTC	percutaneous transhepatic cholangiography (After injection of a contrast medium through the skin into the liver's biliary system, an x-ray examination of the bile ducts is performed.)
S&D	stomach and duodenum
TE	tracheoesophageal
UGI	upper gastrointestinal

15.13 Putting It All Together

Exercise 15-1   SHORT ANSWER

1. Name three functions of the digestive tract.

   _____

   _____

2. Name six major structures of the gastrointestinal tract and four accessory organs.

   _____

   _____

   _____

   _____

   _____

3. Describe the location of the:
   (a) lower esophageal sphincter

   _____

   (b) pyloric sphincter

   _____

4. Name the sections of the large intestine, in sequence, starting from the ileocecal valve.

   _____

   _____

5. Name the sections of the small intestine, proximal to distal.

   _____

   _____

6. Name the three salivary glands.

   _____

   _____

7. What is the function of salivary amylase?

   _____

   _____

8. List six functions of the liver.

   _____

   _____

   _____

9. Name two hormones secreted by the pancreas. What is their function?

_____

_____

10. Define: parietal peritoneum, visceral peritoneum, and peritoneal cavity.

_____

_____

11. Define hepatic duct, cystic duct, and common bile duct.

_____

_____

Exercise 15-2   MATCHING

Match the structure in Column A with its function in Column B.

Column A	Column B
_____ 1. uvula	A. mastication
_____ 2. rugae	B. prevents aspiration of food into the trachea
_____ 3. papillae	C. produces bile
_____ 4. villi	D. increase the surface area of the small intestine
_____ 5. large intestine	E. closes off the nasal passages during swallowing
_____ 6. teeth	F. increase the surface area of the stomach
_____ 7. plicae circulares	G. defecation
_____ 8. liver	H. absorption of digested foodstuffs
_____ 9. epiglottis	I. stores bile
_____ 10. gallbladder	J. contain taste buds

Exercise 15-3   DEFINITIONS

Define the following component parts.

1. bucc/o   _____

2. cec/o   _____

3. cheil/o   _____

4. cholangi/o _____

5. cholecyst/o _____

6. choledoch/o _____

7. odont/o   _____

8. enter/o _____

9. gingiv/o _____

10. gloss/o _____

11. hepat/o _____

12. ile/o _____

13. jejun/o _____

14. labi/o _____

15. lapar/o _____

16. lingu/o _____

17. lith/o _____

18. orex/i _____

19. proct/o _____

20. sial/o _____

21. sialaden/o _____

22. steat/o _____

23. stomat/o _____

24. or/o _____

25. viscer/o _____

26. -chalasia _____

27. -grade _____

28. -emesis _____

29. -phagia _____

30. -pepsia _____

31. -plakia _____

32. -prandial _____

33. peri- _____

34. -emia _____

Exercise 15-4   BUILDING MEDICAL TERMS

Build the medical term.

1. pertaining to the anus and rectum _____

2. pertaining to around the anus _____

3. surgical removal of the appendix _____

4. inflammation of the appendix   _____

5. surgical fixation of the cecum   _____

6. pertaining to the ventricles and
   peritoneum   _____

7. surgical repair of the lips   _____

8. suturing of the lip   _____

9. abnormal condition of the lips   _____

10. inflammation of the colon   _____

11. hernia repair   _____

12. creation of a new opening between
    the colon and the abdomen   _____

13. creation of a new opening between
    two segments of the colon   _____

14. pertaining to liver cells   _____

15. bile stones   _____

16. tumor of the liver   _____

17. displacement of intestines through
    the inguinal canal   _____

18. excessive vomiting   _____

19. vomiting of blood   _____

20. black vomit   _____

21. no eating   _____

22. difficulty in eating   _____

23. excessive eating   _____

Exercise 15-5   IDENTIFYING SURGICAL AND CLINICAL PROCEDURES

Mark an **X** beside the terms indicating surgical or clinical procedures.

1. perianal   _____

2. cheiloplasty   _____

3. cecopexy   _____

4. cholecystitis   _____

5. edentulous   _____

6. orthodontist   _____

7. gastroesophageal reflux   _____

8. esophageal atresia   _____

9. gastrotomy   _____

10. postprandial   _____

11. choledocholithotripsy   _____

12. proctoclysis   _____

13. dyspepsia   _____

14. visceroptosis   _____

15. endoscopy   _____

Exercise 15-6   ADJECTIVAL FORMS

Mark an **X** beside the adjectival forms found in the list below.

1. anus   _____

2. biliary   _____

3. cecum   _____

4. duodenal   _____

5. colon   _____

6. periodontist   _____

7. esophageal   _____

8. anorexia   _____

9. pylorus   _____

10. salivary   _____

Exercise 15-7   SPELLING PRACTICE

Circle any misspelled words in the list below and correctly spell them in the space provided.

1. iliocecal valve   _____

2. melanemesis   _____

3. colecystitis   _____

4. cholitis   _____

5. gingivobuccal   _____

6. chielorhaphy   _____

7. pancreatitis   _____

8. saliviary   _____

9. visceroptosis   _____

10. vomitting   _____

Exercise 15-8 PATHOLOGY

Match the following terms with their descriptions. Some terms are used more than once. Not all terms are used.

antibiotics

cecopexy

cholecystolithiasis

Crohn's disease

esophageal atresia

gastrectomy

Helicobacter pylori

labial

melanemesis

ostomy

peptic

staphylococcus aureus

steatorrhea

stomatitis

ulcers

1. disease that might cause obstruction of intestinal contents _____

2. open sore created by wearing away of the mucous membrane lining _____

3. pertaining to digestion _____

4. inflammatory bowel disease _____

5. black vomit _____

6. treatment for Crohn's disease _____

7. might be the cause of ulcers _____

8. a treatment for duodenal ulcers _____

9. creation of an artificial opening _____

10. might be caused by overuse of nonsteroidal anti-inflammatory drugs _____

15.14 Review of Vocabulary

In the following tables, the medical terms are organized into these categories: anatomy, pathology, diagnostics, and medical and surgical procedures. Define each term and decide into which category the word belongs. This will help you associate the term with its purpose, and thus help you remember its meaning.

TABLE 15-1

REVIEW OF ANATOMICAL TERMS

1. alveolus	2. biliary tract	3. buccal mucosa
4. deglutition	5. dentin	6. duodenal
7. endodontist	8. epiglottis	9. frenulum
10. gastroenterologist	11. gastrointestinal	12. gingivobuccal
13. hepatocellular	14. jejunal	15. labial
16. labioglossopharyngeal	17. oral	18. orthodontist
19. perianal	20. periodontist	21. pharyngeal
22. retroperitoneal	23. salivary	24. sphincter of Oddi
25. uvula		

TABLE 15-2

REVIEW OF PATHOLOGIC TERMS

1. achalasia	2. anorexia	3. aphagia
4. cholecystitis	5. cholecystolithiasis	6. choledocholithiasis
7. cholelith	8. colitis	9. Crohn's disease
10. dental caries	11. dyspepsia	12. dysphagia
13. edentulous	14. esophageal atresia	15. femoral hernia
16. gastroenteritis	17. gastroesophageal reflux	18. gingivitis
19. hematemesis	20. hepatitis	21. hepatoma
22. hiatal hernia	23. hyperemesis	24. leukoplakia
25. melanemesis	26. pancreatitis	27. peritonitis
28. polyphagia	29. pyloric stenosis	30. pylorospasm
31. rectostenosis	32. sialadenitis	33. sialolith
34. steatorrhea	35. stomatitis	36. ulcer
37. visceroptosis		

TABLE 15-3

REVIEW OF DIAGNOSTIC TERMS

1. cholangiogram	2. cholangiopancreatography	3. laparoscopy
4. laparotomy	5. retrograde	6. sigmoidoscopy

TABLE 15-4

REVIEW OF MEDICAL AND SURGICAL TERMS

1. appendectomy	2. cecopexy	3. cheiloplasty
4. cheilorrhaphy	5. cholecystectomy	6. choledocholithotripsy
7. choledochotomy	8. colocolostomy	9. colostomy
10. gastrectomy	11. gastrotomy	12. glossectomy
13. herniorrhaphy	14. ileostomy	15. ileotomy
16. litholytic agents	17. lithotripsy	18. nasogastric tube
19. postprandial	20. proctoclysis	21. pyloromyotomy
22. ventriculoperitoneal shunt		

....

15.15 Medical Terms in Context

After you read the Discharge Summary, answer the questions that follow it. Use your text, medical dictionary, or other references if necessary.

DISCHARGE SUMMARY

CLINICAL HISTORY: This 42-year-old woman was admitted for elective resection of her Crohn's disease. She has a five-year history of Crohn's disease for which she was treated medically. Examination revealed severe stenosis in her terminal ileum with an area of approximately 15 cm of severe Crohn's disease with an ileal-sigmoid fistula. In recent months, she has had increased weight loss and diarrhea.

PAST HISTORY: Pyloromyotomy

MEDICATIONS: Prednisone and Flagyl

PHYSICAL EXAMINATION: Examination of the abdomen revealed a tender mass in the right lower quadrant. The rest of the examination was normal.

INVESTIGATIONS: Urinalysis was normal. Her electrolytes were normal.

RBCs were 4.0 million per microliter.

TREATMENT AND PROGRESS: The patient was taken to the operating room two days after admission for a right hemicolectomy and closure of the ileal-sigmoid fistula.

Pathology report revealed Crohn's disease of the terminal ileum and ascending colon.

Her postoperative course was uneventful. She was discharged home seven days after admission.

MOST RESPONSIBLE DIAGNOSIS: CROHN'S DISEASE WITH ILEAL-SIGMOID FISTULA.

QUESTIONS ON THE DISCHARGE SUMMARY

1. The patient was admitted with a(n):

    a. colostomy

    b. displacement of the terminal ileum

    c. inflammatory bowel disease

    d. wearing away of the mucous membrane of the small bowel

2. Examination revealed:

   a. inflammation of the rectum

   b. narrowing of the distal small intestine

   c. stenosis of the descending colon

   d. pain of the terminal colon

3. The patient is admitted for:

   a. partial excision of the colon

   b. pyloromyotomy

   c. suturing of the hernia

   d. none of the above

4. The fistula (abnormal passage between two organs) is between the:

   a. ascending colon and sigmoid

   b. proximal and distal segment of the large bowel

   c. proximal and distal segments of the small bowel

   d. segments of the small and large bowels

5. The ileum refers to the:

   a. ascending colon

   b. descending colon

   c. distal portion of the small intestine

   d. proximal portion of the small intestine

6. Sigmoid refers to the:

   a. ascending colon

   b. descending colon

   c. distal portion of the large intestine

   d. proximal portion of the small intestine

16 CHAPTER

The Urinary and Male Reproductive Systems

CHAPTER ORGANIZATION

This chapter will help you learn about the urinary and male reproductive systems. It is divided into the following sections:

16.1	Urinary System
16.2	Additional Word Parts
16.3	Term Analysis and Definition Pertaining to the Urinary System
16.4	Common Diseases of the Urinary System
16.5	Abbreviations Pertaining to the Urinary System
16.6	Male Reproductive System
16.7	Term Analysis and Definition Pertaining to the Male Reproductive System
16.8	Common Diseases of the Male Reproductive System
16.9	Abbreviations Pertaining to the Male Reproductive System
16.10	Putting It All Together
16.11	Review of Vocabulary Pertaining to the Urinary System
16.12	Review of Vocabulary Pertaining to the Male Reproductive System
16.13	Medical Terms in Context

CHAPTER OBJECTIVES

On completion of this chapter, you will be able to do the following:

1. Name and locate the organs of the urinary system
2. Describe the function of the urinary system
3. Describe the structure and functions of the kidney, ureters, bladder, and urethra
4. Describe glomerular filtration, tubular reabsorption, and tubular secretion
5. Name and locate the organs of the male reproductive system
6. Describe the functions of the male reproductive system
7. Analyze, define, pronounce, and spell common terms of the urinary and male reproductive systems
8. Describe common diseases
9. Define common abbreviations of the urinary and male reproductive systems

INTRODUCTION

In this chapter, you will learn about the terminology associated with the male and female urinary systems, as well as basic structure and function. Because some structures of the male urinary system also function in the reproductive system, that system is dealt with here as well. The female reproductive system is discussed in Chapter 17.

16.1   Urinary System

The urinary system, as illustrated in Figure 16-1, consists of two **kidneys**, two tubes called **ureters** (yoo-**REE**-ters), a sac called the **urinary bladder**, and another tube called the **urethra** (yoo-**REE**-thra). The ureters drain fluid called **urine** from the kidneys into the urinary bladder. From there, the urine travels through the urethra and is excreted from the body. The only difference between male and female systems is that the male has a longer urethra, because it extends through the penis.

Memory Key	The urinary system consists of:
	two kidneys a urinary bladder
	two ureters a urethra

The body's cells are surrounded by fluid called **extracellular fluid**. This fluid contains minerals such as sodium (Na^+), calcium (Ca^{++}), potassium (K^+), and chloride (Cl^-), referred to as **electrolytes** (ee-**LECK**-troh-lights). Electrolytes are important to cellular functions. Extracellular fluid also contains waste products such as **urea** (you-**REE**-ah), **uric acid**, and **creatinine** (kree-**AT**-ih-neen). When the level of extracellular fluid is too high, some of the fluid seeps through capillary walls into the blood and lymph systems, carrying with it any excess electrolytes and wastes. This fluid is then transported to the kidneys. There, the fluid and electrolytes are either excreted or reabsorbed if the body now needs them. In this way, the urinary system maintains fluid and electrolyte balance and rids the body of wastes. This is another example of how the body maintains **homeostasis** (hoh-mee-oh-**STAY**-sis). Death comes quickly if fluid and electrolyte homeostasis is not maintained.

Memory Key	The urinary system maintains homeostasis of extracellular fluid by filtering out electrolytes and waste products and excreting them with excess fluid. The excretion is called urine.

THE KIDNEYS

The kidneys are bean-shaped, fist-sized organs lying on each side of the lumbar vertebrae. Their location is **retroperitoneal** (ret-roh-**per**-ih-toh-**NEE**-al), which means they are behind the peritoneal membrane. Each kidney is covered with tissue called the **renal** (**REE**-nal) **capsule** and is encased in a layer of **perirenal** (per-ih-**REE**-nal) **fat**, held in place by a thin membrane called the **renal fascia** (**REE**-nal **FASH**-ee-ah). These coverings prevent movement. The indented medial region of the kidney is called the **hilum** (**HIGH**-lum), the area of entry and exit for nerves, the renal artery, and the renal vein.

FIGURE 16-1
Anatomy of the urinary system

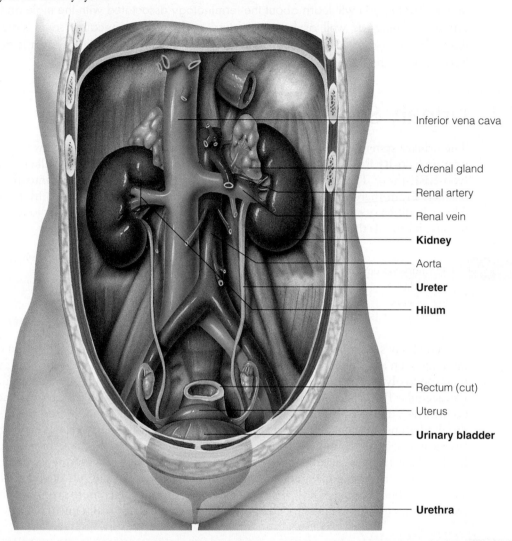

Inferior vena cava

Adrenal gland

Renal artery

Renal vein

Kidney

Aorta

Ureter

Hilum

Rectum (cut)

Uterus

Urinary bladder

Urethra

Memory Key	• The kidneys lie retroperitoneally on each side of the lumbar area.
	• The outer covering of the kidney is the renal capsule, covered by perirenal fat and the renal fascia.
	• The nerves, renal artery, and renal vein enter and exit at the hilum.

The internal structure of the kidney is illustrated in Figure 16-2. Underlying the renal capsule is a layer called the **cortex** (**KOR**-tecks). Extensions of the cortex called **renal columns** lie between the **renal pyramids**, which are pyramid-shaped structures constituting the next layer, the **renal medulla** (meh-**DULL**-lah). The tip of each renal pyramid is called the **renal papilla** (pah-**PILL**-ah). This structure secretes urine into a small cavity called a **minor calyx** (**KAL**-icks) (pl. **calyces**). From there, the urine drains into larger cavities called **major calyces** (**KAL**-ih-sees), and then into ducts leading to the **renal pelvis**, which is the dilated, proximal portion of the ureter.

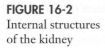

FIGURE 16-2
Internal structures
of the kidney

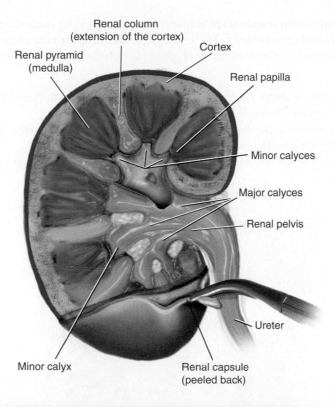

Renal column
(extension of the cortex)

Cortex

Renal pyramid
(medulla)

Renal papilla

Minor calyces

Major calyces

Renal pelvis

Ureter

Minor calyx

Renal capsule
(peeled back)

Memory Key
- Under the renal capsule is the cortex, which projects inward in columns.
- Between the columns are the renal pyramids of the renal medulla, tipped with renal papilla, which drain urine into minor calyces.
- The urine then flows into the major calyces and then drains through ducts into the renal pelvis.

THE URETERS, URINARY BLADDER, AND URETHRA

The ureters are long, narrow tubes connecting the kidney to the bladder. Urine is moved along each ureter by peristalsis (per-ih-**STAL**-sis), the same type of muscle contraction that moves food through the digestive tract. The ureters empty into an expandable sac called the **urinary bladder,** which, along with associated structures, is illustrated in Figure 16-3. Note the **trigone** (**TRI**-gohn) area of the bladder, defined by the triangle formed by the two ureteral openings and the opening into the urethra.

The urethra is the tube that carries urine out of the body from the urinary bladder. The external opening of the urethra is called the urethral **meatus** (**MEE**-ah-tus) or orifice (Figure 16-1). In females, the urethra is 1.6 inches (4.1 cm) long. In males, the urethra is 7.9 inches (20 cm) long. It runs along the length of the penis and also serves as part of the reproductive tract for the transport of semen. The first 1.6 inches (4 cm) of the male urethra passes through the prostate gland (Figure 16-3).

When sufficient urine has collected in the bladder, muscle fibers in the wall of the bladder contract, causing urine to pass into the urethra. This is called urination or micturition (**mick**-too-**RISH**-un). For urination to take place, two sphincter muscles must be relaxed.

The **internal urethral sphincter** is found where the bladder joins the urethra (Figure 16-3) and is controlled involuntarily. The **external urethral sphincter** surrounds the urethra distal to the internal urethral sphincter (Figure 16-3) and can be controlled voluntarily.

Memory Key • Urine empties from the renal pelvis of each kidney into the ureters and is pushed along by peristalsis to the trigone of the urinary bladder.
• Muscle contraction pushes the urine out of the bladder into the urethra, from which it is voided from the body.

FIGURE 16-3
Ureters, urinary bladder,
and urethra

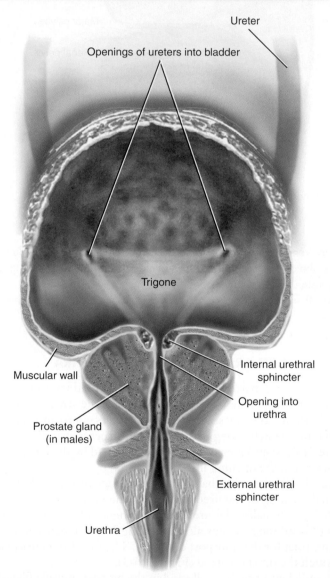

URINE PRODUCTION IN THE KIDNEY

Within each kidney are approximately one million nephrons (Figure 16-4). These tiny structures are responsible for producing urine. In very general terms, they do so by filtering out excess electrolytes and waste products from the blood. Filtration of the blood occurs in a network of capillaries known as glomerular capillaries. Each cluster of glomerular capillaries is called a **glomerulus** (gloh-**MER**-yoo-lus). The walls of these capillaries allow

FIGURE 16-4

(A) Kidney, ureters, and bladder; (B) the nephron includes the glomerulus, Bowman's capsule, and renal tubule. The renal tubule itself includes: the proximal convoluted tubule, Henle's loop, and the distal convoluted tubule. Note the capillary net surrounding the renal tubule.

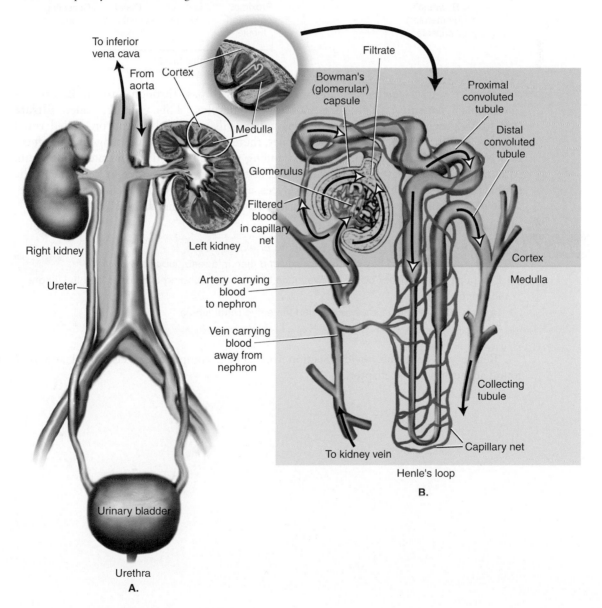

FIGURE 16-5

Exchange of substances between nephron and blood

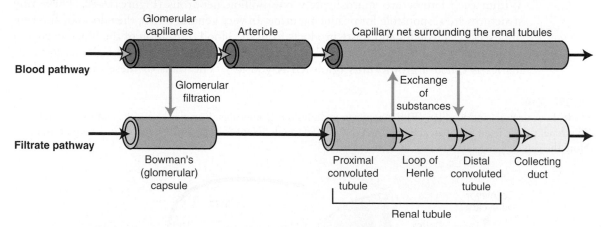

a mixture of water, electrolytes, and waste products to pass through into the **Bowman's** (glomerular) **capsule**, which surrounds the glomerulus. This mixture, called **filtrate** (**FIL**-trayt), then flows into long twisting tubes, still part of the nephron, called **renal tubules**. As filtrate travels along renal tubules, there is a continuous exchange of substances between the blood in the capillaries surrounding the tubules and the filtrate inside them. After the filtrate has traveled its entire course, urine is left, which is then excreted out of the nephron into collecting ducts, onto the calyces, and into the ureters. Figure 16-5 is a schematic drawing of the nephron and capillaries surrounding the nephron.

Memory Key
• Blood is filtered in the glomerular capillaries or glomerulus.
• The filtrate passes into Bowman's capsules and then into renal tubules.
• Exchange of substances occurs between the blood in surrounding capillaries and the filtrate in the renal tubules.
• Urine is left after the filtrate has traveled the entire renal tubule.

Before you continue, review Section 16.1. Then, complete Exercises 16-1 and 16-2 found at the end of the chapter.

16.2   Additional Word Parts

The following roots, suffixes, and prefix will also be used in this chapter to build medical terms.

Root	Meaning
bacteri/o	bacteria
crypt/o	hidden
noct/o	night
protein/o	protein
spermat/o	sperm

Suffix	Meaning
-cidal	to kill
-continence	to stop

Prefix	Meaning
trans-	through; across

16.3   Term Analysis and Definition Pertaining to the Urinary System

ROOTS

	calic/o; calyc/o	calix; calyx
Term	**Term Analysis**	**Definition**
caliceal (calyceal) (**kal**-ih-**SEE**-al)	-eal = pertaining to	pertaining to the calyces (calices)
caliectasis (calyectasis) (**kal**-ee-**ECK**-tah-sis)	-ectasis = dilation; stretching	dilation of the calyx

Term	catheter/o Term Analysis	something inserted Definition
catheterization (**kath**-eh-ter-eye-**ZAY**-shun)	-ion = process	the process of inserting a flexible tube into a body cavity, such as the urinary tract, for the purpose of removing fluid
	corpor/o	**body**
extracorporeal (**ecks**-trah-kor-**POR**-ee-al)	-eal = pertaining to extra- = outside	pertaining to outside the body
	cortic/o	**cortex; outer layer**
cortical (**KOR**-tih-kal)	-al = pertaining to	pertaining to the cortex or outer layer of the kidney
	cyst/o	**bladder**
cystitis (sis-**TYE**-tis)	-itis = inflammation	inflammation of the bladder
cystoscope (**SIS**-toh-skope)	-scope = instrument used to visually examine	instrument used to visually examine the bladder
cystoscopy (sis-**TOS**-koh-pee)	-scopy = process of visual examination	process of visually examining the bladder (Figure 16-6)
	glomerul/o	**glomerulus**
glomerulonephritis (glow-**mer**-yoo-low-neh-**FRY**-tis)	-itis = inflammation **nephr/o** = kidney	inflammation of the glomeruli of the kidney
glomerulosclerosis (gloh-**mer**-yoo-loh-skleh-**ROH**-sis)	-sclerosis = hardening	hardening of the glomerulus
	lith/o	**stone**
lithotripsy (**LITH**-oh-**trip**-see)	-tripsy = crushing	surgical crushing of kidney stones *NOTE*: A procedure such as **extracorporeal shock wave lithotripsy** (ESWL) utilizes ultrasound to break up the stones into small pieces, that are then transported out of the body in urine (Figure 16-7).

FIGURE 16-6
Cystoscopy

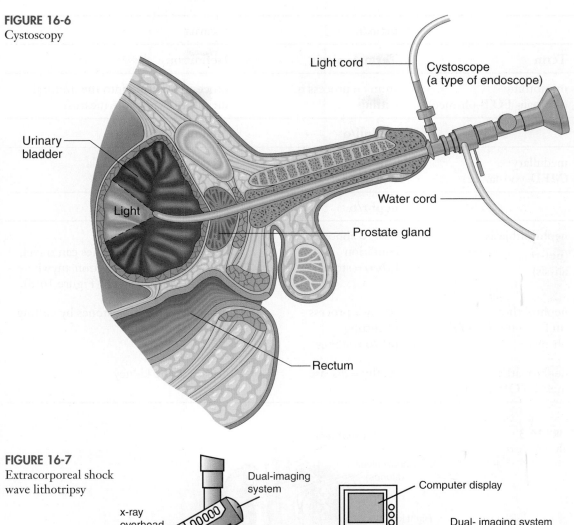

Light cord

Cystoscope
(a type of endoscope)

Urinary
bladder

Light

Water cord

Prostate gland

Rectum

FIGURE 16-7
Extracorporeal shock
wave lithotripsy

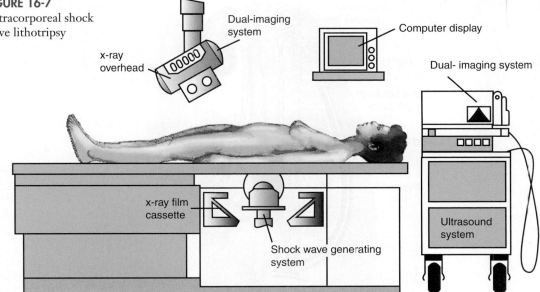

Dual-imaging
system

x-ray
overhead

Computer display

Dual- imaging system

x-ray film
cassette

Shock wave generating
system

Ultrasound
system

	meat/o	meatus
Term	**Term Analysis**	**Definition**
meatotomy (**mee**-ah-**TOT**-oh-mee)	-tomy = process of cutting	process of cutting into the urethral meatus (to widen the meatus)
	medull/o	**medulla**
medullary (**MED**-yoo-lar-ee)	-ary = pertaining to	pertaining to the medulla
	nephr/o	**kidney**
nephrolithiasis (**nef**-roh-lih-**THIGH**-ah-sis)	-iasis = abnormal condition **lith/o** = stones	kidney stones *NOTE:* The kidney stones can travel, causing urinary obstruction anywhere along the urinary tract (Figure 16-8).
nephrolithotomy (**nef**-roh-lih-**THOT**-oh-mee)	-tomy = process of cutting **lith/o** = stones	process of removing stones by cutting into the kidney
nephropathy (neh-**FROP**-ah-thee)	-pathy = disease	disease of the kidney

FIGURE 16-8
Nephrolithiasis

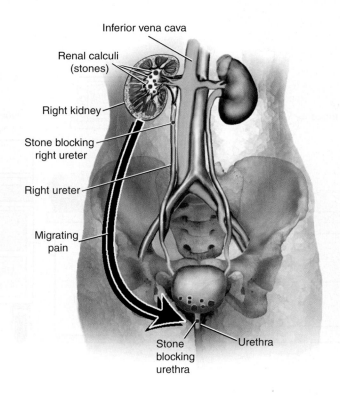

Inferior vena cava

Renal calculi (stones)

Right kidney

Stone blocking right ureter

Right ureter

Migrating pain

Stone blocking urethra

Urethra

Term	Term Analysis	Definition
nephropexy (**NEF**-roh-**peck**-see)	-pexy = surgical fixation	surgical fixation of the kidney
nephroptosis (**nef**-rop-**TOH**-sis)	-ptosis = drooping; prolapse; sagging	drooping kidney
nephrotomography (**nef**-roh-toh-**MOG**-rah-fee)	-graphy = process of recording; producing images **tom/o** = cut	procedure that utilizes x-rays to show the renal tissue at various depths. *NOTE:* Tomography gives different "cuts" or views of the kidney.
hydronephrosis (**high**-droh-neh-**FROH**-sis)	-osis = abnormal condition **hydr/o** = water	accumulation of fluid in the renal pelvis due to the obstruction of the normal urinary pathway (Figure 16-9)

FIGURE 6-9
Hydronephrosis

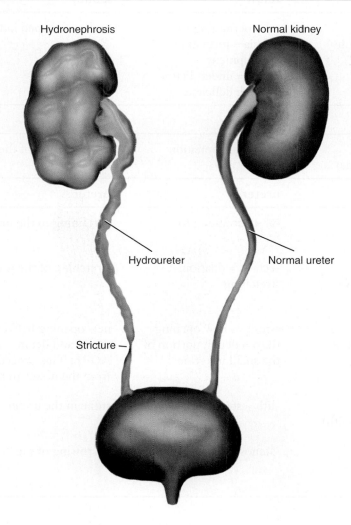

Term	Term Analysis	Definition
nephroblastoma (**nef**-roh-blas-**TOH**-mah)	-oma = tumor; mass -blast = immature; a growing thing	malignant tumor of the kidney, usually occurring in children; also known as Wilm's tumor
	pyel/o	**renal pelvis (dilated upper portion of ureter)**
pyelogram (**PYE**-eh-loh-gram)	-gram = record	record of the ureters and kidneys, particularly the renal pelvis
pyelonephritis (pye-eh-loh-neh-**FRY**-tis)	-itis = inflammation **nephr/o** = kidney	inflammation of the renal pelvis and kidney
	ren/o	**kidney**
renal hypoplasia (**REE**-nal **high**-poh-**PLAY**-zee-ah)	-al = pertaining to -plasia = formation; development hypo- = under; below normal; deficient	underdeveloped kidney
	trigon/o	**trigone**
trigonitis (**trig**-oh-**NIGH**-tis)	-itis = inflammation	inflammation of the trigone
	ureter/o	**ureter**
ureteral (yoo-**REE**-ter-al)	-al = pertaining to	pertaining to the ureter
ureterectasis (yoo-**ree**-ter-**ECK**-tah-sis)	-ectasis = dilation; stretching	stretching of the ureters
ureteroileostomy (yoo-**ree**-ter-oh-**il**-ee-**OS**-toh-mee)	-stomy = new opening **ile/o** = ileum; portion of the small intestine	new opening between the ureter and ileum *NOTE:* This procedure diverts urine from the ureter to the ileum.
ureterolith (yoo-**REE**-ter-oh-lith)	-lith = stone	stone in the ureter
ureterostenosis (yoo-**ree**-ter-oh-steh-**NOH**-sis)	-stenosis = narrowing	narrowing of the ureter

	urethr/o	**urethra**
Term	**Term Analysis**	**Definition**
cystourethrography (**sis**-toh-yoo-ree-**THROG**-rah-fee)	-graphy = process of recording; producing images **cyst/o** = bladder	process of producing an image of the bladder and urethra using x-rays. If this procedure is performed as the patient is discharging urine, it is called a **voiding** cystourethrography (VCUG).
transurethral (**trans**-yoo-**REE**-thral)	-al = pertaining to trans- = across; through	pertaining to through the urethra
urethrorrhagia (yoo-**ree**-throh-**RAY**-jee-ah)	-rrhagia = bursting forth; hemorrhage	hemorrhaging from the urethra
urethroplasty (yoo-**REE**-throh-**plas**-tee)	-plasty = surgical repair; surgical reconstruction	surgical repair of the urethra
	urin/o	**urine**
urinary (**YOO**-rih-**nar**-ee)	-ary = pertaining to	pertaining to urine
	ur/o	**urinary tract; urine; urination**
uremia (you-**REE**-mee-ah)	-emia = blood condition	accumulation of waste products in the blood due to loss of kidney function; azotemia
urogram (**YOO**-roh-gram)	-gram = record	record of the urinary tract *NOTE:* One type of urogram is (a) **excretory urogram**, an x-ray examination of the urinary tract following injection of a contrast medium into a vein, also known as intravenous urogram (IVU), or intravenous pyelogram (IVP). In Figure 16-10, note the kidneys and ureters as seen on an excretory urogram. Another type of urogram is (b) **retrograde urogram**, in which a contrast medium is injected into the ureters through a cystoscope and allowed to flow backward, highlighting the urinary structures; also known as retrograde pyelogram.

FIGURE 16-10
Excretory urogram

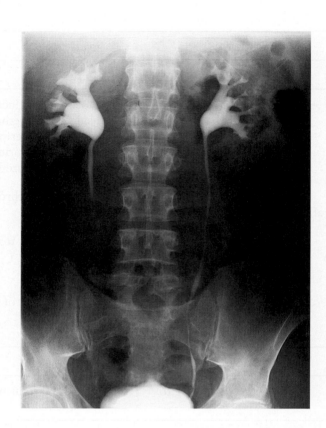

Term	Term Analysis	Definition
urologist (yoo-**ROL**-oh-jist)	-logist = specialist	specialist in the study of the urinary system in females and the urinary and reproductive systems in males
	vesic/o	**bladder**
vesicosigmoidostomy (**ves**-ih-koh-**sig**-moi-**DOS**-toh-mee)	-stomy = new opening	new opening between bladder and sigmoid colon
vesicoureteral reflux (**ves**-ih-koh-yoo-**REE**-ter-al **REE**-flucks)	-al = pertaining to **ureter/o** = ureter -flux = flow re- = back	backward flow of urine from bladder to ureter

SUFFIXES

	-lysis	separate; breakdown; destruction
Term	**Term Analysis**	**Definition**
dialysis (dye-**AL**-ih-sis)	dia- = through; complete	mechanical replacement of kidney function when the kidney is dysfunctional *NOTE:* Types include: hemodialysis (HD), in which the blood is passed through a kidney machine for waste removal; and peritoneal dialysis (PD), in which fluid is injected into the peritoneal cavity. Wastes flow out of the blood into the fluid, and the fluid is removed (see Figures 16-11 and 16-12).
	urin/o	**urine**
urinalysis (**yoo**-rih-**NAL**-ih-sis)	-lysis = breakdown; separate; destruction ana- = apart	laboratory analysis of urine *NOTE:* A urinalysis is one of the most common tests performed to evaluate the general health of a person. The urine is analyzed for the presence of such elements as albumin (a protein), bacteria, bilirubin, blood, ketones, glucose, pus, white blood cells, and casts (clumps of cellular matter that have formed as if in a mold). The color, pH (balance between acids and bases), and specific gravity (the amount of wastes, minerals, and other substances) are also noted in urine.
	-uria	**urine; urination**
anuria (ah-**NOO**-ree-ah)	an- = no; not; lack of	no urine formation; also known as suppression
bacteriuria (back-**teer**-ee-**YOO**-ree-ah)	**bacteri/o** = bacteria	bacteria in the urine
dysuria (dis-**YOO**-ree-ah)	dys- = painful; difficult; bad	painful urination
hematuria (**hem**-ah-**TOO**-ree-ah)	**hemat/o** = blood	blood in the urine

Term	Term Analysis	Definition
nocturia (nock-**TOO**-ree-ah)	**noct/o** = night	frequent urination at night
oliguria (**ol**-ih-**GOO**-ree-ah)	oligo- = deficient; few; scanty	decreased urination
proteinuria (**pro**-teen-**YOO**-ree-ah)	**protein/o** = protein	excessive amounts of protein in the urine; albuminuria
pyuria (pye-**YOO**-ree-ah)	**py/o** = pus	pus in the urine

PREFIXES

	in-	no; not
Term	**Term Analysis**	**Definition**
incontinence (in-**KON**-tih-nens)	-continence = to stop	no control of excretory functions such as urination
	poly-	**many**
polyuria (**pol**-ee-**YOO**-ree-ah)	-uria = urine; urination	excretion of large amounts of urine
polycystic kidneys (**pol**-ee-**SIS**-tick)	-ic = pertaining to **cyst/o** = sac; cysts	kidney with many cysts *NOTE:* Cysts are cavities or sacs filled with fluid, semifluid, or solid.

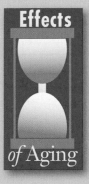

Effects *of Aging*

The kidneys slowly become smaller and less efficient as we age. The ability to filtrate waste products is impaired by a reduction in the number of glomeruli. More water might be excreted, leading to dehydration. Reabsorption of nutrients and electrolytes decreases. Usually, however, these changes do not significantly affect health due to the overcapacity of the kidneys. The impaired inability to filter does lead to increased sensitivity to medication, requiring dosage adjustment with increasing age.

Controlling urination becomes more difficult because of changes in the urinary tract. The bladder shrinks and its muscles weaken, causing more frequent urination and decreased ability to empty the bladder. The urinary sphincter muscle also weakens, causing impaired ability to delay urination when the urge to urinate is felt. This can ultimately result in urinary incontinence, which is an inability to control urination.

16.4 Common Diseases of the Urinary System

RENAL FAILURE

Renal failure is loss of kidney function. It can be acute (sudden onset), chronic (gradual onset), or end-stage renal disease (ESRD).

Acute Renal Failure

In acute renal failure (ARF), over a period of hours to days, the kidneys are unable to filter waste products from the blood, and the amount of urine excreted is decreased (oliguria). Without adequate filtration, the waste products build up in the blood and death occurs because of uremia. Acute renal failure is reversible.

There are many causes of acute renal failure. The most common is an inadequate blood flow to the kidneys. This can be caused by severe hemorrhaging or shock (reduced blood pressure). Fluid replacement to increase blood pressure and maintain normal fluid balance is vital for survival.

Chronic Renal Failure

Chronic renal failure (CRF) can become irreversible renal failure. This condition usually develops over a long period of time. Chronic diseases such as polycystic kidneys, diabetes, and hypertension damage the renal tissue, resulting in loss of renal function. Waste products are not filtered, resulting in uremia and death.

End-stage Renal Disease

The final stage of renal failure is called end-stage renal disease. At this point, the kidneys function at less than 10% of their normal capacity. They cannot filter blood or its waste products. The result is uremia and, without treatment, death.

Renal dialysis is a procedure that replaces normal kidney function when kidney failure prevents the kidney from filtering substances from the blood. Two common types of dialysis are **hemodialysis** (HD) and ambulatory **peritoneal dialysis** (PD).

In hemodialysis, the blood is passed through an artificial kidney machine that filters unwanted material from the blood. The blood is then returned to the body (Figure 16-11).

In peritoneal dialysis, a solution is placed in the abdominal cavity through a small tube (Figure 16-12). Over time, the solution draws the waste products from the blood. The fluid is drained through a catheter (flexible tube) to the outside of the body. Peritoneal dialysis can be performed continuously throughout the day, or at night while the patient sleeps.

There is no cure for CRF or ESRD. Renal dialysis and kidney transplants might be necessary.

VOIDING DISORDERS

Urinary Incontinence

Urinary incontinence (in-**KON**-tih-nens) is involuntary (no control) outflow of urine. **Stress incontinence** occurs when there is pressure on the bladder from coughing or laughing. **Urge incontinence** is the inability to stop the flow of urine once the urge has been felt.

FIGURE 16-11
Hemodialysis

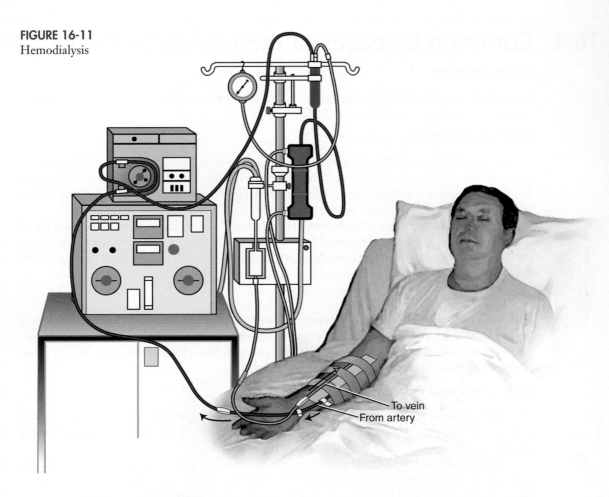

To vein
From artery

Urinary Retention

Urinary retention is inability of the bladder to empty completely during urination. The kidney continues to produce urine.

In men, a common cause of urinary retention is an enlarged prostate. It squeezes on the urethra, restricting the flow of urine. In women, pressure against the urethra from a displaced rectum can cause urinary retention. Other causes include spinal cord injuries and neurological diseases.

If urine must be removed from the bladder before an effective treatment has been established, catheterization is performed.

FIGURE 16-12
Peritoneal dialysis

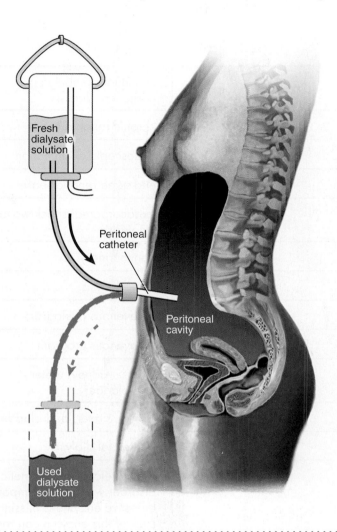

16.5   Abbreviations Pertaining to the Urinary System

Abbreviation	Meaning
ARF	acute renal failure
BUN	blood urea nitrogen (test that measures amount of urea nitrogen, a waste product, in the blood; increased amounts indicate glomerular dysfunction)

continued on page 21

continued from page 20

CAPD	continuous ambulatory peritoneal dialysis
CRF	chronic renal failure
cysto	cystoscopic examination
ESRD	end-stage renal disease
ESWL	extracorporeal shock wave lithotripsy
GU	genitourinary
HD	hemodialysis
IVP	intravenous pyelogram
IVU	intravenous urogram
KKUB	kidney, kidney, ureter, and bladder
KUB	kidney, ureter, and bladder
PD	peritoneal dialysis
PKU	phenylketonuria (A genetic disorder whereby an important digestive enzyme is missing. Lack of this enzyme can result in mental retardation if not treated promptly.)
QNS	quantity not sufficient
RP	retrograde pyelogram
UA	urinalysis
UTI	urinary tract infection
VCUG	voiding cystourethrography

16.6   Male Reproductive System

The kidneys can be thought of as manufacturing centers for the product urine. The urinary tract is the distribution network. The male reproductive system can be viewed in a similar way. The **testes** (**TEST**-tees), or **testicles** (**TEST**-ick-els), are the manufacturing centers for the product **sperm**, and the **reproductive tract** is the distribution network. The other components are the **accessory reproductive organs** and the **external genitalia**, all illustrated in Figure 16-13.

Memory Key	The male reproductive system consists of the:
	testes accessory reproductive organs
	reproductive tract external genitalia

FIGURE 16-13
Anatomy of the male reproductive system

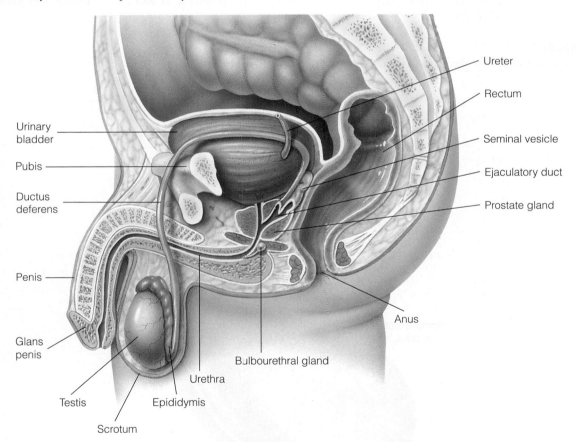

The testes are located in an external skin sac called the **scrotum** (**SKROH**-tum). Sperm production is called **spermatogenesis** (**sper**-mah-toh-jen-**EE**-sis) and takes place within tiny tubes inside the testes called **seminiferous tubules** (Figure 16-14). **Interstitial (Leydig) cells** in the testes produce the hormone **testosterone** (tes-**TOS**-ter-own), which is essential for spermatogenesis and the development of secondary male gender characteristics such as facial hair and pubescent voice change.

Memory Key	• The testes lie in the scrotum.
	• Sperm production (spermatogenesis) takes place in seminiferous tubules in the testes.
	• The sex hormone testosterone is produced in interstitial cells in the testes.

The reproductive tract begins with the **epididymis** (**ep**-ih-**DID**-ih-mis), a coiled tube on the superior surface of each testicle. The epididymis stores sperm and leads into a duct called the **ductus deferens** or **vas deferens** (vas-**DEF**-er-enz), which circles the urinary bladder and joins a duct from the **seminal vesicle** (**SEM**-ih-nal **VES**-ih-kal) to form the **ejaculatory duct**. This duct leads through the **prostate** (**PROS**-tayt) **gland** and joins the urethra.

FIGURE 16-14
Internal structures of the testes. The path sperm travels is indicated by the arrow.

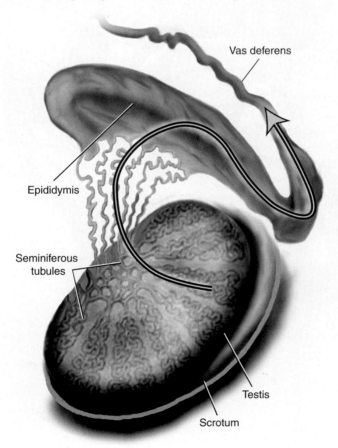

Vas deferens

Epididymis

Seminiferous tubules

Testis

Scrotum

| Memory Key | The reproductive tract starts at the epididymis, and then continues to the ductus (vas) deferens, where it joins the seminal vesicle to form the ejaculatory duct, and then continues through the prostate gland to join the urethra. |

The accessory organs are the **seminal vesicles**, **prostate**, and **bulbourethral** (**bul-boh-you-REE**-thral), or **Cowper's glands**. These glands secrete substances that together form the fluid in which sperm is ejaculated, called **semen**. This substance nourishes and protects sperm.

| Memory Key | The accessory organs are the seminal vesicles, prostate, and bulbourethral (Cowper's) glands, which together secrete semen. |

The scrotum and the penis are the external genitalia. The tip of the penis is called the **glans penis** (glanz **PEE**-nis), which contains the opening for urination and ejaculation, the **urethral orifice**, also called the urinary **meatus**. The glans is covered with loose skin called **foreskin** or **prepuce** (**PRE**-pyoos), which is often removed by a surgical process called **circumcision** (ser-kum-**SIZH**-un).

| Memory Key | • The external genitalia includes the penis and scrotum.
• The glans penis is the tip of the penis.
• The meatus is the urethral opening.
• The prepuce is excess skin covering the glans penis. |

Before you continue, review Section 16.6. Then, complete Exercise 16-3 found at the end of the chapter.

16.7 Term Analysis and Definition Pertaining to the Male Reproductive System

ROOTS

	andr/o	male
Term	**Term Analysis**	**Definition**
androgenic (**an**-droh-**JEN**-ick)	-genic = producing	producing masculinizing effects
	balan/o	**glans penis**
balanitis (**bal**-ah-**NIGH**-tis)	-itis = inflammation	inflammation of the glans penis

Term	Term Analysis	Definition
balanorrhea (**bal**-an-oh-**REE**-ah)	-rrhea = flow; discharge	discharge from the glans penis
	epididym/o	**epididymis**
epididymitis (**ep**-ih-did-ih-**MY**-tis)	-itis = inflammation	inflammation of the epididymis
	orchid/o; orchi/o	**testicle; testis**
cryptorchidism (krip-**TOR**-kih-**diz**-um)	-ism = process **crypt/o** = hidden	undescended testicles *NOTE:* During fetal development, the testicles fail to descend into the scrotum, remaining instead in the abdominal cavity. This condition can result in sterility if not treated.
orchidopexy (**OR**-kid-oh-**peck**-see)	-pexy = surgical fixation	surgical fixation of the testicle onto the scrotum *NOTE:* A treatment for cryptorchidism.
orchitis (or-**KYE**-tis)	-itis = inflammation	inflammation of the testicle
	prostat/o	**prostate**
prostatitis (**pros**-tah-**TYE**-tis)	-itis = inflammation	inflammation of the prostate *NOTE:* Do not confuse prostate with prostrate (**PROS**-trayt) meaning stretched out with face on the ground.
prostatectomy (**pros**-tah-**TECK**-toh-mee)	-ectomy = excision; surgical removal	excision of the prostate
	sperm/o; spermat/o	**spermatozoa; sperm**
aspermatogenesis (ay-**sper**-mah-toh-**JEN**-eh-sis)	-genesis = production; formation a- = no; not; lack of	no production of spermatozoa *NOTE:* Singular of spermatozoa is spermatozoon.
oligospermia (**ol**-ih-goh-**SPER**-mee-ah)	oligo- = deficient; scanty; few	deficient number of spermatozoa

Term	Term Analysis	Definition
spermatic cord (sper-**MAT**-ick)	-ic = pertaining to cord = a long, rounded, slender structure	structure extending from the inguinal canal to the testis, containing blood vessels, nerves, and vas deferens, enclosed by a fibrous covering
spermatocidal (**sper**-mah-toh-**SYE**-dal)	-cidal = to kill	to kill or destroy spermatozoa; spermicidal
	testicul/o	**testicle; testis**
testicular (tes-**TICK**-yoo-lar)	-ar = pertaining to	pertaining to the testicle
	vas/o	**vas deferens**
vasectomy (vah-**SECK**-toh-mee)	-ectomy = excision; surgical removal	excision of the vas deferens or a portion of it (Figure 16-15)

SUFFIXES

	-cele	**hernia**
Term	Term Analysis	Definition
hematocele (**HEE**-mah-toh-**seel**)	**hemat/o** = blood	accumulation of blood around the testicles
hydrocele (**HIGH**-droh-seel)	**hydr/o** = water	accumulation of fluid around the testicles (Figure 16-16)
spermatocele (**SPER**-mah-toh-**seel**)	**spermat/o** = sperm	accumulation of a milky fluid in the testicles or epididymis

FIGURE 16-15
Vasectomy

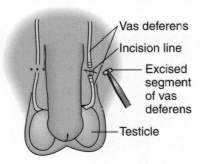

FIGURE 16-16
Hydrocele

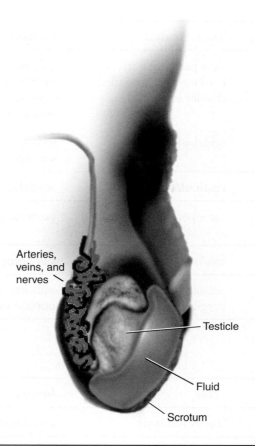

Arteries, veins, and nerves

Testicle

Fluid

Scrotum

Term	Term Analysis	Definition
varicocele (**VAR**-ih-koh-**seel**)	**varic/o** = varicose veins; dilated, twisted veins	dilatation of testicular veins inside the scrotum (Figure 16-17)
	-potence	**power**
impotence (**IM**-poh-tens)	in(m) = no; not	inability to achieve and maintain an erection; erectile dysfunction

Memory Key -in changes to -im before word elements starting with *p.*

FIGURE 16-17
Varicocele

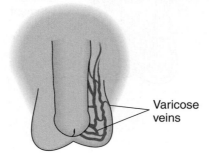

Varicose veins

	–spadias	opening; tear
Term	**Term Analysis**	**Definition**
epispadias (**ep**-ih-**SPAY**-dee-as)	epi- = on; upon; above	congenital opening of the meatus on the dorsum (top side) of the penis (Figure 16-18)
hypospadias (**high**-poh-**SPAY**-dee-as)	hypo- = under	congenital opening of the meatus on the ventral (underside) of the penis (Figure 16-19)

PREFIXES

	circum-	around
Term	**Term Analysis**	**Definition**
circumcision (**ser**-kum-**SIZH**-un)	-ion = process **cis/o** = to cut	removal of the prepuce or foreskin

FIGURE 16-18
Epispadias

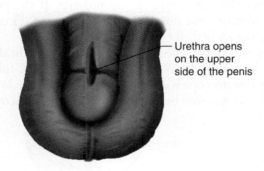

Urethra opens on the upper side of the penis

FIGURE 16-19
Hypospadias

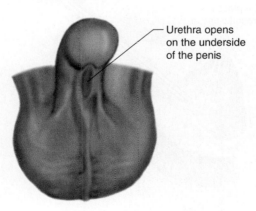

Urethra opens on the underside of the penis

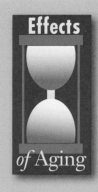

Aging affects the reproductive system, but less significantly in males than in females. Fertility remains in males, although sperm levels decrease. A reduction in testosterone levels might reduce sex drive. The prostate might enlarge, impeding urinary elimination. Erectile dysfunction, also is much more common.

16.8   Common Diseases of the Male Reproductive System

BENIGN PROSTATIC HYPERPLASIA

Benign prostatic hyperplasia (BPH) is a non-cancerous enlargement of the prostate. The male urethra goes through a hole in the prostate. If the prostate enlarges, it squeezes the urethra and obstructs the flow of urine. This causes urinary retention. This condition more commonly occurs in men over 50 years of age.

   If surgery is necessary, a procedure called **transurethral resection of the prostate (TURP)** might be performed. A resectoscope (ree-**SECK**-toh-skohp) is inserted through the urethra. The resectoscope is equipped with a cystoscope to visualize the prostate. Some, but not all, of the prostate can be cut away with the resectoscope (Figure 16-20).

FIGURE 16-20
Transurethral resection

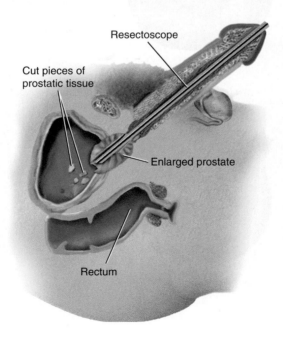

When larger prostates need to be excised, the surgery might involve a **prostatectomy** (**pros**-tah-**TECK**-tah-mee). With this operation, the chances of impotence and incontinence increase. The prostate is removed through a lower abdominal incision just above the pubic bone.

Several newer procedures to treat BPH have been developed using different forms of high-intensity heat, such as electrical currents to vaporize tissue. Lasers and microwave heat therapy are also used.

CANCER OF THE PROSTATE

Cancer of the prostate is a malignant tumor of the prostate that primarily affects men over 50.

A digital rectal examination (DRE) is useful in detecting early prostatic cancer. A normal prostate feels solid and smooth. A cancerous prostate is **indurated** (hard).

Prostatic-specific antigen (PSA) is a laboratory test that measures the level of PSA in the blood. PSA is a protein produced by the prostate gland. Although most PSA is removed from the body in semen, a small amount enters the bloodstream and can be measured. An elevated PSA might indicate prostatic cancer.

Radiation therapy, hormonal deprivation therapy, and prostatectomy are used to treat prostate cancer. Radiation therapy uses radioactive substances to irradicate cancer cells. Hormonal deprivation therapy includes the use of anti-androgen drugs to block the production of testosterone (an androgen), which normally stimulates the growth of prostatic cells.

16.9   Abbreviations Pertaining to the Male Reproductive System

Abbreviation	Meaning
BPH	benign prostatic hypertrophy
DRE	digital rectal exam
PSA	prostatic-specific antigen
TUR	transurethral resection
TURP	transurethral resection of the prostate

16.10 Putting It All Together

Exercise 16-1   MATCHING

Match the term in Column A with its definition in Column B.

Column A	Column B
_____ 1. renal medulla	A. filter blood
_____ 2. renal pelvis	B. triangular area of the bladder
_____ 3. trigone	C. innermost portion of the kidney
_____ 4. renal fascia	D. membrane surrounding the kidney
_____ 5. glomeruli	E. dilated, upper portion of the ureter

Exercise 16-2   SHORT ANSWER—URINARY SYSTEM

1. Name, in the proper sequence, the structures through which urine passes. Start at the kidney.

   _____

   _____

2. Name three electrolytes. Why are electrolytes important?

   _____

   _____

3. How does the kidney help maintain homeostasis?

   _____

   _____

Exercise 16-3   SHORT ANSWER—MALE REPRODUCTIVE SYSTEM

1. Name, in the proper sequence, the structures through which sperm passes. Start at the testicles.

   _____

   _____

2. Write one function of the following structures:

   a. epididymis _____

   b. accessory organs _____

   c. seminiferous tubules _____

   d. Leydig cells _____

Exercise 16-4   IDENTIFICATION

Write the suffix; root, and/or prefix for the following terms:

1. glans penis _____

2. calix _____

3. bladder _____

4. stone _____

5. kidney _____

6. testicle _____

7. renal pelvis _____

8. vas deferens _____

9. urine _____

10. urinary tract _____

11. hernia _____

12. opening; tear _____

13. around _____

14. outside _____

15. hardening _____

16. narrowing _____

17. crushing _____

18. process of cutting _____

19. abnormal condition _____

20. blood condition _____

21. surgical fixation _____

22. drooping _____

23. record _____

24. deficient; scanty _____

25. to kill _____

26. across _____

27. varicose vein _____

28. through; complete _____

29. night _____

30. disease _____

Exercise 16-5   BUILDING MEDICAL TERMS

Build the medical term for the following definitions:

1. pertaining to outside the body _____

2. instrument used to visually examine
   the bladder _____

3. crushing of stones _____

4. accumulation of fluid in the renal
   pelvis due to the obstruction of the
   normal urinary pathway _____

5. undescended testicles _____

6. deficient numbers of spermatozoa _____

7. hemorrhaging from the urethra _____

8. new opening between the bladder and
   sigmoid colon _____

9. new opening between the ureter
   and ileum _____

10. process of cutting into the
    urinary meatus _____

11. surgical repair of the urethra _____

Exercise 16-6   BUILDING TERMS

I. Use -cele to build terms for the following definitions:

1. accumulation of blood around
   the testicles _____

2. accumulation of fluid around
   the testicles _____

3. accumulation of a milky fluid in
   the testicles or epididymis _____

4. dilation of testicular veins inside
   the scrotum _____

II. Use -uria to build terms for the following definitions:

5. no urine formation _____

6. bacteria in the urine _____

7. painful urination _____

8. blood in the urine _____

9. frequent urination at night _____

10. decreased urination

    _____

11. excessive amounts of protein in
    the urine

    _____

12. pus in the urine

    _____

III. Use **nephr/o** to build terms for the following definitions:

13. kidney stones

    _____

14. process of removing stones by
    cutting into the kidney

    _____

15. disease of the kidney

    _____

16. surgical fixation of the kidney

    _____

17. drooping kidney

    _____

18. procedure that utilizes x-rays to
    show renal tissue at various depths

    _____

19. malignant tumor of the kidney,
    made up of undeveloped material

    _____

Exercise 16-7 IDENTIFICATION

Place an **X** beside the terms indicating a surgical or clinical procedure.

1. androgenic   _____

2. glomerulosclerosis   _____

3. lithotripsy   _____

4. nephrolithiasis   _____

5. nephrolithotomy   _____

6. cryptorchidism   _____

7. orchidopexy   _____

8. renal hypoplasia   _____

9. vasectomy   _____

10. cystourethrography   _____

11. urinary   _____

12. vesicoureteral reflux   _____

13. epispadias   _____

14. circumcision   _____

Exercise 16-8 ADJECTIVES

Write the adjective for the following terms.

1. cortex _____

2. calyx _____

3. glomerulus _____

4. testicle _____

5. ureter _____

6. urethra _____

Exercise 16-9 PLURALS

Write the plural for the following terms. Use the dictionary if necessary.

1. cortex _____

2. calix; calyx _____

3. epididymis _____

4. glomerulus _____

5. meatus _____

6. testis _____

7. kidney pelvis _____

8. testicle _____

9. spermatozoon _____

10. ureter _____

Exercise 16-10 SPELLING

Circle any misspelled words in the following list and correctly spell them in the space provided.

1. balanorhea _____

2. orchitis _____

3. cysitis _____

4. epididymus _____

5. caliseal _____

6. prostratectomy _____

7. trigonitis _____

8. ureterorrhagia _____

9. incontinance _____

10. extracorporeal _____

Exercise 16-11 PATHOLOGY

I. Match the treatment with the diseases listed. More than one treatment might be used for each condition.

catheterization

hemodialysis

hormonal deprivation therapy

peritoneal dialysis

prostatectomy

radiation therapy

transurethral resection of the prostate

1. benign prostatic hypertrophy _____

2. cancer of the prostate _____

3. chronic renal failure _____

4. urinary retention _____

II. Define the following:

1. indurated _____

_____

2. stress incontinence _____

_____

3. urge incontinence _____

_____

4. peritoneal dialysis _____

_____

III. Name one cause of the following diseases:

1. renal failure _____

2. urinary retention _____

16.11 Review of Vocabulary Pertaining to the Urinary System

In the following tables, the medical terms are organized into these categories: anatomy, pathology, diagnostics, and clinical and surgical procedures. Define each term and decide into which category the word belongs. This will help you associate the term with its purpose and help you remember its meaning.

TABLE 16-1

REVIEW OF ANATOMICAL TERMS PERTAINING TO THE URINARY SYSTEM

1. bladder	2. caliceal	3. cortical
4. extracorporeal	5. kidneys	6. medullary
7. nephron	8. renal pelvis	9. transurethral
10. ureteral	13. urethra	12. urinary

TABLE 16-2

REVIEW OF PATHOLOGIC TERMS PERTAINING TO THE URINARY SYSTEM

1. anuria	2. bacteriuria	3. caliectasis
4. cystitis	5. dysuria	6. glomerulonephritis
7. glomerulosclerosis	8. hematuria	9. hydronephrosis
10. incontinence	11. nephroblastoma	12. nephrolithiasis

continued on page 38

Table 16-2 *continued from page 37*

13. nephropathy	14. nephroptosis	15. nocturia
16. oliguria	17. polycystic kidneys	18. polyuria
19. proteinuria	20. pyelonephritis	21. pyuria
22. renal hypoplasia	23. trigonitis	24. uremia
25. ureterectasis	26. ureterolith	27. ureterostenosis
28. urethrorrhagia	29. vesicoureteral reflux	

TABLE 16-3

REVIEW OF DIAGNOSTIC TERMS PERTAINING TO THE URINARY SYSTEM

1. cystourethrography	2. nephrotomography	3. pyelogram
4. urinalysis	5. urogram	

TABLE 16-4

REVIEW OF CLINICAL AND SURGICAL PROCEDURES PERTAINING TO THE URINARY SYSTEM

1. catheterization	2. cystoscope	3. cystoscopy
4. dialysis	5. lithotripsy	6. meatotomy
7. nephrolithotomy	8. nephropexy	9. ureteroileostomy
10. urethroplasty	11. vesicosigmoidostomy	

16.12 Review of Vocabulary Pertaining to the Male Reproductive System

In the following tables, the medical terms are organized into these categories: anatomy, physiologic, pathology, and surgical procedures. Define each term and decide into which category the word belongs. This will help you associate the term with its purpose and help you remember its meaning.

TABLE 16-5

REVIEW OF ANATOMICAL AND PHYSIOLOGICAL TERMS PERTAINING TO THE MALE REPRODUCTIVE SYSTEM

1. androgenic	2. testes	3. Cowper's gland
4. semen	5. prepuce	6. vas deferens
7. seminiferous tubules	8. interstitial cells of Leydig	

TABLE 16-6

REVIEW OF PATHOLOGIC TERMS PERTAINING TO THE MALE REPRODUCTIVE SYSTEM

1. aspermatogenesis	2. balanitis	3. balanorrhea
4. benign prostatic hypertrophy	5. cryptorchidism	6. epididymitis
7. epispadias	8. hematocele	9. hydrocele
10. hypospadias	11. impotence	12. oligospermia
13. orchitis	14. prostatitis	15. spermatocele
16. spermatocidal	17. varicocele	

TABLE 16-7

REVIEW OF SURGICAL PROCEDURES PERTAINING TO THE MALE REPRODUCTIVE SYSTEM

1. circumcision	2. orchidopexy	3. prostatectomy
4. transurethral resection	5. vasectomy	

....

16.13 Medical Terms in Context

After you read the Diagnostic Imaging Report and the Operative Report, answer the questions that follow. Use your text, medical dictionary, or other references if necessary.

DIAGNOSTIC IMAGING REPORT

EXCRETORY UROGRAM WITH NEPHROTOMOGRAPHY: On the preliminary film, multiple surgical clips are present in the right upper quadrant, presumably related to previous cholecystectomy. There are also multiple surgical clips in the epigastric region. No organomegaly or radiopaque calculi are seen.

Following the intravenous injection of contrast media, there is prompt and equal excretion bilaterally. Renal outlines, calyces, and ureters are normal. Bladder is normal in size, shape, and position and empties normally.

IMPRESSION: NORMAL UPPER URINARY TRACT

OPERATIVE REPORT

OPERATION PERFORMED: Transurethral resection of prostate

PROCEDURE: After spinal anesthesia was achieved, the patient was placed in the lithotomy position. The lower abdomen was prepared and draped in the usual manner. A resectoscope was passed per urethra. Twenty grams of benign-appearing prostatic tissue was resected from the prostate. Following the resection, bleeding was well controlled, and a catheter was inserted per urethra.

DIAGNOSIS: BENIGN PROSTATIC HYPERPLASIA.

QUESTIONS ON THE DIAGNOSTIC IMAGING AND OPERATIVE REPORTS

Fill in the blanks with the most appropriate answer.

1. CT scan was done on the _____.

2. The organ that the preliminary film shows to have been previously removed is the _____.

3. Why is contrast medium given? _____

_____

4. The urogram showed normal excretion of the contrast medium on both sides. In the report, the medical word used to mean both sides is _____.

5. In the Diagnostic Imaging Report, a diagnosis of *normal upper urinary tract* was made by studying which structures? _____

_____

6. What is a resectoscope? _____

_____

7. Define resection. _____

_____

8. Following the transurethral resection of the prostate, how is the patient expected to urinate? _____

_____

9. Explain what is meant by transurethral resection. _____

_____

10. Define spinal anesthesia. _____

_____

17

CHAPTER

The Female Reproductive System and Obstetrics

CHAPTER ORGANIZATION

This chapter will help you learn about the female reproductive system and obstetrics. It is divided into the following sections:

17.1 Structures of the Female Reproductive System

17.2 Menstrual Cycle

17.3 Menopause

17.4 Additional Word Parts

17.5 Term Analysis and Definition Pertaining to the Female Reproductive System

17.6 Common Diseases of the Female Reproductive System

17.7 Abbreviations Pertaining to the Female Reproductive System

17.8 Obstetrics

17.9 Term Analysis and Definition Pertaining to Obstetrics

17.10 Common Obstetrical Conditions

17.11 Abbreviations Pertaining to Obstetrics

17.12 Putting It All Together

17.13 Review of Vocabulary Pertaining to the Female Reproductive System

17.14 Review of Vocabulary Pertaining to Obstetrics

17.15 Medical Terms in Context

CHAPTER OBJECTIVES

On completion of this chapter, you will be able to do the following:

1. Name, locate, and describe the structures of the female reproductive system

2. Describe the menstrual, ovulatory, and secretory periods

3. Describe the terms related to pregnancy and parturition

4. Analyze, define, pronounce, and spell common terms of the female reproductive system and obstetrics

5. Describe common diseases of gynecology and obstetrics

6. Define common abbreviations of the female reproductive system and obstetrics

INTRODUCTION

The female reproductive system consists of the **ovaries** (**OH**-vah-rees), the **uterus** (**YOO**-ter-us), the **uterine** or **fallopian** (fal-**LOH**-pee-an) **tubes**, the **vagina** (vah-**JIGH**-nah) the **external genitalia**, and the **mammary glands**. Figure 17-1 has two illustrations of these structures (except the mammary glands).

> **Memory Key**   The female reproductive system consists of ovaries, uterus, uterine (fallopian) tubes, vagina, external genitalia, and mammary glands.

....

17.1   Structures of the Female Reproductive System

THE OVARIES

The almond-shaped ovaries are glands. They are located in the pelvic cavity, one on each side of the uterus. They are held in place by ligaments (broad, ovarian, and suspensory) (Figure 17-1B). Their functions are to discharge the **egg** or **ovum** (pl. ova), and to produce various hormones. The ovaries of a newborn female contain a lifetime supply of immature eggs. Puberty brings on egg release. In approximately 28-day cycles, alternating from ovary to ovary, one egg is released. This process is called **ovulation** (ov-yoo-**LAY**-shun).

> **Memory Key**   The ovaries are glands that discharge ova and produce sex hormones. The process of egg release is called ovulation.

The ovaries regulate the menstrual cycle (discussed in the following) by the release of the sex hormones **estrogen** (**ES**-troh-jen) and **progesterone** (pro-**JES**-ter-ohn). Estrogen is important in the development of secondary female characteristics such as the breasts and pubic hair growth. Progesterone stimulates the growth of blood vessels in the uterus, which will be needed to supply blood if the egg is fertilized. The estrogen stimulates the thickening of the lining of the uterus to prepare for the implantation of a fertilized egg. If no fertilization takes place, this buildup of tissue is sloughed off in a process called **menstruation** (men-stroo-**AY**-shun) or **menses** (**MEN**-seez). Sometime between the ages of 45 and 55, all of the eggs either have been discharged or have degenerated. The reproductive cycle then ceases, and the woman is in **menopause** (**MEN**-oh-pawz), discussed in a following section.

> **Memory Key**   Stimulated by the hormones estrogen and progesterone, the lining of the uterus becomes thicker and more vascular to prepare for implantation of a fertilized egg. Menstruation follows if fertilization does not occur.

FIGURE 17-1

Structures of the female reproductive system: (A) female reproductive organs in relation to the urinary and digestive tracts; (B) uterus, ovaries, fallopian tubes, and related structures

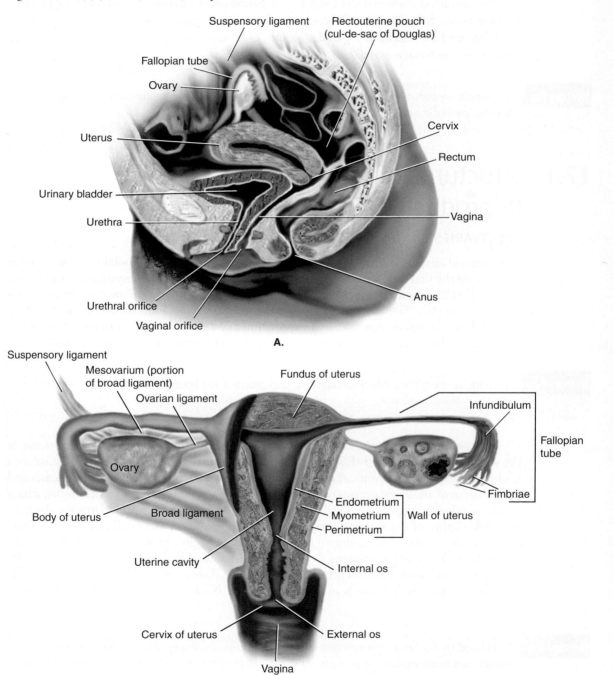

THE FALLOPIAN TUBES

The two fallopian tubes can be seen in Figure 17-1B. They link the ovaries and the uterus. The distal end of each tube is funnel-shaped and is called the **infundibulum** (**in**-fun-**DIB**-yoo-lum). It is equipped with tiny fingerlike projections called **fimbriae** (**FIM**-bree-ee), which sweep back and forth, creating waves in the fluid surrounding the ovary. This action pulls the ovum into the tube for transport to the uterus. If the ovum is fertilized, it begins to grow and is called a **zygote** (**ZYE**-goht). If it is not fertilized, it breaks down within 48 hours.

> **Memory Key**
> - The fallopian tubes link the ovaries and uterus.
> - Fingerlike fimbriae in the funnel-shaped distal end of the tubes create waves that pull the ovum into the tube and down to the uterus.
> - A fertilized egg is called a zygote.

THE UTERUS

The uterus is a muscular, thick-walled organ, hollow and shaped like an inverted pear. It is held in place in the pelvic cavity by ligaments. The superior, rounded portion is called the **fundus** (**FUN**-dus). The middle portion is the **body**. The inferior portion is the **cervix uteri** (**SER**-vicks **YOO**-ter-eye), which projects into the vagina. The superior and inferior openings of the cervix are called the **internal os** and the **external os**, respectively (Figure 17-1B). Lying between the uterus and the rectum is the lowest point of the abdominal cavity, the **rectouterine** (reck-toh-**YOO**-ter-in) **pouch**, also called the **cul-de-sac of Douglas** (Figure 17-1A). This is a gathering place for microorganisms and is therefore prone to an infection called **pelvic inflammatory disease** (PID).

> **Memory Key**
> - The uterus consists of the:
>   fundus
>   body
>   cervix uteri
> - The superior and inferior openings of the cervix are the internal os and the external os.

THE VAGINA

The vagina is a muscular tube leading from the cervix to the exterior. It is approximately 6-inches long and is lined with mucous membrane. The entrance to the vagina, the **introitus** (in-**TRO**-ih-tus) is covered by the hymen (**HIGH**-men), a fold of mucous membrane.

> **Memory Key**   The muscular vagina leads from the cervix to the exterior. The opening is the introitus.

THE EXTERNAL GENITALIA

The **external genitalia**, or **vulva** (**VUL**-vah), are illustrated in Figure 17-2. Included are the **clitoris** (**KLIT**-oh-ris), the **labia** (**LAY**-bee-a) **majora, labia minora, mons pubis**, and **Bartholin's** (**BAR**-toh-linz) **glands**, which secrete lubricant for intercourse. The area from the vulva to the anus is called the **perineum** (per-ih-**NEE**-um).

FIGURE 17-2
External genitalia

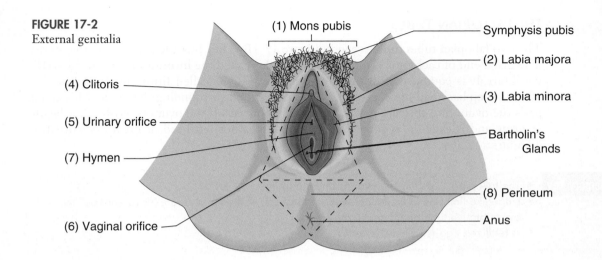

(1) Mons pubis

Symphysis pubis

(2) Labia majora

(4) Clitoris

(3) Labia minora

(5) Urinary orifice

Bartholin's
Glands

(7) Hymen

(8) Perineum

Anus

(6) Vaginal orifice

Memory Key
- The external genitalia consist of the:
  clitoris   mons pubis
  labia majora   Bartholin's glands
  labia minora
- The area from the vulva to the anus is the perineum.

THE BREASTS

Figure 17-3 illustrates the structures of the **breast** or mammary gland. The **nipple** is surrounded by a darker ring of skin called the **areola**. The mammary glands produce milk after childbirth. The milk is stored in **lactiferous** (lack-**TIF**-er-us) **sinuses** and travels through the **lactiferous ducts** to tiny openings in the nipple. Oils produced by glands in the areola help minimize drying out of the skin around the nipple due to breastfeeding.

Memory Key The breast includes:
  nipple
  areola
  lactiferous sinuses
  lactiferous ducts

FIGURE 17-3
Breast

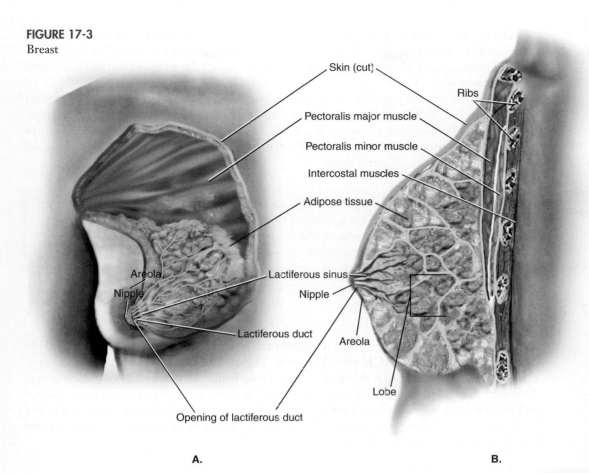

Skin (cut)

Ribs

Pectoralis major muscle

Pectoralis minor muscle

Intercostal muscles

Adipose tissue

Areola

Nipple

Lactiferous sinus

Nipple

Lactiferous duct

Areola

Lobe

Opening of lactiferous duct

A.   **B.**

17.2 Menstrual Cycle

The time of life when the **menstrual cycle** first begins is called **menarche** (men-**AR**-kee). It is continuous for approximately 40 years except during pregnancy. The average length of the menstrual cycle is 28 days and consists of three periods: the **menstrual period**, the **ovulatory period**, and the **secretory period**.

> **Memory Key**
> - Menarche is when the menstrual cycle first begins.
> - The menstrual cycle consists of the menstrual, ovulatory, and secretory periods.

The menstrual period lasts from 3 to 6 days. The endometrium (the inner lining of the uterus) has become thickened and more vascular, preparing itself for housing a fertilized egg. If pregnancy does not occur, the endometrium is unnecessary and is sloughed off along with blood cells in what is known as a **period**, **menses**, or **menstruation**.

During the ovulatory period, the egg is released from its sac and breaks free from the ovary into the abdominopelvic cavity, where it slowly makes its way to the uterine tubes. This event occurs at midcycle, approximately the fourteenth day of the cycle, and is referred to as **ovulation**.

During the secretory period, the hormones estrogen and progesterone from the ovaries are secreted into the bloodstream. They are responsible for the thickening and vascularization of the endometrium, preparing it for the fertilized egg. When pregnancy does not occur, these hormones decrease, and the endometrium is not maintained and is sloughed off. The menstrual period starts again.

Memory Key	• During the menstrual period, the thickened lining of the uterus is sloughed off. • During the ovulatory period, the egg travels to the uterine tubes. • During the secretory period, estrogen and progesterone are secreted, stimulating the endometrium to thicken and vascularize.

17.3 Menopause

Menopause is the complete stoppage of menses and is commonly known as the change of life or the **climacteric** (kli-**MACK**-ter-ick) period. The usual age of occurrence is 45–55 years. During this time, there is a decrease of hormones from the ovary, and ovulation stops. Although many women pass through this period without difficulty, a significant number will experience hot flashes (involuntary, sudden heat waves involving the chest, neck, and head) and vaginal changes as estrogen levels fall. A woman is in menopause when menses has been absent for at least 12 consecutive months.

Memory Key	Menopause is the complete stoppage of menses.

Before you continue, review Sections 17.1 to 17.3. Then, complete Exercise 17-1 found at the end of the chapter.

17.4 Additional Word Parts

The following roots, suffixes, and prefixes will also be used in this chapter to build medical terms.

Root	Meaning
men/o	menstruation; menses; month
tub/o	tube; fallopian tube
versi/o	tilting; turning; tipping

Suffix	Meaning
-an	pertaining to
-ine	pertaining to
-pause	stoppage; cessation

Prefix	Meaning
nulli-	none
oxy-	sharp
primi-	first
secundi-	second

17.5 Term Analysis and Definition Pertaining to the Female Reproductive System

ROOTS

	cervic/o	cervix; neck of uterus; cervix uteri
Term	**Term Analysis**	**Definition**
cervicitis (ser-vih-**SIGH**-tis)	-itis = inflammation	inflammation of the cervix
cervical polyp (**SER**-vih-kal **POL**-up)	-al = pertaining to polyp = protruding growth from the mucous membrane	growth extending from the mucous membrane of the cervix uteri into the uterine cavity (Figure 17-12)
	colp/o	**vagina**
colporrhaphy (kol-**POR**-ah-fee)	-rrhaphy = suture	suture of the vagina
colposcopy (kol-**POS**-ka-pee)	-scopy = process of visually examining	process of visually examining the vagina

	culd/o	cul-de-sac
Term	**Term Analysis**	**Definition**
culdocentesis (**kul**-doh-sen-**TEE**-sis)	-centesis = surgical puncture to remove fluid	surgical puncture to remove fluid from the cul-de-sac of Douglas
culdoscope (**KUL**-doh-skohp)	-scope = instrument used to visually examine	instrument used to visually examine the cul-de-sac of Douglas
	episi/o	**vulva; external genitalia; pudendum**
episiotomy (eh-**piz**-ee-**OT**-oh-mee)	-tomy = process of cutting	process of cutting the vulva, between the vagina and anus (perineum) *NOTE:* An episiotomy is used to assist delivery of the fetus by enlarging the vaginal opening.
episiorrhaphy (eh-**piz**-ee-**OR**-ah-fee)	-rrhaphy = suture	suturing the vulva and perineum
	fibr/o	**fibers; fibrous tissue**
uterine fibroid (**YOO**-ter-in **FYE**-broid)	-oid = resembling -ine = pertaining to **uter/o** = uterus	benign, smooth muscle tumor of the uterus; also known as leiomyoma (Figure 17-12)
	galact/o	**milk**
galactorrhea (gah-**lack**-toh-**REE**-ah)	-rrhea = discharge; flow	discharge of milk from the breast after breastfeeding has stopped
	gynec/o	**woman**
gynecologist (**guy**-neh-**KOL**-oh-jist)	-logist = specialist	specialist in the study of diseases and treatment of the female genital tract
gynecology (**guy**-neh-**KOL**-oh-jee)	-logy = study of	the study of diseases and treatment of the female genital tract

	hyster/o	uterus
Term	**Term Analysis**	**Definition**
hysterectomy (**hiss**-ter-**ECK**-toh-mee)	-ectomy = excision; surgical removal	surgical removal of the uterus through the abdomen (abdominal hysterectomy) or the vagina (vaginal hysterectomy) *NOTE:* Types of hysterectomies include total hysterectomy, in which the uterus plus the cervix are removed, and subtotal, in which the cervix is left intact.
hysterotomy (**his**-ter-**OT**-oh-mee)	-tomy = process of cutting	process of cutting into the uterus (usually to remove the fetus)
	labi/o	**lips**
labial (**LAY**-bee-al)	-al = pertaining to	pertaining to the lips
	lact/o	**milk**
lactogenesis (**lack**-toh-**JEN**-ih-sis)	-genesis = production; formation	production and secretion of milk from the breast
	lapar/o	**abdomen**
laparoscopy (**lap**-ar-**OS**-koh-pee)	-scopy = process of visually examining	process of visually examining the abdominal cavity *NOTE:* A laser may be used with a laparoscope to remove or destroy tissue without opening the abdominal cavity (Figure 17-4).
	ligati/o	**binding; tying**
tubal ligation (**TOO**-bal lye-**GAY**-shun)	-ion = process -al = pertaining to **tub/o** = tube; fallopian tube	method of sterilization whereby the lumen of the fallopian tube is blocked by tying the tube with a threadlike material (Figure 17-5)
	mamm/o; mast/o	**breast**
mammary (**MAM**-ah-ree)	-ary = pertaining to	pertaining to the breast
mammography (mam-**OG**-rah-fee)	-graphy = process of recording; producing images	x-ray of the breast to diagnose abnormalities that may not show up on a typical physical examination (Figure 3-4)

FIGURE 17-4
Laparoscopy

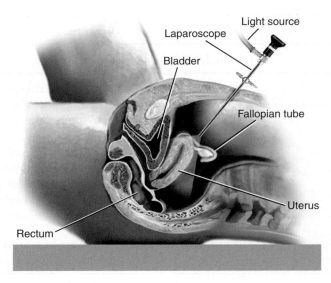

Light source

Laparoscope

Bladder

Fallopian tube

Uterus

Rectum

FIGURE 17-5
Tubal Ligation

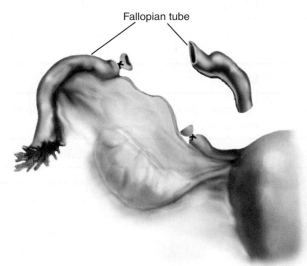

Fallopian tube

Term	Term Analysis	Definition
mammoplasty (**MAM**-oh-**plas**-tee)	-plasty = surgical repair; surgical reconstruction	surgical reconstruction of the breast *NOTE:* Includes post-mastectomy reconstruction and breast enlargement.
mastectomy (mas-**TECK**-toh-mee)	-ectomy = excision; surgical removal	excision of the breast
mastopexy (**MAS**-toh-**peck**-see)	-pexy = surgical fixation	surgical fixation of the breast *NOTE:* A mastopexy is performed to improve breast shape when the breast is sagging.

	men/o	menses; menstruation; month
Term	**Term Analysis**	**Definition**
amenorrhea (ah-**men**-oh-**REE**-ah)	-rrhea = discharge; flow a- = no; not; lack of	no menstruation
dysmenorrhea (**dis**-men-oh-**REE**-ah)	dys- = painful; difficult; bad	painful menstruation
menopause (**MEN**-oh-pawz)	-pause = stoppage; cessation	stoppage of menstruation usually occurring at about 45–55 years of age
menorrhea (**men**-oh-**REE**-ah)	-rrhea = discharge; flow	normal menstruation
menorrhagia (**men**-oh-**RAY**-jee-ah)	-rrhagia = burst forth	excessive uterine bleeding during menstruation
oligomenorrhea (**ol**-ih-goh-**men**-oh-**REE**-ah)	-rrhea = discharge; flow oligo- = diminished; scanty; deficient; few	diminished or infrequent menstruation
menometrorrhagia (**men**-oh-**met**-roh-**RAY**-jee-ah)	-rrhagia = bursting forth **metr/o** = uterus	excessive uterine bleeding during menstruation and at variable intervals

	metr/o	uterus
endometriosis (**en**-doh-**mee**-tree-**OH**-sis)	-osis = abnormal condition endo- = within	endometrial tissue found at sites other than the uterus (Figure 17-12)
endometrium (**en**-doh-**MEE**-tree-um)	-ium = structure endo- = within	inner wall of the uterus (Figure 17-1B)
metroptosis (**meh**-troh-**TOH**-sis)	-ptosis = falling	displacement of the uterus through the vaginal canal; uterine prolapse
metrorrhagia (**meh**-troh-**RAY**-jee-ah)	-rrhagia = burst forth	uterine bleeding at times other than at the regular menstrual period
myometrium (**my**-oh-**MEE**-tree-um)	-ium = structure **my/o** = muscle	muscular wall of the uterus (Figure 17-1B)
parametrium (**par**-ah-**MEE**-tree-um)	-ium = structure para- = near; beside	structures located beside the uterus such as supporting ligaments
perimetrium (**per**-ih-**MEE**-tree-um)	-ium = structure peri- = around	the outermost wall of the uterus (Figure 17-1B)

	o/o; ov/o	egg
Term	**Term Analysis**	**Definition**
oocyte (**OH**-oh-sight)	-cyte = cell	egg cell; the developing ovum
ovoid (**OH**-void)	-oid = resembling	resembling an egg shape
	oophor/o	**ovary**
oophororrhagia (oh-**of**-oh-**RAY**-jee-ah)	-rrhagia = bursting forth	hemorrhaging from the ovary
	ovari/o	**ovary**
ovarian cyst (oh-**VAR**-ree-an **SIST**)	-an = pertaining to cyst = a closed sac or cavity that contains fluid, solid, or semisolid material	cyst formed on an ovary (Figure 17-12)
	perine/o	**perineum (area from the vulva to anus)**
colpoperineoplasty (**kol**-poh-**per**-in-**EE**-oh-**plas**-tee)	-plasty = surgical reconstruction; surgical repair **colp/o** = vagina	surgical reconstruction of the vagina and perineum
perineorrhaphy (**per**-ih-nee-**OR**-ah-fee)	-rrhaphy = suture	suture of the perineum
	salping/o	**fallopian tube; uterine tube**
hysterosalpingectomy (**his**-ter-oh-**sal**-pin-**JECK**-toh-mee)	-ectomy = excision; surgical removal **hyster/o** = uterus	excision of the uterus and fallopian tubes
hysterosalpingogram (**his**-ter-oh-sal-**PING**-oh-gram)	-gram = record **hyster/o** = uterus	record of the uterus and fallopian tubes by the use of x-rays after injection of a contrast medium
salpingopexy (sal-**PING**-oh-**peck**-see)	-pexy = surgical fixation	surgical fixation of the fallopian tubes
salpingo-oophorectomy (sal-**ping**-goh-**oh**-of-oh-**RECK**-toh-mee)	-ectomy = excision; surgical removal **oophor/o** = ovary	excision of the fallopian tubes and ovaries; may be bilateral or unilateral

	thel/o	nipple
Term	**Term Analysis**	**Definition**
polythelia (**pol**-ee-**THEE**-lee-ah)	-ia = condition poly- = many	more than one nipple present on the breast
thelitis (thee-**LYE**-tis)	-itis = inflammation	inflammation of the nipple

	uter/o	uterus
intrauterine (**in**-trah-**YOO**-ter-in)	-ine = pertaining to intra- = within	pertaining to within the uterus
rectouterine (**reck**-toh-**YOO**-ter-in)	-ine = pertaining to **rect/o** = rectum	pertaining to the rectum and uterus
uterovesical (**yoo**-ter-oh-**VES**-ih-kal)	-al = pertaining to **uter/o** = uterus	pertaining to the uterus and bladder

	vagin/o	vagina
vaginitis (**vaj**-ih-**NIGH**-tis)	-itis = inflammation	inflammation of the vagina
vaginomycosis (**vaj**-in-oh-mye-**KOH**-sis)	-osis = abnormal condition **myc/o** = fungus	fungal infection of the vagina

	vulv/o	**vulva; external genitalia; pudendum**
vulvectomy (vul-**VECK**-toh-mee)	-ectomy = excision; surgical removal	excision of the vulva
vulvorectal (**vul**-voh-**RECK**-tal)	-al = pertaining to **rect/o** = rectum	pertaining to the vulva and rectum

SUFFIXES

	-arche	**beginning**
Term	**Term Analysis**	**Definition**
menarche (men-**AR**-kee)	**men/o** = menses; menstruation; month	beginning of the regular menstrual cycle occurring at approximately 13 years of age

	-cele	hernia (protrusion of an organ from the structure that normally contains it)
Term	**Term Analysis**	**Definition**
cystocele (**SIS**-toh-seel)	**cyst/o** = bladder	hernia of bladder against the vaginal wall (Figure 3-1)
rectocele (**RECK**-toh-seel)	**rect/o** = rectum	hernia of the rectum against the vaginal wall (Figure 3-2)
	-logy	**the study of**
cytology (sigh-**TOL**-oh-jee)	**cyt/o** = cells	the study of cells. A cytology commonly performed is the **Papanicolaou** (pap-ah-**nick**-oh-**LAY**-ooh) **smear**, or **Pap smear**, which differentiates normal cells from precancerous and cancerous cells of the cervix uteri.
	-opsy	**to view**
biopsy (**BYE**-op-see)	**bi/o** = life	living tissue is excised from the body and viewed under a microscope *NOTE:* Common biopsies on the cervix uteri are **conization** (**kon**-ih-**ZAY**-shun), in which a piece of cervix, shaped like a cone, is surgically removed for the purposes of microscopic examination; and **punch biopsy**, which removes a circular piece of tissue for microscopic examination.
	-salpinx	**fallopian tube; uterine tube**
hematosalpinx (**hem**-ah-toh-**SAL**-pinks)	**hemat/o** = blood	accumulation of blood in the fallopian tube
hydrosalpinx (**high**-droh-**SAL**-pinks)	**hydr/o** = water	accumulation of a watery fluid in the fallopian tube
pyosalpinx (**pye**-oh-**SAL**-pinks)	**py/o** = pus	accumulation of pus in the fallopian tube

PREFIXES

	ante-	before
Term	**Term Analysis**	**Definition**
anteflexion (**an**-tee-**FLECK**-shun)	-ion = process **flex/o** = bending	bending forward of a part of an organ *NOTE*: Anteflexion describes the position of the uterus as it bends forward over the bladder (Figure 17-6).
anteversion (**an**-tee-**VER**-zhun)	-ion = process **versi/o** = turning; tilting; tipping	tilting forward of an organ *NOTE*: Anteversion describes the position of the uterus as it tilts over the bladder. Considered a malposition of the uterus (Figure 17-7).

FIGURE 17-6
Anteflexion

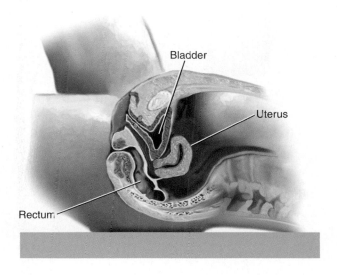

FIGURE 17-7
Anteversion

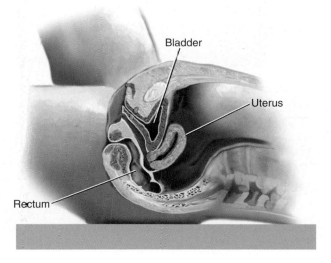

	retro-	back; behind
Term	**Term Analysis**	**Definition**
retroflexion (**ret**-roh-**FLECK**-shun)	-ion = process **flex/o** = bending	bending back of a part of an organ *NOTE*: Retroflexion describes the malpositioned uterus as it bends backward toward the rectum (Figure 17-8).
retroversion (**ret**-roh-**VER**-zhun)	-ion = process **versi/o** = turning; tilting; tipping	tilting backward of an organ *NOTE*: Retroversion describes a malpositioned uterus as it tilts backward toward the rectum (Figure 17-9).

FIGURE 17-8
Retroflexion

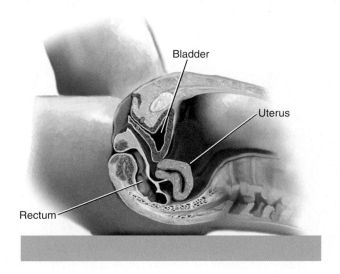

FIGURE 17-9
Retroversion

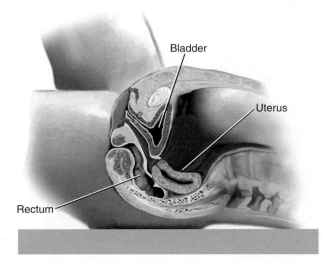

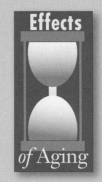

Effects

of Aging

Menopause causes several changes in the female reproductive organs. Hormone levels decrease and no more eggs are released from the ovaries. Pregnancy is no longer possible. The ovaries and uterus decrease in size due to decreased hormone levels. The vaginal tissues become less elastic, and there may be complaints of vaginal dryness. The breasts become less firm, and therefore sag. Sexual activity is not significantly impaired.

17.6   Common Diseases of the Female Reproductive System

BREAST CANCER

Breast cancer is a malignant tumor of the breast. If untreated, breast cancer can metastasize (meh-**TAS**-tah-size), or spread to the surrounding breast tissue and then to other parts of the body through the blood and lymph.

The exact cause is unknown. Breast cancer is associated with several risk factors: high estrogen levels, age, alcohol and tobacco use, and a family history of breast cancer. Two breast cancer genes have been identified, **BRCA1** and **BRCA2**. Inherited defects in either one of these genes, although rare, increase the chance of breast cancer.

Treatment includes surgical removal of the tumor by **lumpectomy**. The cancerous tissue is removed, but the remainder of the breast tissue is left intact. At the same time, lymph nodes are checked to see if the cancer has spread beyond the breast. This is followed by **radiation therapy** to kill any cancer cells.

Another surgical procedure is **mastectomy**, the surgical removal of the breast. This involves excising the entire breast. The most common mastectomies are **modified radical mastectomy** and **simple mastectomy**. In a modified radical mastectomy, the breast and axillary lymph nodes are removed. The chest muscles are left intact for purposes of breast reconstruction. With a simple mastectomy, the axillary lymph nodes are not removed. Mastectomy is followed by chemotherapy and radiation therapy.

UTERINE (ENDOMETRIAL) CANCER

Endometrial cancer is a malignant tumor of the endometrium. Uterine cancer is the most common cancer of the reproductive organs.

Uterine cancer is thought to be linked to high levels of estrogen circulating in a woman's body. Common sources of increased estrogen are estrogen-replacement therapy, obesity (fat cells produce estrogen), early menarche, or late menopause. Another factor is a family history of breast or ovarian cancer.

A combination of **surgery**, **radiation therapy**, **hormonal therapy** and **chemotherapy** is the most common treatment. Different surgeries are done, depending on how far the cancer has spread. A **hysterectomy** may be done. In some cases, a **total abdominal hysterectomy** with bilateral salpingo-oophorectomy (TAH-BSO) is necessary. If the cancer has spread even further, a **radical hysterectomy** may be performed. This includes removal of the nearby lymph nodes.

SEXUALLY TRANSMITTED DISEASES

Sexually transmitted diseases (STDs) include any disease that has been transmitted through any type of sexual activity, including vaginal, oral, and anal sex. AIDS is also a sexually transmitted disease. (Details about AIDS are in Chapter 13, Blood and Immune Systems). The most common types of STDs are chlamydia, genital warts, genital herpes, gonorrhea, and syphilis.

Chlamydia

Chlamydia (klah-**MID**-ee-ah) is caused by the bacteria *Chlamydia trachomatis*. In women, it can damage the cervix and urethra. In men, it can cause discharge from the penis. In most patients, chlamydia is asymptomatic (there are no symptoms) for several weeks, and because of this, it can cause permanent damage before the patient knows he or she is infected. Chlamydia is treated with antibiotics.

Genital Herpes

Genital herpes is caused by herpes simplex viruses 1 or 2 (HSV-1, HSV-2). It causes painful vesicles (blisters) in the genital and anorectal areas. It occurs in males and females. There is no cure for genital herpes. The virus remains in the body forever and the vesicles can erupt at any time. Antiviral medication can be taken to reduce the symptoms and appearance of vesicles.

Gonorrhea

Gonorrhea (gon-oh-**REE**-ah) is caused by *Neisseria gonorrhoeae*, a bacterium. It can infect the urethra, cervix, rectum, pharynx, or eyes. Treatment is antibiotics.

Human Papillomaviruses

There are over 100 different human papillomaviruses (**pap-**ih-**LOH**-mah-**vye**-rus-ez) (HPV). Since over 30 of them can be transmitted through sexual contact, infection with these viruses is considered to be the most common sexually transmitted disease.

Many of the sexually transmitted papillomaviruses are strongly associated with cervical cancer, and are thus referred to as "high-risk". Many others cause warts. At least two of these cause warts in the genital area (penis, vulva, cervix, urethra, and anorectal area). These types are called low-risk because they are not commonly associated with cervical cancer. Some infected people do not develop warts at all, and because there are no other symptoms, these people can spread the disease without knowing it.

There is no cure for HPV, but symptoms can be treated. Topical therapy is one approach. This involves the application of medication directly to the warts. Cryotherapy is another treatment. It involves destruction of the wart using extreme cold.

Recently, a vaccine has been designed to prevent cervical cancer by stopping the high-risk HPV from infecting cervical tissue. The vaccine is recommended for girls 11 to 12 years old, but is applicable to all ages.

Syphilis

Syphilis (**SIF**-ih-lis) is caused by *Treponema pallidum*. It is an infection that enters through the skin or mucous membranes and spreads throughout the body, affecting any organ. In the early stages of the disease, a lesion called a **chancre** appears in the genital and anorectal regions. Skin rashes, lymphadenopathy, and organ damage occur in later stages of the disease. It is fatal if not treated with antibiotics.

17.7   Abbreviations Pertaining to the Female Reproductive System

Abbreviation	Meaning
BSO	bilateral salpingo-oophorectomy
D&C	dilation and curettage (a type of operation in which the uterus is dilated and the surface of the endometrium is scraped, or curetted)
Gyn; gyne	gynecology
HPV	human papillomavirus
HRT	hormone replacement therapy
HSG	hysterosalpingogram
IUD	intrauterine device (a type of contraceptive device)
LMP	last menstrual period
Pap smear	Papanicolaou smear
PID	pelvic inflammatory disease
TAH	total abdominal hysterectomy
STD	sexually transmitted disease
VD	venereal disease

17.8   Obstetrics

PREGNANCY

If fertilization does occur in the uterine tube, the fertilized egg (the zygote) travels to the uterus and implants in the uterine wall. The uterus begins to enlarge. The zygote is referred to as the **embryo** (**EM**-bree-oh) from the second to the eighth week of pregnancy. For the remainder of the **gestation** period the name **fetus** (**FEE**-tus) is used. Gestation is the length of time from conception (fertilization) to birth, on the average, 40 weeks.

Memory Key	The zygote becomes the embryo, which becomes the fetus.

At the beginning of pregnancy, the placenta develops and attaches to the uterine wall. The placenta is the organ that allows for the exchange of nutrients and waste products between the developing embryo and the mother. The placenta is made up of embryonic tissue: the **chorion**, the outermost layer surrounding the embryo, and the **amnion**, the innermost layer (Figure 17-10). The amnion forms the amniotic cavity, which holds the embryo floating in **amniotic fluid**. Thus, the embryo (and later the fetus) develops in a protective environment, the amniotic fluid, which acts as a shock absorber. Near the time of birth, the amnion ruptures, releasing its fluid, and signaling the onset of labor. After delivery, the placenta detaches from the uterus, hence the term **afterbirth**.

During placental development, fingerlike projections called chorionic villi form and extend from the chorion into the endometrial tissue of the mother. This arrangement allows the vessels of the embryo (chorionic villi) to lie side by side with the mother's blood vessels. At no time during gestation does the fetal blood mix with the maternal blood, yet nutrients and waste products are exchanged.

Materials that are exchanged must be transported to and from the embryo. This transport is made possible by the **umbilical** (um-**BILL**-ih-kahl) **cord**. The umbilical cord contains two arteries and one vein, which become the lifelines between the mother and the baby, carrying nutrients and waste products to and from the developing embryo.

FIGURE 17-10
Amniotic sac

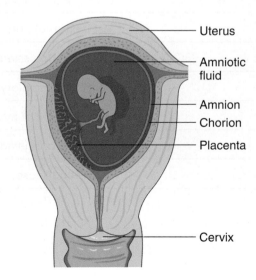

Uterus

Amniotic fluid

Amnion

Chorion

Placenta

Cervix

The placenta secretes **human chorionic gonadotropin (HCG)**. This is a **hormone** secreted early in the pregnancy. It confirms pregnancy when tested for in women who suspect they are pregnant. HCG stimulates the release of estrogen and progesterone. These hormones maintain the uterine wall—an important contribution to fetal development. Low levels of these hormones can lead to a spontaneous abortion, or miscarriage.

Memory Key
- During pregnancy, the placenta exchanges nutrients and waste products between the embryo and the mother.
- Placenta is made up of the amnion and chorion.
- Human chorionic gonadotropin is a hormone secreted by the placenta early in pregnancy.

Detection of fetal abnormalities can be determined by two diagnostic procedures: **amniocentesis** and **chorionic villus sampling (CVS)**, as seen in Figure 17-11. Amniocentesis withdraws amniotic fluid from the amniotic sac for laboratory analysis at 15 to 18 weeks' gestation. Chorionic villus sampling removes placental tissue for chemical and microscopic examination at 9 to 11 weeks' gestation.

PARTURITION

The birth process is known as **parturition (par-**tyoo-**RISH**-un). At about 9 months, the uterine muscles begin to contract. This marks the beginning of labor, which has three stages: **cervical dilatation** (dil-ah-**TAY**-shun), **fetal delivery**, and **placental delivery**. During cervical dilatation, the cervix begins to dilate, ultimately reaching approximately 4 inches (10.2 cm) in diameter. During fetal delivery, uterine contractions move the infant through the cervix and vagina to the outside world. The umbilical cord connecting the infant to the placenta is severed once the baby is out. The placenta is expelled from the uterus during placental delivery.

Memory Key The birth process is called parturition. The stages of labor are cervical dilatation, fetal delivery, and placental delivery.

The fetus is delivered head first. If the buttocks present first, it is in a **breech** position. In such cases, or when the fetus is too large for vaginal delivery, a surgical procedure known as **cesarean** (seh-**ZER**-ree-an) **section (CS)** may be used. This involves removal of the fetus through an incision in the abdomen and uterus.

Memory Key If the fetus is too large or in breech position, delivery may be by cesarean section.

The condition of the newborn is evaluated within one minute of birth and again 15 minutes later. A numerical rating called an **Apgar score** is obtained by evaluating each of the following on a 2-point scale, 2 being the highest: heart rate, respiration, muscle tone, reflex response, and color. The highest rating is therefore 10.

FIGURE 17-11
(A) chorionic villi sampling (9 to 11 weeks); (B) amniocentesis (15 to 18 weeks)

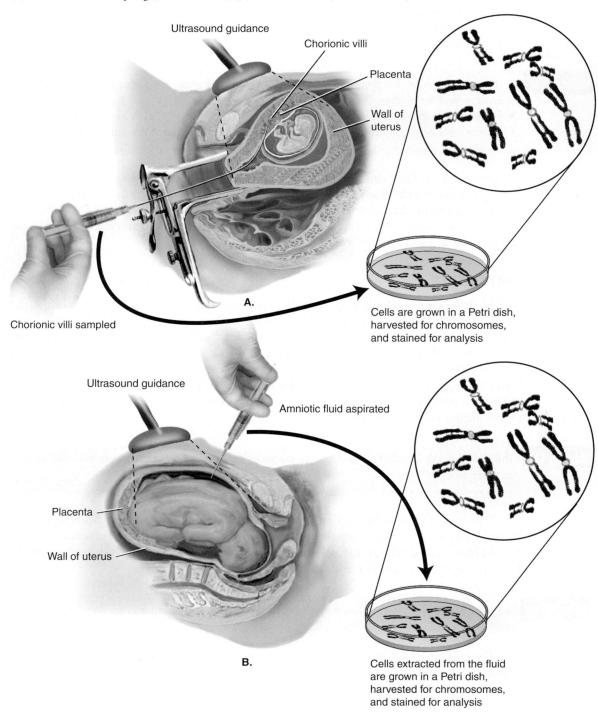

Ultrasound guidance

Chorionic villi

Placenta

Wall of uterus

Chorionic villi sampled

A.

Cells are grown in a Petri dish, harvested for chromosomes, and stained for analysis

Ultrasound guidance

Amniotic fluid aspirated

Placenta

Wall of uterus

B.

Cells extracted from the fluid are grown in a Petri dish, harvested for chromosomes, and stained for analysis

> **Memory Key**
> - Apgar scoring rates heart rate, respiration, muscle tone, reflex response, and color, each out of a highest possible score of 2.
> - The best possible score is 10.

The 6 to 8 weeks following parturition are known as the **postpartum period**. During this period, the uterus returns to normal size, a process known as **involution**, and the mammary glands are stimulated to produce milk; the production of milk is called lactation. During the first few days, the mammary glands produce **colostrum** (kuh-**LOS**-trum), which is a highly nourishing fluid containing antibodies to protect the infant.

> **Memory Key**
> Colostrum is produced by the mammary glands during the first few days of the postpartum period.

The terms **gravida** (**GRAV**-ih-dah) and **para** are used to describe a woman's obstetrical history. *Gravida* refers to a pregnant woman, whereas *para* refers to a woman whose pregnancy has resulted in viable offspring, regardless of whether the child was alive at birth. So, for example, a woman who is **primigravida** (pregnant for the first time) is described as gravida I, para 0 before the birth. If a viable child is born, the woman is then described as gravida I, para I, whether she has a single child, twins, or triplets, because *para* refers only to the number of occasions a woman has given birth to a viable child and not to the number of children born on any of those occasions. During her next pregnancy, this same woman would be described as gravida II, para I. If she gives birth to viable offspring, she is gravida II, para II. If she does not, she will remain gravida ll, para l.

> **Memory Key**
> - *Gravida* refers to a pregnant woman.
> - *Para* refers to a woman whose pregnancy has resulted in viable births.

Before you continue, review Section 17.8. Then, complete Exercise 17-2 found at the end of the chapter.

17.9 Term Analysis and Definition Pertaining to Obstetrics

ROOTS

	amni/o	amnion; sac in which the fetus lies in the uterus
Term	**Term Analysis**	**Definition**
amniocentesis (**am**-nee-oh-sen-**TEE**-sis)	-centesis = surgical puncture	surgical puncture to withdraw or aspirate fluid from the amniotic sac for analysis (Figure 17-11)

	nat/o	birth
Term	**Term Analysis**	**Definition**
postnatal period (pohst-**NAY**-tal)	-al = pertaining to post- = after	pertaining to the period after birth (referring to the newborn)
prenatal (pree-**NAY**-tal)	-al = pertaining to pre- = before	pertaining to before birth (referring to the fetus); antenatal
	top/o	place
ectopic pregnancy (eck-**TOP**-ick **PREG**-nan-see)	-ic = pertaining to ec- = out	pregnancy occurring in a place other than the uterus, such as in the fallopian tube (Figure 17-12)

FIGURE 17-12
Ectopic pregnancy, endometriosis, leiomyoma, ovarian cyst, cervical polyp

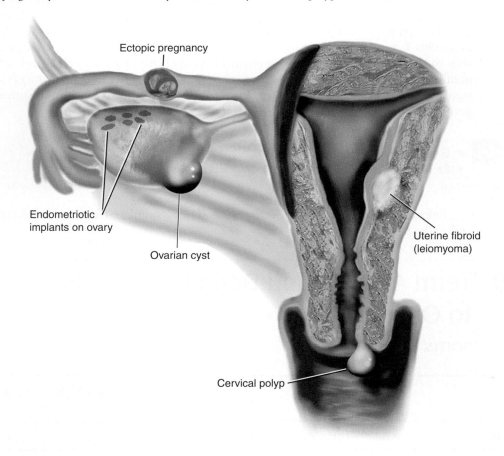

SUFFIXES

	-cyesis	pregnancy
Term	**Term Analysis**	**Definition**
pseudocyesis (**soo**-doh-sigh-**EE**-sis)	pseudo- = false	false pregnancy
	-emesis	**vomit**
hyperemesis gravidarum (**high**-per-**EM**-eh-sis **grav**-ih-**DAR**-um)	hyper- = excessive; above normal gravidarum = pregnancy	excessive vomiting during pregnancy
	-gravida	**pregnancy**
multigravida (**mul**-tih-**GRAV**-ih-dah)	multi- = multiple	a woman who has been pregnant two or more times (written gravida II, gravida III, gravida IV, etc., or as GII, GIII, GIV, etc.)
nulligravida (**nul**-ih-**GRAV**-ih-dah)	nulli- = none	a woman who has never been pregnant
primigravida (**prih**-mih-**GRAV**-ih-dah)	primi- = first	a woman who is pregnant for the first time (written gravida I or GI)
secundigravida (see-**kun**-dih-**GRAV**-ih-dah)	secundi- = second	a woman pregnant for the second time (written gravida II or GII)
	-metry	**process of measuring**
pelvimetry (pel-**VIM**-eh-tree)	**pelv/i** = pelvis	process of measuring the dimensions of the mother's pelvis to determine if its dimensions will allow the passage of the fetus through the birth canal
	-para	**to bear; give birth; part with child**
multipara (mul-**TIP**-ah-rah)	multi- = multiple	a woman who has given birth to viable offspring two or more times (written as para II, para III, para IV, etc., or as PII, PIII, PIV, etc.)
nullipara (nul-**LIP**-ah-rah)	nulli- = none	a woman who has never given birth to viable offspring

Term	Term Analysis	Definition
primipara (prye-**MIP**-ah-rah)	primi- = first	a woman who has given birth to viable offspring for the first time (written para I or PI)
secundipara (see-kun-**DIP**-ah-rah)	secundi- = second	a woman who has given birth to viable offspring twice (written para II or PII)
	-partum	**labor; delivery; childbirth**
antepartum (an-tee-**PAR**-tum)	ante- = before	before birth (referring to the mother)
postpartum (pohst-**PAR**-tum)	post- = after	the period after birth (referring to the mother)
	-tocia; -tocin	**labor**
dystocia (dis-**TOH**-see-ah)	dys- = painful; difficult; bad	difficult labor
oxytocin (**ock**-see-**TOH**-sin)	oxy- = sharp	hormone secreted from the posterior pituitary that initiates uterine contractions, starting childbirth

PREFIXES

	ultra-	**excess; beyond**
Term	**Term Analysis**	**Definition**
pelvic ultrasonography (**PEL**-vick **ul**-trah-son-**OG**-rah-fee)	-graphy = process of recording **son/o** = sound pelvic = pertaining to the pelvis	visualization of organs in the pelvic area by recording high-frequency sound waves as they bounce off the tissues *NOTE:* This procedure may be used to determine fetal size and position.

17.10 Obstetrical Conditions

PLACENTA PREVIA

Placenta previa (**PREH**-vee-ah) is the attachment of the placenta near the cervix uteri instead of high up on the uterine wall. This can cause hemorrhaging and premature labor that places mother and baby at risk. Cesarean section (the removal of the fetus through an incision in the abdominal and uterine wall) is necessary.

PRE-ECLAMPSIA AND ECLAMPSIA

Pre-eclampsia (pree-eh-KLAMP-see-ah) is a condition that can occur between the 20th week of pregnancy and the 1st week postpartum. It is signified by high blood pressure, albuminuria (protein in the urine), and excessive edema (accumulation of fluid in body tissues). If left untreated, convulsions and coma might result, and the condition is then called **eclampsia**, which can be fatal. Treatment includes medication and delivery of the fetus.

UTERINE INERTIA

Uterine inertia (YOO-ter-een ih-**NER**-shah) is weak or sluggish uterine contractions during labor.

When labor seems to have slowed down or ceased, uterine contractions may be induced (brought on) using an injection of the hormone oxytocin (Syntocinon).

17.11 Abbreviations Pertaining to Obstetrics

Abbreviation	Meaning
AB	abortion (termination of the pregnancy before the embryo or fetus is outside the uterus)
CPD	cephalopelvic disproportion
CS; C-section; C-S	cesarean section (incision into the uterus to remove the fetus)
CVS	chorionic villus sampling
DOB	date of birth
EDC	expected date of confinement
FHS	fetal heart sound
G	gravida
HCG	human chorionic gonadotropin (hormone secreted by the placenta)
NB	newborn
Ob; OB	obstetrics
P	para
UC	uterine contractions

···

17.12 Putting It All Together

Exercise 17-1   MATCHING

Match the word in Column A with its definition in Column B.

Column A

_____ 1. estrogen

_____ 2. fundus

_____ 3. parturition

_____ 4. progesterone

_____ 5. introitus

_____ 6. fimbriae

_____ 7. Bartholin's glands

_____ 8. lactiferous sinuses

_____ 9. placenta

_____ 10. perineum

Column B

A. fingerlike projections at the distal ends of the fallopian tubes

B. secrete lubricant for intercourse

C. store milk produced by mammary glands

D. birth process

E. provides fetus with nourishment

F. stimulates development of secondary female characteristics

G. entrance to the vagina

H. area from the vulva to the anus

I. superior rounded portion of the uterus

J. stimulates the growth of blood vessels in the uterus

Exercise 17-2   MATCHING OBSTETRICAL TERMS AND DEFINITIONS

Match the definitions with the terms listed below. Not all terms are used.

amnion

chorion

colostrum

estrogen

gravida

human chorionic gonadotropin

involution

luteinizing hormone

para

parturition

postpartum

progesterone

1. The outermost layer of the placenta surrounding the embryo   _____

2. Birth process   _____

3. Hormone that forms the basis of
   pregnancy tests because it is secreted
   in urine early in the pregnancy   _____

4. Fluid that is secreted from mammary
   glands and contains antibodies   _____

5. The innermost layer of the placenta
   surrounding the embryo   _____

6. A pregnant woman   _____

7. A woman whose pregnancy has
   resulted in viable offspring   _____

8. Return of the uterus to its normal size
   following delivery of the fetus   _____

Exercise 17-3   IDENTIFICATION

Write the suffix, root, or prefix for the medical term for each of the following word or phrases.

1. vagina	_____	9. fallopian tube	_____
2. external genitalia	_____	10. place	_____
3. woman	_____	11. beginning	_____
4. milk	_____	12. pregnancy	_____
5. breast	_____	13. to bear; give birth	_____
6. menstruation	_____	14. labor	_____
7. birth	_____	15. before	_____
8. ovary	_____		

Exercise 17-4   BUILDING MEDICAL TERMS

Build the medical term for each of the following definitions.

1. inflammation of the neck of the uterus   _____

2. suturing the vulva   _____

3. surgical puncture to remove fluid from
   the cul-de-sac of Douglas   _____

4. specialist in the study of diseases and
   treatment of the female genital tract   _____

5. surgical removal of the uterus   _____

6. pertaining to the breast   _____

7. excision of the breast   _____

8. resembling an egg shape   _____

9. excision of the fallopian tubes
   and ovaries   _____

10. more than one nipple present on
    the breast   _____

11. pregnancy occurring in a place other
    than the uterus   _____

12. fungal infection of the vagina   _____

13. hernia of the bladder against
    the vaginal wall   _____

14. false pregnancy   _____

15. the period after birth, referring to
    the mother   _____

16. accumulation of pus in the
    fallopian tube   _____

17. difficult labor   _____

18. bending back of an organ   _____

Exercise 17-5   ADJECTIVES

Write the adjective for each of the following. Use a medical dictionary if necessary.

1. cervix   _____

2. uterus   _____

3. ovary   _____

4. perineum   _____

5. vagina   _____

Exercise 17-6   BUILDING TERMS

I. Use **men/o** to build terms for the following definitions.

1. no menstruation   _____

2. painful menstruation   _____

3. stoppage of menstruation at about
   45 to 55 years of age   _____

4. normal menstruation   _____

5. excessive uterine bleeding at time
   of menstruation   _____

6. diminished or infrequent
   menstruation _____

7. excessive uterine bleeding during
   menstruation and at variable intervals _____

II. Use **metr/o** to build terms for the following definitions.

8. uterine prolapse _____

9. uterine bleeding at times other than
   at the regular menstrual period _____

10. muscular wall of the uterus _____

11. outermost wall of the uterus _____

12. innermost wall of the uterus _____

III. Use -gravida to build terms for the following definitions.

13. a woman who has been pregnant
    two or more times _____

14. a woman who has never been
    pregnant _____

IV. Use -para to build terms for the following definitions.

15. a woman who has given birth for
    the first time _____

16. a woman who has given birth to
    viable offspring twice _____

Exercise 17-7   IDENTIFICATION

Place an **X** beside the terms indicating a surgical or clinical procedure.

1. lactogenesis _____

2. menarche _____

3. colporrhaphy _____

4. oophororrhagia _____

Exercise 17-8   PLURALS

Write the plural for each of the following terms. Use a medical dictionary if necessary.

1. uterus _____

2. ovary _____

Exercise 17-9   SPELLING

Circle any misspelled words in the following list and correctly spell them in the space provided.

1. cervixitis _____

2. mamography _____

3. oligomenorrhea _____

4. perimetrium _____

5. dismenorrhea _____

6. ocyte _____

7. colpoperineoplasty _____

8. salpingo-oophorectomy _____

9. polythilea _____

10. extopic _____

11. vulvoectomy _____

12. pseudocyesis _____

13. secundigravida _____

14. retroflextion _____

15. episiotomy _____

Exercise 17-10   PATHOLOGY

Match the disease listed with its definition. Not all terms are used.

BRCA1

breast cancer

chlamydia

eclampsia

genital warts

gonorrhea

pre-eclampsia

syphilis

uterine inertia

1. caused by human papillomavirus _____

2. caused by *Treponema pallidum* _____

3. metastasizes through lymphatic channels _____

4. characterized by high blood pressure, albuminuria, and edema _____

5. weak uterine contractions during labor _____

. . . .

17.13 Review of Vocabulary Pertaining to the Female Reproductive System

In the following tables, the medical terms are organized into these categories: anatomy, physiology, pathology, diagnostics, clinical procedures, surgical instruments. Define each term and decide into which category the word belongs. This will help you associate the term with its purpose and help you remember its meaning.

TABLE 17-1

REVIEW OF ANATOMICAL AND PHYSIOLOGICAL TERMS OF THE FEMALE REPRODUCTIVE SYSTEM

1. endometrium	2. estrogen	3. fallopian tube
4. fimbriae	5. gynecology	6. internal os
7. intrauterine	8. introitus	9. labial
10. lactogenesis	11. mammary	12. menarche
13. menopause	14. menorrhea	15. myometrium
16. oocyte	17. ovary	18. ovoid
19. parametrium	20. perimetrium	21. perineum

continued on page 35

Table 17-1 *continued from page 34*

22. progesterone	23. rectouterine	24. uterovesical
25. vulvorectal		

TABLE 17-2

REVIEW OF PATHOLOGIC TERMS PERTAINING TO THE FEMALE REPRODUCTIVE SYSTEM

1. amenorrhea	2. anteflexion	3. anteversion
4. cervical polyp	5. cervicitis	6. chlamydia
7. cystocele	8. dysmenorrhea	9. endometriosis
10. galactorrhea	11. hematosalpinx	12. hydrosalpinx
13. menometrorrhagia	14. menorrhagia	15. metroptosis
16. metrorrhagia	17. oligomenorrhea	18. oophororrhagia
19. ovarian cyst	20. polythelia	21. pyosalpinx
22. rectocele	23. retroflexion	24. retroversion

continued on page 36

Table 17-2 *continued from page 35*

25. syphilis	26. thelitis	27. uterine fibroids
28. vaginitis	29. vaginomycosis	

TABLE 17-3

REVIEW OF DIAGNOSTIC TERMS OF THE FEMALE REPRODUCTIVE SYSTEM

1. cytology	2. hysterosalpingogram	3. mammography
4. Pap smear (Papanicolaou)		

TABLE 17-4

REVIEW OF CLINICAL PROCEDURES OF THE FEMALE REPRODUCTIVE SYSTEM

1. colpoperineoplasty	2. colporrhaphy	3. colposcopy
4. conization biopsy	5. culdocentesis	6. episiorrhaphy
7. episiotomy	8. hysterectomy	9. hysterosalpingectomy
10. hysterotomy	11. laparoscopy	12. mammoplasty
13. mastectomy	14. mastopexy	15. perineorrhaphy

continued on page 37

Table 17-4 *continued from page 36*

16. punch biopsy	17. salpingo-oophorectomy	18. salpingopexy
19. tubal ligation	20. vulvectomy	

....

17.14 Review of Obstetrical Vocabulary

In the following tables, common obstetrical terms are listed. Define each term in the space provided.

TABLE 17-5		
REVIEW OF OBSTETRICAL TERMS		
1. antenatal	2. antepartum	3. dystocia
4. ectopic pregnancy	5. hyperemesis gravidarum	6. multigravida
7. multipara	8. nulligravida	9. nullipara
10. oxytocin	11. prenatal	12. postnatal
13. postpartum	14. primigravida	15. primipara
16. pseudocyesis	17. secundigravida	18. secundipara

TABLE 17-6		
REVIEW OF DIAGNOSTIC TERMS PERTAINING TO OBSTETRICS		
1. amniocentesis	2. pelvimetry	3. ultrasonography

17.15 Medical Terms in Context

After you read the following Discharge Summary, answer the questions that follow it. Use your text, medical dictionary, or other references if necessary.

DISCHARGE SUMMARY

ADMISSION DIAGNOSIS: GRADE 1 ENDOMETRIAL CARCINOMA OF THE UTERUS.

CLINICAL HISTORY: This 48-year-old gravida 2, para 1 was brought in for a total abdominal hysterectomy and bilateral salpingo-oophorectomy. Investigations done in the office, including endometrial biopsy for vaginal bleeding, revealed grade 1 endometrial carcinoma.

The patient had a left mastectomy eight years ago for breast cancer. Because of recurrence, she was placed on Tamoxifen.

INVESTIGATIONS: Hemoglobin was 13.4, platelets 186, white count 5.4. Her postoperative hemoglobin was 11.45.

TREATMENT AND PROGRESS: The patient was taken to the operating room. A vertical midline incision was made; a total abdominal hysterectomy and bilateral salpingo-oophorectomy were performed without complications. Total blood loss was approximately 210 ml.

Postoperatively, she did well and remained afebrile throughout. Peritoneal washing revealed benign cytology. Final pathology revealed bilateral adnexa showing salpingitis with no malignancy. The uterus showed a grade 1 adenocarcinoma. The endometrium also showed focal hyperplasia with leiomyomas.

The patient was discharged home on Tylenol #3. She will be followed up in the office in four weeks' time.

MOST RESPONSIBLE DIAGNOSIS: GRADE 1 ADENOCARCINOMA OF THE UTERUS

QUESTIONS ON THE DISCHARGE SUMMARY

1. Adnexa includes:

    a. fallopian tubes

    b. leiomyomas

    c. uterus

    d. all the above

2. The malignancy involved which of the following:

    a. uterus

    b. fallopian tubes

    c. ovaries

    d. vagina

3. The patient's obstetrical history includes:

    a. one pregnancy, one set of twins

    b. two pregnancies, one viable birth

    c. one pregnancy, two viable births

    d. two viable births, one pregnancy

4. A biopsy was performed on the:

    a. inner lining of the uterus

    b. muscle layer of the uterus

    c. outer lining of the uterus

    d. vagina

5. Surgery during this admission included removal of:

    a. fallopian tubes

    b. both ovaries

    c. uterus

    d. all the above

6. Thrombocyte count was:

    a. 13.4

    b. 5.4

    c. 11.45

    d. 186

7. After the operation, it was noted that the patient:

   a. was emotional

   b. had a fever

   c. was alert

   d. none of the above

8. Focal means:

   a. centralized area

   b. margin

   c. periphery

   d. side

9. The pathology report indicated a(n):

   a. increase in the number of normal cells

   b. benign tumor of smooth muscle

   c. inflammation of the fallopian tubes

   d. all the above

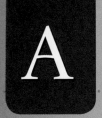
Word Part to Definition

WORD ELEMENT	DEFINITION
a(n)-	inadequate; no; not; lack of
ab-	away from
abdomin/o	abdomen
-ac	pertainin g to
acetabul/o	acetabulum; hip socket
acr/o	extremity; top
acromi/o	acromion
ad-	toward
aden/o	gland
adenoid/o	adenoids
adip/o	fat
adren/o	adrenal gland
adrenal/o	adrenal gland
-al	pertaining to
albin/o	white
albumin/o	albumin (a blood protein)
-algia	pain
alveol/o	air sacs; alveolus
ambly/o	dull; dim
amni/o	amnion; sac in which the fetus lies in the uterus
ana-	apart; up
an/o	anus
andr/o	male; man
angi/o	vessel
anis/o	unequal
ankyl/o	fusion of parts; bent; crooked
ante-	before
anter/o	front
anti-	against
aort/o	aorta
append/o	appendix
aque/o	water
-ar	pertaining to
-arche	beginning

WORD ELEMENT	DEFINITION
arteri/o	artery
arthr/o	joint
articul/o	joint
-ary	pertaining to
-assay	analysis of a mixture to identify its contents
-asthenia	no strength
ather/o	fatty debris; fatty plaque
-ation	process
atri/o	atria (upper chambers of the heart)
audi/o	hearing
audit/o	hearing
aur/o	ear
auto-	self
axill/o	armpit
bacteri/o	bacteria
balan/o	glans penis (tip of the penis)
bi/o	life
bil/i	bile
bilirubin/o	bilirubin (a bile pigment)
-blast	immature, growing thing
blephar/o	eyelid
brachi/o	arm
brady-	slow
bronch/o	bronchus
bronchi/o	bronchus
bronchiol/o	bronchioles; small bronchi
bucc/o	cheek
burs/o	bursa (sac filled with synovial fluid located around joints)
calc/o	calcium
calcane/o	heel

WORD ELEMENT	DEFINITION
calic/o; calyc/o	calix; calyx
-capnia	carbon dioxide
capsul/o	capsule
carcin/o	cancer; cancerous
cardi/o	heart
carp/o	wrist
cartilagin/o	cartilage
catheter/o	something inserted
caud/o	tail
cec/o	cecum
-cele	hernia (protrusion of an organ from the structure that normally contains it)
cellul/o	cell
-centesis	surgical puncture to remove fluid
cephal/o	head
cerebell/o	cerebellum
cerebr/o	brain
cervic/o	cervix; neck; neck of uterus; cervix uteri
-chalasia	relaxation
cheil/o	lips
chol/e	bile; gall
cholangi/o	bile ducts
cholecyst/o	gallbladder
choledoch/o	common bile duct
cholesterol/o	cholesterol
chondr/o	cartilage
chori/o	choroid
chrom/o	color
-cidal	to kill
cili/o	hair
-clasis	surgical fracture or refracture
-clast	breakdown
clavicul/o	clavicle; collarbone
-clonus	turmoil
-clysis	washing; irrigation
coagulati/o	to condense; to clot
coccyg/o	coccyx; tailbone
cochle/o	cochlea
col/o	colon; large intestine
colon/o	colon
colp/o	vagina
coni/o	dust
conjunctiv/o	conjunctiva
constrict/o	to draw together; narrowing
-continence	to stop
-conus	cone-shaped
core/o	pupil
corne/o	cornea

WORD ELEMENT	DEFINITION
coron/o	crown
corpor/o	body
cortic/o	cortex; outer covering; outer layer
cost/o	ribs
crani/o	skull
crin/o	to secrete
-crine	to secrete
-crit	separate
cry/o	cold
crypt/o	hidden
culd/o	cul-de-sac
-cusis	hearing
cutane/o	skin
cycl/o	ciliary body
-cyesis	pregnancy
cyst/o	bladder; sac
cyt/o	cell
-cyte	cell
-cytosis	increase in the number of cells
dacry/o	tears
dacryocyst/o	lacrimal sac
de-	lack of; removal
dent/o	tooth
derm/o	skin
-derma	skin
dermat/o	skin
-dermis	skin
-desis	surgical binding; surgical fusion
di-	two
dia-	complete; through
diaphor/e	profuse sweating
dilat/o	dilation; dilatation; to expand; widen
dipl/o	double
-dipsia	thirst
don/o	donates
dors/o	back
dorsi-	back
duct/o	to draw
duoden/o	duodenum (proximal portion of small intestine)
dur/o	dura mater (outermost membrane surrounding the brain)
-dynia	pain
dys-	bad; difficult; painful; poor
e-	out; outside; outward; without
-eal	pertaining to

WORD ELEMENT	DEFINITION
ec-	out
ech/o	sound
-ectasis	dilation; (dilatation) stretching; widen; to expand
ecto-	outward
-ectomy	excision; surgical removal
-edema	accumulation of fluid
electr/o	electric
embol/o	plug
-emesis	vomit; vomiting
-emia	blood condition
emmetr/o	in proper measure
en-	inward
encephal/o	brain
endo-	with; within
enter/o	small intestine; intestine
epi-	above; on; upon
epididym/o	epididymis
episi/o	vulva; external genitalia; pudendum
epitheli/o	covering
-er	specialist; one who specializes; specialist in the study of
erythemat/o	red
erythr/o	red
eso-	inward
esophag/o	esophagus
-esthesia	sensation
estr/o	female
ethm/o	ethmoid bone; sieve
eu-	normal; good
ex-	out; outside; outward
exo-	out; outside; outward
extra-	out; outside; outward
faci/o	face
fasci/o	fascia
femor/o	femur; thigh bone
fibr/o	fibers; fibrous tissue
fibul/o	fibula (bone of lower leg)
flex/o	bending
fluor/o	luminous
-flux	flow
front/o	frontal bone
galact/o	milk
gastr/o	stomach
-gen	producing
-genesis	development; production
-genic	producing; produced by
gingiv/o	gums
glen/o	socket; pit; glenoid cavity
gli/o	glue

WORD ELEMENT	DEFINITION
glomerul/o	glomerulus
gloss/o	tongue
gluc/o	sugar
glycogen/o	glycogen (storage form of sugar)
gonad/o	gonads; sex glands
goni/o	angle (of the anterior chamber)
-grade	to step; to go
-gram	record; writing
granul/o	granules
-graph	instrument used to record
-graphy	process of recording; producing images
-gravida	pregnancy
gynec/o	female; woman
hem/o	blood
hemat/o	blood
hemi-	half
hepat/o	liver
herni/o	hernia
hiat/o	hiatus, opening
hidr/o	sweat
hist/o	tissue
histi/o	tissue
home/o	same
humer/o	humerus; upper arm
hydr/o	water
hyper-	abnormal increase; above; above normal; excessive
hypo-	abnormal decrease; below; below normal; under
hyster/o	uterus
-ia	condition; state of
-iasis	abnormal condition; process
-ic	pertaining to
-ician	specialist; one who specializes; expert
ile/o	ileum (distal portion of the small intestine)
ili/o	hip
immun/o	immunity; safe
in-	no; not; in; into
-ine	pertaining to
infer/o	below; downward
infra-	within
inguin/o	groin
insulin/o	insulin
inter-	between
intestin/o	intestine
intra-	within
-ion	process

WORD ELEMENT	DEFINITION
-ior	pertaining to
ir/o	iris
irid/o	iris
is/o	equal
isch/o	hold back
ischi/o	ischium (posterior portion of the hip bone)
-ism	condition; process; state of
-ist	specialist; one who specializes; specialist in the study of
-itis	inflammation (the redness, swelling, heat, and pain that occur when the body protects itself from injury)
-ium	structure
jejun/o	jejunum (middle portion of small intestine)
kal/o	potassium
kerat/o	cornea; hard; hornlike
keratin/o	hard; hornlike
kinesi/o	movement; motion
-kinesia	movement; motion
-kinesis	movement; motion
kyph/o	humpback
labi/o	lips
labyrinth/o	inner ear; labyrinth
lacrim/o	lacrimal apparatus; tears
lact/o	milk
lapar/o	abdominal wall; abdomen
laryng/o	larynx; voice box
lei/o	smooth
leuk/o	white
ligati/o	binding; tying
lingu/o	tongue
lip/o	fat
lipid/o	fat
-lith	calculus; stone
lith/o	calculus; stone
lob/o	lobe
-logist	specialist; one who specializes; specialist in the study of
-logy	study of; process of study
lord/o	swayback
lumb/o	lower back; loins
lymph/o	lymph (a clear, watery fluid)
lymphaden/o	lymph glands; lymph nodes
lymphangi/o	lymph vessels

WORD ELEMENT	DEFINITION
-lysis	breakdown; destruction; separation
-lytic	pertaining to destruction, separation, or breakdown
magnet/o	magnet
-malacia	softening
malleol/o	malleolus (bony projection on the distal aspects of the tibia and fibula)
mamm/o	breast
mandibul/o	mandible; lower jaw
mast/o	breast
maxill/o	maxilla; upper jaw
meat/o	meatus
mediastin/o	mediastinum (cavity between the lungs)
medi/o	middle
medull/o	marrow; medulla; inner portion of an organ
-megaly	enlargement
melan/o	black
men/o	menses; menstruation; month
mening/o	membrane; meninges
meta-	change; transformation
metacarp/o	metacarpals (bones of the hand)
metatars/o	metatarsals (bones of the foot)
-meter	instrument used to measure
metr/o	uterus
-metrist	specialist in the measurement of
-metry	process of measuring; to measure; measurement
mi/o	contraction; less
mono-	one
-mortem	death
muc/o	mucus (a bodily secretion of the mucous membrane, sometimes sticky and frequently thick)
multi-	multiple
muscul/o	muscle
my/o	muscle
myc/o	fungus
mydri/o	dilation (dilatation); wide
-myein	to shut
myel/o	bone marrow; spinal cord
myelin/o	myelin sheath
myos/o	muscle
myring/o	tympanic membrane; eardrum
nas/o	nose
nat/i	birth
natr/o	sodium
necr/o	death

WORD ELEMENT	DEFINITION
nephr/o	kidney
neur/o	nerve
noct/o	night
norm/o	normal
nulli-	none
o/o	egg
occipit/o	occiput (back part of the head)
ocul/o	eye
odont/o	teeth; tooth
-oid	resembling
-ole	small
olecran/o	elbow; olecranon
oligo-	deficient; few; scanty
-oma	mass; tumor
onych/o	nail
oophor/o	ovary
ophthalm/o	eye
-opia	visual condition; vision
-opsia	visual condition; vision
-opsy	to view
-opt/o	vision; sight
-or	one who; person or thing that does something
or/o	mouth
orchi/o	testicle; testis
orchid/o	testicle; testis
orex/i	appetite
ortho-	straight
-ory	pertaining to
-ose	pertaining to
-osis	abnormal condition
oste/o	bone
ot/o	ear
-ous	pertaining to
ov/o	egg
ovari/o	ovary
ox/i	oxygen
ox/o	oxygen
oxy-	quick; sharp
palpebr/o	eyelid
pan-	all
pancreat/o	pancreas
papill/o	optic disc; nipple-like
para-	abnormal; beside; near
-para	give birth; near; part with child; to part with
parathyroid/o	parathyroid gland
pariet/o	parietal bone; wall
-partum	labor; delivery; childbirth

WORD ELEMENT	DEFINITION
patell/a	patella; kneecap
patell/o	patella; kneecap
path/o	disease
-pathy	disease; process of disease
-pause	stoppage; cessation
pector/o	chest
ped/o	child
per-	through
pelv/i	pelvis
pelv/o	pelvis
-penia	decrease; deficiency
-pepsia	digestion
peri-	around
perine/o	perineum
peritone/o	peritoneum
-pexy	surgical fixation
phac/o	lens
-phagia	swallow; to eat
phalang/o	phalanx (one of the bones making up the fingers or toes)
phall/o	penis
pharmac/o	drug
pharyng/o	pharynx; throat
-phasia	speech
phleb/o	vein
-phobia	fear; irrational fear
-phonia	voice
-phoresis	transmission; carry
phot/o	light
phren/o	diaphragm
physi/o	nature
-physis	to grow
pil/o	hair
pine/o	pineal gland
pituitar/o	pituitary gland
-plakia	patches
-plasia	development; formation
-plastic	pertaining to formation
-plasty	surgical repair or reconstruction
-plegia	paralysis (loss or impairment of motor function)
pleur/a	pleura; pleural cavity
pleur/o	pleura; pleural cavity
-pnea	breathing
pneum/o	air; respiration; lungs
pneumat/o	air; respiration; lungs
pneumon/o	lungs
-poiesis	production; manufacture; formation
-poietin	a hormone that stimulates the production of various cell types
poikil/o	variation; irregular
polio-	gray

WORD ELEMENT	DEFINITION	WORD ELEMENT	DEFINITION
poly-	many	scapul/o	scapula
-porosis	porous	-schisis	cleft; splitting
post-	after	-sclerosis	hardening
poster/o	back	scoli/o	curved
practition/o	practice	-scope	instrument used to visually examine (a body cavity or organ)
-prandial	meal		
pre-	before; in front of	-scopy	process of visually examining (a body cavity or organ)
presby-	old age		
primi-	first	seb/o	sebum
pro-	before	sect/o	to cut
proct/o	rectum	secundi-	second
pronati/o	pronation	sial/o	saliva
prostat/o	prostate; prostate gland	sialaden/o	salivary glands
proxim/o	near; close	sigmoid/o	sigmoid colon
pseudo-	false	sinus/o	sinuses
-ptosis	downward displacement; drooping; falling; prolapse; sagging	-sis	state of; condition
		skelet/o	skcleton
-ptysis	spitting	somat/o	body
pub/o	pubis (a portion of the hip bone)	son/o	sound
pulmon/o	lungs	-spadias	opening; split; tear
pupill/o	pupil	-spasm	sudden, involuntary contraction
py/o	pus	sperm/o	spermatozoa; sperm
pyel/o	renal pelvis (dilated upper portion of the ureter)	spermat/o	spermatozoa; sperm
		sphen/o	sphenoid bone; wedge
pylor/o	pylorus (distal portion of the stomach); pyloric sphincter	spin/o	spine; spinal column; backbone; spinal cord
		splen/o	spleen
quadri-	four	spondyl/o	vertebra
		staped/o	stapes
radi/o	radius (one of the bones of the lower arm); x-rays	-stasis	standing; stable; stoppage; stopping; controlling
radicul/o	nerve roots	steat/o	fat
re-	back	-stenosis	narrowing; stricture
rect/o	rectum	stern/o	sternum; breastbone
ren/o	kidney	steth/o	chest
reticul/o	network	-stitial	pertaining to a place
retin/o	retina	stomat/o	mouth
retro-	backward; back; behind	-stomy	new opening
rhabd/o	rod-shaped; striped; striated	sub-	under
rhin/o	nose	super/o	above; toward the head
rhythm/o	rhythm	supinati/o	supination
-rrhage	bursting forth	supra-	above; beyond; excessive
-rrhagia	bursting forth	sym-	together; with
-rrhaphy	suture; sew	synovi/o	synovium; synovial membrane
-rrhea	flow; discharge		
-rrhexis	rupture	tachy-	fast
		-taxia	order; coordination
sacr/o	sacrum	tempor/o	temporal bone
salping/o	eustachian tube; fallopian tubes; uterine tubes	ten/o	tendon
		tend/o	tendon
-salpinx	fallopian tube; uterine tube	tendin/o	tendon
-sarcoma	malignant tumor of connective tissue	tenosynovi/o	tendon sheath (covering of a tendon)

WORD ELEMENT	DEFINITION	WORD ELEMENT	DEFINITION
tens/o	stretch	uln/o	ulnar (one of the bones of the lower arm)
tensi/o	tension	ultra-	excess; beyond
test/o	testicle; testis	-um	structure
testicul/o	testicle; testis	ungu/o	nail
tetra-	four	ur/o	urinary tract; urine; urination
thalam/o	thalamus	ure/o	urea (end product of protein breakdown)
thel/o	nipple	ureter/o	ureters
-therapy	treatment	urethr/o	urethra
-thermy	heat	-uria	urine; urination
thorac/o	chest; thorax	urin/o	urine
-thorax	chest	-us	condition; thing
thromb/o	clot	uter/o	uterus
thym/o	thymus; thymus gland	uve/o	uvea (includes the choroid, ciliary body, and iris)
thyr/o	thyroid gland; shield		
thyroid/o	thyroid gland; shield		
tibi/o	tibia; shin	vagin/o	vagina
-tic	pertaining to	valvul/o	valve
-tocia	labor	varic/o	varicose vein; dilated, twisted vein
-tocin	labor	vas/o	vas deferens; ductus deferens; vessel
tom/o	to cut	vascul/o	vessel
-tome	instrument used to cut	ven/o	vein
-tomy	process of cutting; incision	ventr/o	front
ton/o	tension	ventricul/o	ventricles (lower chambers of the heart)
tonsill/o	tonsils		
top/o	place		
trabecul/o	trabecula; meshwork; latticework	versi/o	turning; tilting; tipping
trache/o	trachea; windpipe	vertebr/o	vertebra
trans-	across	vesic/o	bladder
trigon/o	trigone	viscer/o	internal organs
-tripsy	crushing	vitre/o	glasslike; gel-like
-trophic	pertaining to nourishment or growth	vulv/o	external genitalia; pudendum; vulva
-trophy	development; growth; nutrition; nourishment		
-tropia	turning	xer/o	dry
-tropic	stimulating	xiph/o	sword
-tropion	turning		
tub/o	fallopian tube	-y	process; condition
tympan/o	tympanic membrane; eardrum		
-ule	small	zygomat/o	cheekbone

Definition to Word Element

DEFINITION	WORD ELEMENT
abdomen	abdomin/o; lapar/o
abdominal wall	lapar/o
abnormal	para-
abnormal condition	-iasis; -osis
abnormal increase	hyper-
above	epi ; hyper-; super/o; supra-
accumulation of fluid	-edema
acetabulum	acetabul/o
acromion	acromi/o
across	trans-
adenoids	adenoid/o
adrenal gland	adren/o; adrenal/o
after	post-
against	anti-
air	pneum/o; pneumat/o
air sacs	alveol/o
albumin (a blood protein)	albumin/o
all	pan-
alveolus	alveol/o
amnion	amni/o
analysis of a mixture to identify its contents	-assay
angle (of the anterior chamber)	goni/o
anus	an/o
aorta	aort/o
apart	ana-
appendix	append/o
appetite	orex/i
arm	brachi/o
armpit	axill/o
around	circum-; peri-
artery	arteri/o
aspiration	-centesis
atria (lower) chambers of the heart	atri/o

DEFINITION	WORD ELEMENT
away from	ab-
back	dorsi-; dors/o; poster/o; re-; retro-
back part of the head (occiput)	occipit/o
backbone	spin/o
backward	retro-
bacteria	bacteri/o
bad	dys-
bear (to)	-para
before	ante-; pro-; pre-
beginning	-arche
behind	retro-
below	hypo-; infer/o; sub-
below normal	hypo-
bending	flex/o
bent	ankyl/o
beside	para-
between	inter-
beyond	supra-; ultra-
bile	bil/i; chol/e
bile vessel	cholangi/o
bilirubin (a bile pigment)	bilirubin/o
binding	ligati/o
birth	nat/o
black	melan/o
bladder	cyst/o; vesic/o
blood	hem/o; hemat/o
blood condition	-emia
body	corpor/o; somat/o
bone	osse/o; oste/o
bone marrow	myel/o
bony projection on the distal aspects of the tibia and fibula	malleol/o

DEFINITION	WORD ELEMENT	DEFINITION	WORD ELEMENT
brain	cerebr/o; encephal/o	contraction	mi/o
breakdown	-clast; -lysis	controlling	-stasis
breast	mamm/o; mast/o	coordination	-taxia
breastbone	stern/o	cornea	corne/o; kerat/o
breathing	-pnea	cortex	cortic/o
bronchioles	bronchiol/o	covering	epitheli/o
bronchus	bronchi/o; bronch/o	covering of a tendon	tenosynovi/o
bursa	burs/o	crooked	ankyl/o
bursting forth	-rrhage; -rrhagia	crown	coron/o
		crushing	-tripsy
calcium	calc/o	cul-de-sac	culd/o
calculus	-lith; lith/o	curved	scoli/o
calix	calic/o; calyc/o	cut (to)	cis/o; sect/o; tom/o
calyx	calic/o; calyc/o		
cancer	carcin/o	death	necr/o; -mortem
cancerous	carcin/o	decrease	hypo-; -penia
capsule	capsul/o	deficiency	-penia; oligo-; hypo-
carbon dioxide	-capnia	deficient	oligo-; -penia; hypo-
carry	-phoresis	delivery	-partum
cartilage	cartilagin/o; chondr/o	destruction	-lysis
cecum	cec/o	development	-plasia; -trophy; -genesis
cell	cellul/o; cyt/o; -cyte	diaphragm	phren/o
cerebellum	cerebell/o	difficult	dys-
cervix	cervic/o	digestion	-pepsia
cervix uteri	cervic/o	dilated, twisted vein	varic/o
cessation	-pause	dilated upper portion	pyel/o
change	meta-	of the ureter	
cheek	bucc/o	dilation (dilatation)	dilat/o; -ectasis; mydri/o
cheekbone	zygomat/o	dim	ambly/o
chest	pector/o; steth/o;	discharge	-rrhea
	thorac/o; -thorax	disease	path/o; -pathy
child	ped/o	donates	don/o
childbirth	-partum	double	dipl/o
cholesterol	cholesterol/o	downward	infer/o
choroid	chori/o	downward displacement	-ptosis
ciliary body	cycl/o	draw (to)	duct/o
clavicle	clavicul/o	draw together (to)	constrict/o
clear, watery fluid	lymph/o	drooping	-ptosis
cleft	-schisis	drug	pharmac/o
close	proxim/o	dry	xer/o
clot (a)	thromb/o	dull	ambly/o
clot (to)	coagulati/o	ductus deferens	vas/o
coccyx	coccyg/o	duodenum (proximal	duoden/o
cochlea	cochle/o	portion of small	
cold	cry/o	intestine)	
collarbone	clavicul/o	dura mater (outermost	dur/o
colon	col/o; colon/o	membrane surrounding	
color	chrom/o	the brain)	
common bile duct	choledoch/o		
complete	dia-	ear	aur/o; ot/o
condense (to)	coagulati/o	eardrum	myring/o; tympan/o
condition	-ia; -ism; -sis; -y	eat (to)	-phagia
cone-shaped	-conus	egg	o/o; ov/o

DEFINITION	WORD ELEMENT
elbow	olecran/o
electric	electr/o
enlargement	-megaly
epididymis	epididym/o
equal	is/o
esophagus	esophag/o
ethmoid bone	ethm/o
eustachian tube	salping/o
excess	ultra-
excessive	hyper-; supra-
excision	-ectomy
expand (to)	dilat/o; -ectasis
expert	-ician
external genitalia	episi/o; vulv/o
extremity	acr/o
eye	ocul/o; ophthalm/o
eyelid	blephar/o; palpebr/o
face	faci/o
falling	-ptosis
fallopian tube	salping/o; -salpinx; tub/o
false	pseudo-
fascia (band of tissue surrounding a muscle)	fasci/o
fast	tachy-
fat	adip/o; lip/o; lipid/o; steat/o
fatty debris	ather/o
fatty plaque	ather/o
fear	-phobia
female	estr/o; gynec/o
femur	femor/o
few	oligo-
fibers	fibr/o
fibrous tissue	fibr/o
fibula (bone of lower leg)	fibul/o
first	primi-
flow	-flux; -rrhea
formation	-plasia; -poiesis
formed in	-genic
four	quadri-; tetra-
front	anter/o; ventr/o
frontal bone	front/o
fungus	myc/o
fusion of parts	ankyl/o
gall	chol/e
gallbladder	cholecyst/o
gel-like	vitre/o
give birth	-para
gland	aden/o

DEFINITION	WORD ELEMENT
glans penis (tip of penis)	balan/o
glasslike	vitre/o
glenoid cavity	glen/o
glomerulus	glomerul/o
glycogen (storage form of sugar)	glycogen/o
go (to)	-grade
gonads	gonad/o
good	eu-
granules	granul/o
gray	polio-
groin	inguin/o
grow (to)	-physis
growing thing	-blast
growth	-trophy
gums	gingiv/o
hair	cili/o; pil/o
half	hemi-
hard	kerat/o; keratin/o
hardening	-sclerosis; scler/o
head	cephal/o
hearing	audi/o; -cusis
heart	cardi/o
heat	-thermy
heel	calcane/o
hernia (protrusion of an organ from the structure that normally contains it)	-cele; herni/o
hiatus	hiat/o
hidden	crypt/o
hip	ili/o
hip socket	acetabul/o
hold back	isch/o
hormone that stimulates the production of various cell types	-poietin
hornlike	kerat/o; keratin/o
humerus	humer/o
humpback	kyph/o
ileum (distal portion of the small intestine)	ile/o
immature	-blast
immunity	immun/o
in; into	in-
in proper measure	emmetr/o
inadequate	a(n)-

DEFINITION	WORD ELEMENT	DEFINITION	WORD ELEMENT
incision	-tomy	loss or impairment of motor function	-plegia
increase in the number of cells	-cytosis	lower back	lumb/o
inflammation (redness, swelling, heat, and pain that occur when the body protects itself from injury)	-itis	lower jaw	mandibul/o
		luminous	fluor/o
		lungs	pneum/o; pneumon/o; pulmon/o
in front of	pre-	lymph (clear, watery fluid)	lymph/o
inner ear	labyrinth/o	lymph glands	lymphaden/o
instrument used to cut	-tome	lymph node	lymphaden/o
instrument used to measure	-meter	lymph vessels	lymphangi/o
instrument used to record	-graph	magnet	magnet/o
instrument used to visually examine (a body cavity or organ)	-scope	male	andr/o
		malignant tumor of connective tissue	-sarcoma
insulin	insulin/o	malleolus	malleol/o
internal organ	viscer/o	man	andr/o
intestine	enter/o; intestin/o	mandible (lower jaw)	mandibul/o
inward	en-; eso-	manufacture	-poiesis
iris	irid/o; ir/o	many	poly-
irrational fear	-phobia	marrow	medull/o
irregular	poikil/o	mass	-oma
irrigation	-clysis	maxilla (upper jaw)	maxill/o
ischium	ischi/o	meal	-prandial
		measure (to)	-metry
		meatus	meat/o
jejunum (middle portion of small intestine)	jejun/o	mediastinum	mediastin/o (cavity between the lungs)
joint	arthr/o; articul/o	medulla	medull/o
		membrane	chori/o; mening/o
kidney	nephr/o; ren/o	meninges	mening/o
kill (to)	-cidal	menses	men/o
kneecap	patell/a; patell/o	menstruation	men/o
		meshwork	trabecul/o
labor	-partum; -tocia; -tocin	metacarpals (bones of the hand)	metacarp/o
labyrinth	labyrinth/o	metatarsals (bones of the foot)	metatars/o
lack of	de-		
lacrimal apparatus	lacrim/o	middle	medi/o
lacrimal sac	dacryocyst/o	milk	galact/o; lact/o
large intestine	col/o	month	men/o
larynx	laryng/o	motion	-kinesia; -kinesis; kinesi/o
lattice work	trabecul/o	mouth	or/o; stomat/o
lens	phac/o; phak/o	movement	-kinesia; -kinesis; kinesi/o
less	mi/o	mucus (a bodily secretion, of the mucous membrane, sometimes sticky and frequently thick)	muc/o
life	bi/o		
light	phot/o		
lips	cheil/o; labi/o		
little bronchi	bronchiol/o		
liver	hepat/o	multiple	multi-
lobe	lob/o	muscle	muscul/o; myos/o
loins	lumb/o	myelin sheath	myelin/o

DEFINITION	WORD ELEMENT	DEFINITION	WORD ELEMENT
nail	onych/o; ungu/o	penis	phall/o
narrowing	-stenosis	perineum	perine/o
nature	physi/o	peritoneum	peritone/o
near	proxim/o; para-	person or thing that does something	-or
neck	cervic/o	pertaining to	-ac; -al; -ar; -ary; -eal; -ic; -ine; -ior; -or; -ory; -ose; -ous, -tic
neck of uterus	cervic/o		
nerve	neur/o		
nerve roots	radicul/o		
network	reticul/o	pertaining to a place	-stitial
new opening	-stomy	pertaining to destruction, separation, or breakdown	-lytic
night	noct/o		
nipple	thel/o	pertaining to formation	-plastic
nipple-like	papill/o	pertaining to nourishment or growth	-tropic
no	a(n)-; in-		
no strength	-asthenia	phalanges (one of the bones making up the fingers or toes)	phalang/o
none	nulli-		
normal	eu-; norm/o		
nose	nas/o; rhin/o	pharynx	pharyng/o
not	a(n)-; -in	pineal gland	pine/o
nourishment	-trophy	pit	glen/o
nutrition	-trophy	pituitary gland	pituitar/o
		place	top/o
occiput (back part of the head)	occipit/o	pleura	pleur/a; pleur/o
		pleural cavity	pleur/a; pleur/o
old age	presby-	plug	embol/o
olecranon	olecran/o	poor	dys-
on	epi-	porous	-porosis
one	mono-	posterior portion of the hip bone	ischi/o
one who	-or		
one who specializes; specialist	-er; -or; -ician; -ist; logist	potassium	kal/o
		practice	practition/o
opening	-spadias; hiat/o	pregnancy	-cyesis; -gravida
optic disc	papill/o	process	-iasis; -ation; -ion; -ism; -y
order	-taxia	process of cutting	-tomy
out	e-; ec-; ex-; exo-; extra-	process of disease	-pathy
outer layer	cortic/o	process of measuring	-metry
outside	e-; ec-; ecto-; ex-; exo-; extra-	process of producing images	-graphy
		process of recording	-graphy
outward	e-; ec-; ex-; exo-; extra-	process of study	-logy
ovary	oophor/o; ovari/o	process of visually examining (a body cavity or organ)	-scopy
oxygen	ox/o; ox/i		
		produced by	-genic
pain	-algia; -dynia	producing	-gen; -genic
painful	dys-	producing images	-graphy
pancreas	pancreat/o	production	genesis; -poiesis
paralysis	-plegia	profuse sweating	diaphor/e
parathyroid gland	parathyroid/o	prolapse	-ptosis
parietal bone	pariet/o	pronation	pronati/o
part with child	-para	prostate	prostat/o
patches	-plakia	protrusion	-cele
patella	patell/a; patell/o	pubis (a portion of the hip bone)	pub/o
pelvis	pelv/i; pelv/o		

DEFINITION	WORD ELEMENT	DEFINITION	WORD ELEMENT
pudendum	episi/o; vulv/o	skin	cutane/o; derm/o;
pupil	core/o; pupill/o		-derma; dermat/o;
pus	py/o		-dermis
pyloric sphincter	pylor/o	skull	crani/o
pylorus	pylor/o	small	-ole; -ule
quick	oxy-	small bronchi	bronchiol/o
		small intestine	enter/o
radius (bone of	radi/o	smooth	lei/o
lower arm)		socket	glen/o
reconstruction	-plasty	sodium	natr/o
record	-gram	softening	-malacia
rectum	proct/o; rect/o	something inserted	catheter/o
red	erythemat/o; erythr/o	sound	ech/o; son/o
relaxation	-chalasis	specialist	-ician; -logist
removal	de-	specialist in the	-metrist
renal pelvis	pyel/o	measurement of	
resembling	-oid	specialist in the study of;	-er; -or; -ician; -ist;
respiration	pneumat/o; pneum/o	one who specializes;	-logist
retina	retin/o	specialist	
rhythm	rhythm/o	speech	-phasia
ribs	cost/o	spermatozoa (sperm)	sperm/o; spermat/o
rod-shaped	rhabd/o	sphenoid bone	sphen/o
rupture	-rrhexis	spinal column	spin/o
		spinal cord	myel/o; spin/o
sac	cyst/o	spine	spin/o
sac filled with	burs/o	spitting	-ptysis
synovial fluid located		spleen	splen/o
around joints		split	-spadias
sac in which the fetus	amni/o	splitting	-schisis
lies in the uterus		stable	-stasis
sagging	-ptosis	standing	-stasis
saliva	sial/o	stapes	staped/o
salivary gland	sialaden/o	state of	-ia; -ism; -sis
same	home/o	step (to)	-grade
scanty	oligo-	sternum	stern/o
scapula	scapul/o	stimulating	-tropic
sebum	seb/o	stomach	gastr/o
second	secundi-	stone	-lith; lith/o
secrete (to)	crin/o; -crine	stop (to)	-continence
self	auto-	stoppage	-pause; -stasis
sensation	-esthesia	straight	ortho-
separate	-crit; -lysis	stretching	-ectasis
sew	-rrhaphy	striated	rhabd/o
sex glands	gonad/o	stricture	-stenosis
sharp	oxy-	striped	rhabd/o
shield	thyr/o; thyroid/o	structure	-ium; -um
shin bone	tibi/o	study of	-logy
shut (to)	-myein	sudden, involuntary	-spasm
sieve	ethm/o	contraction	
sight	opt/o	sugar	gluc/o
sigmoid colon	sigmoid/o	supination	supinati/o
sinuses	sinus/o	surgical binding	-desis
skeleton	skelet/o		

DEFINITION	WORD ELEMENT	DEFINITION	WORD ELEMENT
surgical fixation	-pexy	trabecula	trabecul/o
surgical fracture	-clasis	toward the head	super/o
surgical fusion	-desis	trachea	trache/o; windpipe
surgical puncture to remove fluid	-centesis	transformation	meta-
		transmission	-phoresis
surgical reconstruction	-plasty	treatment	-therapy
surgical refracture	-clasis	trigone	trigon/o
surgical removal	-ectomy	tube	tub/o
surgical repair	-plasty	tumor	-oma
suture (to sew)	-rrhaphy	turmoil	-clonus
swallow	-phagia	turning	-tropia; -tropion; versi/o
swayback	lord/o	two	di-
sweat	hidr/o	tying	ligati/o
sword	xiph/o	tympanic membrane	tympan/o; myring/o
synovial membrane	synovi/o		
synovium	synovi/o	ulna (bone of lower arm)	uln/o
		umbilicus	umbilic/o
tail	caud/o	under	hypo-; sub-
tailbone	coccyg/o	unequal	anis/o
tears	dacry/o; lacrim/o	up	ana
tear	-spadias	upon	epi-
teeth	odont/o	upper arm	humer/o
temporal bone	tempor/o	upper jaw	maxill/o
tendon	tend/o; tendin/o	urea (end product of protein breakdown)	ure/o
tendon sheath	tenosynovi/o		
tension	tensi/o; ton/o	ureter	ureter/o
testicle	orchi/o; orchid/o; test/o; testicul/o	urethra	urethr/o
		urinary tract	ur/o
testis	orchi/o; orchid/o; test/o; testicul/o	urination	ur/o; -uria
		urine	ur/o; -uria; urin/o
tetra-	four	uterine tube	salping/o; -salpinx
thalamus	thalam/o	uterus	uter/o; hyster/o; metr/o
thigh bone	femor/o		
thing	-us	uvea	uve/o
thirst	-dipsia		
thorax	thorac/o	vagina	colp/o; vagin/o
throat	pharyng/o	valve	valvul/o
through	per-	variation	poikil/o
thymus gland	thym/o	varicose vein	varic/o
thyroid gland	thyr/o; thyroid/o	vas deferens	vas/o
tibia (shin bone)	tibi/o	vein	phleb/o; ven/o
tilting	versi/o	ventricles (lower chambers of the heart)	ventricul/o
tip of penis	balan/o		
tipping	versi/o	vertebra	vertebr/o; spondyl/o
tissue	hist/o; histi/o	vessel	angi/o; vas/o; vascul/o
together	sym-	view (to)	-opsy
tone	ton/o	vision	-opia; -opsia; opt/o
tongue	gloss/o; lingu/o	visual condition	-opia; -opsia
tonsils	tonsill/o	voice	-phonia
tooth	dent/o; odont/o	voice box	laryng/o
top	acr/o	vomit	-emesis
toward	ad-		

DEFINITION	WORD ELEMENT	DEFINITION	WORD ELEMENT
vulva	episi/o; vulv/o	windpipe	trache/o
wall	pariet/o	with	endo-; sym-
washing	-clysis	within	endo-; infra-; intra-
water	aque/o; hydr/o	without	e-
wedge	sphen/o	woman	gynec/o
white	albin/o; leuk/o	wrist	carp/o
wide	mydri/o	writing	-gram
widen	dilat/o		
		x-rays	radi/o

A

a-, 63
ab-, 54, 67
AB blood type, 313
abbreviations
  body organization, 85
  cardiovascular system, 299–300
  digestive system, 393–394
  endocrine system, 268
  eyes and ears, 228–229, 237
  female reproductive system, 467
  immune system, 328
  integumentary system, 105
  lymphatic system, 328
  male reproductive system, 435
  muscular system, 170
  nervous system, 200
  respiratory system, 358
  skeletal system, 146
  urinary system, 425–426
abdominal, 380
abdominal cavity, 74–75
abdomin/o, 26, 380
abdominocentesis, 43
abdominopelvic cavity, 74–75,
    79–80, 378
abdominoplasty, 102–103
abduction, 54, 167–168
abductor, 163
A blood type, 313
abrasion, 97
absorption, 369
-ac, 46
accessory reproductive organs, 427
acetabular, 134
acetabul/o, 134
acetabuloplasty, 134
acetabulum, 122
achalasia, 390
achondroplasia, 130
acr/o, 34, 261
acromegaly, 261
acrophobia, 38
acute renal failure, 423
ad-, 54, 67
Adam's apple, 341
adduction, 54, 167–168
adductor, 163
adenitis, 6
aden/o, 9, 21, 261
adenocarcinomas, 104
adenohypophysis, 266
adenoidectomy, 345
adenoid/o, 24, 345
adenoids, 325

adenoma, 98, 261
adip/o, 18, 93
adipocyte, 45
adipose, 93
adjectival suffixes, 46–47
adrenal cortex, 260
adrenalectomy, 262
adrenal glands, 252, 253, 257
adrenaline, 257, 260
adrenal medulla, 260
adrenal/o, 262
adren/o, 21, 262
adrenocorticotropic hormone (ACTH),
    255, 259, 266
afterbirth, 468
age-related macular degeneration
    (ARMD), 228
age spots, 103
aging effects
  on cardiovascular system, 298
  on digestive system, 392
  on endocrine system, 267
  on eyes and ears, 226, 236
  on female repodutive system, 465
  on immune system, 327
  on integumentary system, 103
  on male reproductive system, 434
  on muscular system, 169
  on nervous system, 198
  on respiratory system, 356
  on skeletal system, 144
  on urinary system, 422
agranular leukocytes, 312
-aise, 53
-al, 83
albinism, 93
albin/o, 93
albumin, 311
aldosterone, 255, 260
-algia, 35, 46
alpha waves, 190
alveolar ducts, 343, 345
alveoli, 343, 356
alveolitis, 345
alveol/o, 25, 345
Alzheimer's disease, 198
ambly/o, 215
amblyopia, 223
amenorrhea, 459
amni/o, 471
amniocentesis, 469, 471
amnion, 468
amniotic fluid, 468
an-, 63
-an, 455

ana-, 65, 68
anal canal, 375
anatamoy, 65
anatomical position, 75–76
anatomical roots, 18–29
anatomy, 16
andr/o, 429
androgenic, 429
androgens, 257, 262
anemia, 63, 316
anesthesia, 195
aneurysm, 298
angiectasis, 297
angi/o, 23, 289
angiogram, 290
angiography, 289
angioplasty, 290–291
angiospasm, 291
anhidrosis, 95
anis/o, 313
anisocoria, 217
anisocytosis, 316
annulus fibrosus, 121
an/o, 380
anorectal, 380
anorexia, 387
anoxia, 347
ante-, 54–55, 67, 463
anteflexion, 463
antenatal, 54
antepartum, 474
anterior, 76, 78, 84
anterior lobes, 255
anterior pituitary gland, 255–256, 259
anter/o, 82
anteversion, 463
anti-, 63, 67
antibiotic, 63
antibodies, 89, 313
antidiuretic hormone, 254–255,
    259, 264
antigens, 313
antrum, 372–373
anuria, 421
anus, 450
aorta, 280, 287
aortic semilunar valve, 280, 287
aort/o, 291
aortostenosis, 291
aortotomy, 291
apex, 343
Apgar score, 469, 471
aphagia, 390
aphakia, 220
aphasia, 197

aphonia, 353
apnea, 354
appendectomy, 380
appendicitis, 380
appendic/o, 380
appendicular skeleton, 118, 122–126,
        132–135
appendix, 375
append/o, 380
aque/o, 216
aqueous humor, 210, 211, 216
-ar, 53
-arche, 461
areola, 452–453
arrythmia, 295
arteries, 278, 284–285, 286
arteri/o, 23, 292
arteriography, 292
arterioles, 284, 292
arteriosclerosis, 39, 292
arteriostenosis, 292
arthralgia, 35, 135
arthritis, 6, 136–137
arthr/o, 19, 135
arthrocentesis, 140
arthrodesis, 43, 140
arthropathy, 137
arthroplasty, 137–138, 144
arthroscopy, 138–139
articular cartlidge, 126, 144
articul/o, 135
-ary, 46
ascending colon, 375
aseptic, 63
aspermatogenesis, 430
asphyxia, 355
aspiration pneumonia, 357
-assay, 265
-asthenia, 166
asthma, 356
astigmatism, 227
ataxia, 198
atherectomy, 292
ather/o, 292
atheroma, 292
atherosclerosis, 292
atonic, 166
atria, 278–279
atri/o, 292
atrioventicular node (AV node), 282, 283
atrioventricular (AV) valves, 278–279
atrioventricular bundle (AV bundle), 282
atrophy, 169
audi/o, 232
audiogram, 232
audiometry, 232
audit/o, 232
auditory, 232
aural, 232
auricle, 229

aur/o, 232
auto-, 65
autoimmune disease, 326
autoimmunodeficiency syndrome
        (AIDS), 327
autopsy, 65
avascular, 296
axial skeleton, 117–121, 125, 129–132
axillary nodes, 321, 324
axill/o, 18
axons, 180, 198

B

bacteri/o, 413
bacteriuria, 421
balanitis, 429
balan/o, 429
balanorrhea, 430
barrel chest, 356
Bartholin's glands, 451–452
basal cell carcinoma, 98–99, 104
basal cell layer, 88
basal pneumonia, 357
basophils, 312
B blood type, 313
benign prostatic hyperplasia (BPH),
        434–435
beta waves, 190
bi-, 64
biceps brachii, 160
bicuspids, 370–371
bicuspid valve, 279, 280, 287
bilateral, 64
bile, 376
bil/i, 380
biliary, 380
biliary tract, 376
bilirubin/o, 313
bi/o, 18, 93
biopsy, 42, 462
-blast, 140, 316
blephar/o, 21, 216
blepharochalasis, 223
blepharopexy, 216
blepharoplasty, 103, 216
blepharoptosis, 38, 39
blepharospasm, 40
blind spot, 211
blood, 310–319
        abbreviations, 319
        common diseases of, 318–319
        effects of aging on, 318
        formation, 312
        formed elements, 310–312
        plasma, 310, 311
        term analysis and definition, 314–318
blood-brain barrier (BBB), 185
blood glucose, 267
blood pressure, 284

blood types, 313
blood vessels, 278, 284–286
B lymphocytes (B cells), 319–320
body organization, 73–86
        abbreviations, 85
        body parts, 74–75
        cavities, 74–75
        directional teminology, 75–80
        levels of, 16
        planes of the body, 81–82
        term analysis and definition, 83–84
body parts, arrangment of, 74–75
body systems, 16–17
bolus, 371
bone cancers, 144
bone density, 144
bone function, 116
bone marrow transplantation, 318
bones
        See also skeletal system
        anatomy and physiology of, 116
        cranial, 118–119, 129–130
        facial, 118–119, 129–130
        general terminology, 128–129
        major, 142–143
bone structure, 116
bony labyrinth, 231
Bowman's capsule, 412
brachial, 133
brachi/o, 133
brachiocephalic, 133
brady-, 65, 68
-brady, 298
bradycardia, 65, 298
bradykinesia, 168, 197
bradypnea, 354
brain, 178, 179, 182–184
        See also nervous system
brain stem, 182
brain tumors, 199
brain waves, 190–191
BRCA1, 465
BRCA2, 465
breast cancer, 465
breasts, 452–453
breathing, 338
breathing patterns, 354
breech position, 469
bronchi, 342
bronchial asthma, 342
bronchial tree, 342
bronchiectasis, 345
bronchi/o, 25, 345
bronchioles, 46, 338, 342
bronchiolitis, 346
bronchiol/o, 25, 346
bronchitis, 345
bronch/o, 25, 345
bronchodilators, 346, 356
bronchogenic carcinoma, 346

bronchography, 353
bronchopneumonia, 357
bronchoscope, 42
bronchoscopy, 43, 346
bronchospasm, 346
buccal mucosa, 370, 380
bucc/o, 380
bulbourethral gland, 429
bundle branches, 282
bundle of His, 282
burns, 104
bursa, 127
bursae, 127
bursectomy, 139
bursitis, 127, 139
burs/o, 139

C

calcaneal, 134
calcane/o, 134
calcaneus, 123–124
calcitonin, 257, 259
calc/o, 262
caliceal, 413
calic/o, 413
caliectasis, 413
calyc/o, 413
canal of Schlemm, 213
cancer
    bone, 144
    breast, 465
    immune system and, 327
    leukemia, 318–319
    lung, 357
    prostate, 435
    skin, 98–100, 104
    uterine (endometrial), 465–466
canines, 370–371
capillaries, 278, 284, 285, 286, 343, 374
capillary beds, 285
-capnia, 352
carcin/o, 34
carcinogenic, 46
carcinomas, 98–99, 104
cardia, 372–373
cardiac, 46
cardiac arrest, 298
cardiac muscle, 159
cardiac sphincter, 372
cardi/o, 9, 23, 292
cardiograph, 40
cardiologist, 292
cardiology, 6, 8, 293
cardiomegaly, 293
cardiomyopathy, 293
cardiovascular system (CVS), 277–308
    abbreviations, 299–300
    blood pressure, 284
    blood vessels, 284–286

circulation, 286–289
common diseases of, 298–299
conduction system, 282–283
effects of aging on, 298
heart sounds, 284
heart structure, 278–281
term analysis and definition, 289–298
carditis, 6
carpal bones, 122–123
carpal tunnel syndrome (CTS), 169
carpectomy, 133
carp/o, 133
cas/o, 23
cataracts, 226–227
catecholamines, 257, 260
catheterization, 414
catheter/o, 414
cauda equina, 185, 186
caudal, 76, 78, 83
caud/o, 82
cavities, 74–75
cec/o, 380
cecopexy, 380
cecum, 375
-cele, 35–36, 195, 431, 462
cell body, 180
cells, 16, 17
    basal, 88
    blood, 310–312, 319–320
    differentiated, 312
    epithelial, 88, 91
    interstitial, 428
    keratinized, 88, 91
    mast, 89
    memory, 320
    nerve, 178, 180–181
    plasma, 89
    stem, 312
    undifferentiated, 312
cellular immunity, 320
cellul/o, 53
cementum, 370–371
-centesis, 43, 140
central endocrine glands, 252–256
central nervous system (CNS), 178, 179, 182–187
    brain, 182–184
    protective coverings, 185, 187
    spinal cord, 185, 186
cephalgia, 9, 35
cephal/o, 18
cerebellar, 189
cerebellitis, 190
cerebell/o, 189
cerebellum, 182, 183
cerebral angiography, 196
cerebral cortex, 182–184, 190
cerebr/o, 21, 190
cerebromalacia, 37

cerebrospinal, 190
cerebrospinal fluid (CSF), 185, 187
cerebrovascular, 190
cerebrovascular accident (CVA), 297, 299
cerebrum, 182–184
cerumen, 91
ceruminous glands, 91
cervic, 450
cervical, 131
cervical dilatation, 469
cervical nodes, 321, 324
cervical poly, 455
cervical vertebrae, 119–120
cervicitis, 455
cervic/o, 18, 131, 455
cervix uteri, 451
cesarean section (CS), 469
-chalasia, 390
-chalasis, 223
cheil/o, 26, 381
cheiloplasty, 381
cheilorrhaphy, 381
cheilosis, 381
chemotherapy, 318
chlamydia, 466
cholangi/o, 381
cholangiogram, 381
cholangiopancreatography, 381
chol/e, 379
cholecystectomy, 381
cholecystitis, 381
cholecyst/o, 381
cholecystolithiasis, 386
choledoch/o, 381
choledocholithiasis, 386, 387
choledocholithotripsy, 386
choledocotomy, 381
cholelith, 8, 390
cholelithiasis, 387
cholesterol, 311
cholesterol/o, 313
chondr/o, 19
chondrocyte, 130
chondroma, 130
chondromalacia, 37
chondro/o, 130
chondrosarcoma, 141
chordae tendineae, 279
chori/o, 216
chorion, 468
chorionic villus sampling (CVS), 469, 470
chorioretinitis, 216
choroid, 210, 211, 212
choroiditis, 216
choroid/o, 216
chrom/o, 314
chrondromalacia, 140

chrondroplasia, 46
chronic renal failure, 423
chyme, 372
-cidal, 413
cigarette smoking, 356, 357
cilia, 356
ciliary body, 210, 211, 212
ciliary muscles, 210, 211
ciliary process, 210, 211
cili/o, 18
circulation, 286, 287–289
circulatory system, 23
circum-, 55, 67, 433
circumcision, 429, 433
circumduction, 55, 167–168
cis/o, 53
-cispid, 53
-clasis, 140
-clast, 140
clavicles, 122
clavicul/o, 132
cleft palate, 370
climacteric period, 454
clitoris, 451–452
-clonus, 166
closed fracture, 144–145
closed reduction, 145
-clysis, 379
coagulati/o, 215
coccygeal, 131
coccyg/o, 131
coccyx, 120
cochlea, 231
cochlear duct, 231, 232
cochle/o, 232
colitis, 382
collagen, 89, 103
collateral circulation, 287
Colles' fracture, 144–145
col/o, 26, 382
colocolostomy, 382
colon/o, 382
colonoscope, 56, 375
colostomy, 382, 392
colostrum, 471
colp/o, 29, 455
colpoperineoplasty, 460
colporrhaphy, 44, 455
colposcopy, 455
comat/o, 53
combining forms, 9
combining vowels, 7–9
comminuted fracture, 144–145
common bile duct (CBD), 376
computed tomography (CT scan),
    41, 196
conduction system, 282–283
conductive deafness, 236
cones, 210, 211

coni/o, 345
conjunctival membrane, 213–214
conjunctivitis, 216
conjunctiv/o, 216
connective tissue, 89
constipation, 392
constricting, 210
constrict/o, 289
-continence, 413
contra-, 63, 67
contralateral, 63
-conus, 215
conus medullaris, 185, 186
convolutions, 182
core/o, 217
coreometer, 217
cornea, 210, 211
corneal, 217
corne/o, 217
coronal plane, 81–82
coronary arteries, 287–288, 293
coronary veins, 287
coron/o, 293
corpor/o, 414
corpus callosum, 182, 184
cortex, 408–409
cortical, 190, 414
cortic/o, 190, 414
corticospinal, 190
cortisol, 255, 260
cosmetic surgery, 101–103
costal cartilage, 121
cost/o, 19, 130–131
costochondral, 130–131
costosternal, 131
costovertebral joint, 132
Cowper's gland, 429
coxal bones, 122
crania cavity, 74–75
cranial, 76, 78, 83
cranial bones, 118–119
cranial nerves, 187, 188
crani/o, 19, 129–130
craniofacial, 129
craniometer, 41
cranioplasty, 129
craniotomy, 130
creatine, 407
-crine, 265
crin/o, 262
-crit, 316
Crohn's disease, 392
cry/o, 92
cryotherapy, 100
crypt/o, 413
cryptorchidism, 430
cul-de-sac of Douglas, 451
culd/o, 456
culdocentesis, 456

culdoscope, 456
-cusis, 235
cuspids, 370–371
cusps, 279
cutane/o, 18, 93
cuticle, 91
cyan/o, 93
cyanotic, 93
cycl/o, 217
cyclophotocoagulation, 221
cycloplegia, 217
-cyesis, 473
cystic duct, 376
cystitis, 414
cyst/o, 27, 414
cystocele, 35, 462
cystoscope, 414
cystoscopy, 414
cystourethrography, 419
-cyte, 45
cyt/o, 18
cytology, 462
cytopenia, 38
-cytosis, 316

D
-dacry/o, 217
dacryocyst/o, 217
dacryogenic, 217
de-, 198
deafness, 236
debridement, 104
deciduous teeth, 370–371
deep, 76, 79
defecation, 375
deglutition, 371
delta waves, 190
dematologist, 95
demyelination, 198
dendrites, 180
dental caries, 383
dentiform, 8
dentin, 370–371
dent/o, 383
deoxygenated blood, 278, 287
-derma, 98
derma-, 101
dermabrasion, 101
dermatitis, 93, 94
dermat/o, 18, 93
dermatology, 93
dermatomycosis, 96
dermatoplasty, 95
dermis, 88, 89–90
-dermis, 98
derm/o, 18, 93
descending colon, 375
-desis, 43, 140
di-, 64

dia-, 55
diabetes mellitus, 267
diagnosis, 55
diagnostic procedures, suffixes to
    indicate, 40–43
dialysis, 421, 423
diameter, 55
diaphor/e, 95
diaphoresis, 95
diaphragm, 74
diaphysis, 141
diastole, 284
diastolic pressure, 284
diathermy, 169
differentiated cells, 312
digestion, 369
digestive system, 368–405
    abbreviations, 393–394
    accessory organs, 376–377
    common diseases of, 392–393
    common roots, 26
    components of, 369
    effects of aging on, 392
    esophagus, 372
    large intestine, 375
    oral cavity, 370–371
    peritoneum, 378–379
    pharynx, 371
    small intestine, 373–374
    stomach, 372–373
    term analysis and definition, 380–391
digestive tract, 369
digest/o, 53
dilat/o, 289, 345
dipl/o, 215
diplopia, 223
-dipsia, 265
direction, prefixes referring to, 54–62
directional teminology, 75–80
dissection, 64
distal, 76, 79
don/o, 34
dopamine, 199
dorsal, 76, 78, 83
dorsal cavity, 74–75
dorsal vertebrae, 119–120
dorsi-, 163
dorsiflexion, 167–168
dors/o, 82
dorsum, 76, 77, 79
-drome, 53
Duchenne's muscular dystrophy, 170
duct/o, 53, 163
ductus deferens, 428
dudenal, 383
duiplegia, 197
duoden/o, 383
duodenum, 373
dura mater, 185, 187

dur/o, 190
-dynia, 36
dys-, 65, 67
dysesthesia, 196
dyskinesia, 168, 197
dysmenorrhea, 459
dyspepsia, 391
dysphagia, 390
dysphasia, 197
dysphonia, 353
dysplasia, 65
dyspnea, 354
dystocia, 474
dystonia, 166
dystrophy, 169
dysuria, 421

E

e-, 57, 67
-eal, 46
eardrum, 229
ears, 229–237
    abbreviations, 237
    common diseases of, 236
    effects of aging on, 236
    external ear, 229–230
    inner ear (labyrinth), 231
    middle ear, 230–231
    term analysis and definition, 232–235
ech/o, 293
echocardiogram, 293
eclampsia, 475
-ectasis, 297
ecto-, 55
ectogenous, 55
-ectomy, 44
ectopic pregnancy, 472
ectropion, 225
-edema, 215, 314
edentulous, 383
effector, 178
egg, 449
elastin, 89
electr/o, 164
electrocardiogram (ECG), 283, 293
electrocardiograph, 283
electrocochleography, 232
electrocytes, 407
electroencephalogram, 190
electroencephalograph, 191
electroencephalography (EEG), 196
electromyogram, 165
electromyography, 164
electrophoresis, 317
embol/o, 295
embolus, 295
embryo, 468
-emesis, 36, 390, 473
-emia, 316

emmetr/o, 215
emmetropia, 225
emphysema, 356
enamel, 370–371
encephalitis, 191
encephal/o, 21, 190
encephalocele, 36
encephalomalacia, 191
encephalopathy, 191
endarterectomy, 292
endo-, 55, 67, 391
endocardium, 280–281
endocrine glands, 252–260
endocrine hormones, 259–260, 265
endocrine system, 251–276
    abbreviations, 268
    central endocrine glands, 254–256
    common diseases of, 267
    common roots, 22
    effects of aging on, 267
    peripheral endocrine glands, 256–260
    term analysis and definition, 261–266
endocrinologist, 262
endocrinology, 262
endodontist, 387
endolymph, 231
endometrial cancer, 465–466
endometriosis, 459
endometrium, 459
endoscopes, 55–56
endoscopy, 391
endosteum, 129
endotracheal, 352
end-stage renal disease, 423
enteritis, 37
enter/o, 26, 383
entropion, 225
eosinophils, 312
epi-, 57, 67, 68
epicardium, 280–281, 281
epidermis, 88–89, 90, 98
epididymis, 428
epididymitis, 430
epididym/o, 28, 430
epidural, 190
epigastric, 57, 83
epiglottis, 341, 371
epilepsy, 190–191, 199
epinephrine, 257, 260
epiphysis, 141
episi/o, 456
episiorrhaphy, 456
episiotomy, 456
epispadias, 433
epithelial, 95
epithelial cells, 88, 91
epitheli/o, 95
epithelium, 88, 95
eponychium, 91, 96

-er, 45
errors of refraction, 227
erthrocytes, 310
erthyrocytopenia, 317
erythema, 95
erythemat/o, 95
erythematous, 95
erythremia, 316
erythr/o, 95, 315
erythrocytes, 311, 315
erythroderma, 98
erythropoiesis, 310–311, 312, 317
erythropoietin, 318
esophageal atresia, 383
esophageal hiatus, 372
esophag/o, 26, 383
esophagus, 369, 371, 372
esotropia, 225
-esthesia, 195
estr/o, 262
estrogen, 257, 260, 262, 449
ethmoid bone, 118–119
eu-, 261
eupnea, 354
eustachian tubes, 231, 340
euthyroid, 264
eversion, 57
ex-, 57, 67
excision, 57
excretory urogram, 419, 420
exhalation, 338
exo-, 57, 67
exocrine glands, 252, 265
exophthalmia, 219
exotropia, 225
expectoration, 348
expiration, 338
extension, 167–168
external auditory meatus, 229
external ear, 229–230
external genitalia, 427, 449, 451–452
external nare, 339
external os, 451
external sphincters, 375
exto-, 67
extra-, 57, 67
extracapsular cataract extraction
        (ECCE), 226–227
extracellular fluid, 407
extracorporeal, 414
extracorporeal shock wave lithotripsy,
        414–415
extraocular, 57, 219
extravasation, 297
extrinsic ocular muscles, 213–214
eyelids, 213–214
eyes, 210–229
    abbreviations, 228–229
    common diseases of, 226–228

effects of aging on, 226
inner eye, 210–213
outer eye, 213–214
term analysis and definition, 216–225

F
face-lifts, 103
facial bones, 118–119, 129–130
facial renewal, 102
fallopian tubes, 449, 450, 451
farsightedness, 223
fascial, 164
fasciectomy, 164
fasciitis, 164
fasci/o, 164
fasciorrhaphy, 164
fascitis, 164
female reproductive system, 448–467
    See also obstretics
    abbreviations, 467
    common diseases of, 465–467
    common roots, 29
    effects of aging on, 465
    menopause, 454
    menstrual cycle, 453–454
    structures of, 449–453
    term analysis and definition, 455–464
femoral hernia, 384
femor/o, 135
femur, 123
fetal delivery, 469
fetus, 468
fibrinogen, 311, 312, 376
fibr/o, 456
fibroblasts, 89
fibromyalgia, 165
fibula, 123
fibul/o, 135
fibulocalcaneal, 135
fight-or-flight hormones, 257
filtrate, 412
fimbriae, 451
first-degree burns, 104
first heart sound (S$_1$), 284
fissures, 182, 184
flexion, 167–168
flex/o, 163
floating ribs, 121
fluor/o, 34
fluoroscopy, 43
-flux, 379
follicle, 90–91
follicle-stimulating hormone (FSH),
        255, 259
forehead, 118–119
foreskin, 429
-form, 53
formed elements, 310–312
fourth-degree burns, 104

fovea centralis, 210, 211
fractures, 144–145
frenulum, 370
frontal bone, 118–119
frontal lobe, 182
frontal plane, 81–82
fundus, 451
funduscopy, 219, 372–373

G
galacto/o, 456
galactorrhea, 456
gallbladder, 369, 376
gasritis, 6
gastrectomy, 383
gastric, 47
gastric arteries, 287
gastric veins, 287
gastritis, 8
gastr/o, 9, 26, 83, 383
gastrodynia, 36
gastroenteritis, 7, 383
gastroenterologist, 383
gastroesophageal reflux, 383
gastroesophageal sphincter, 372
gastrointestinal, 383
gastrointestinal tract (GIT), 369
gastrojejunostomy, 385
gastrology, 6, 8
gastronomy, 383
gastrorrhagia, 39
gastroscope, 56
-gen, 261
-genesis, 140, 261
-genic, 46
genital herpes, 466
-genous, 54
gestation, 468
gingiva, 370–371
gingivitis, 384
gingiv/o, 384
gingivobuccal, 384
glands
    adrenal, 252, 253, 257
    central endocrine glands, 254–256
    endocrine, 252–260
    exocrine, 252, 265
    hypothalamus, 182, 183, 252, 254–255
    lacrimal, 213–214
    parotoid, 376
    pineal, 258
    pituitary, 252, 254, 255–256, 259
    salivary, 369, 376, 389
    sebaceous, 91, 92, 103
    skin, 91–92
    sweat, 91
    thymus, 320, 322, 323
    thyroid, 252, 253, 256–257, 259
glans penis, 429

glaucoma, 213, 227–228
gli/o, 189
gliomas, 197, 199
globulin, 311
glomerul/o, 414
glomerulonephritis, 414
glomerulosclerosis, 414
glomerulus, 411, 422
glossectomy, 384
gloss/o, 26, 384
glottis, 341
glucagon, 258, 260, 377
gluc/o, 262
glucocorticoids, 257, 260
glucogenesis, 262
gluconeogenesis, 262
glycemia, 36
glyc/o, 34, 262
glycogen/o, 263
glycogenolysis, 263
glycolysis, 262
-gnosis, 54
gonad/o, 263
gonadotropic hormone, 266
gonadotropin, 255, 259
goni/o, 217
gonioscopy, 217
gonorrhea, 466
-grade, 390
-gram, 40
granular leukocytes, 312
granul/o, 314
-graph, 40
-graphy, 41, 196, 353
gravida, 471
-gravida, 473
greater curvature, 372–373
growth hormone (GH), 255, 259
gums, 370–371
gynec/o, 29, 263, 456
gynecologist, 456
gynecology, 456
gynecomastia, 263
gyri, 182, 184

H

hair, 90–91, 103
hair implantation, 102
hard palate, 370
heart, 278
    See also cardiovascular system (CVS)
    effects of aging on, 298
    structure of, 278–281
heart attack, 287, 299
heart sounds, 284
hemangioma, 99
hematemesis, 36, 390
hemat/o, 23, 315
hematocrit, 316

hematologist, 315
hematology, 315
hematoma, 197
hematopoiesis, 46, 312, 318
hematosalpinx, 462
hematuria, 421
hemi-, 64, 67
hemianopia, 223
hemianopsia, 223
hemigastrectomy, 64
hemiplegia, 197
hemispheres, 182
hemithymectomy, 326
hem/o, 23, 315
hemocytoblasts, 312, 316
hemodialysis, 423, 424
hemoglobin (Hgb), 310, 318
hemolysis, 37, 315
hemoptysis, 38, 355
hemorrhage, 39
hemostasis, 44, 318
hemothorax, 355
hepatic ducts, 376
hepatitis, 6, 384
hepat/o, 9, 26, 384
hepatocellular, 384
hepatology, 6, 45
hepatoma, 384
hepatopathy, 9
hermatocele, 431
herniated disc, 121
herni/o, 384
herniorrhaphy, 384
herpes, 466
hiatal hernia, 384, 385
hiat/o, 379
hidr/o, 95
hilum, 407, 408
histamine, 89, 312
histi/o, 18
histiocyte, 45
hist/o, 18
histocyte, 45
home/o, 263
homeostasis, 252, 263, 407
horizontal plane, 81–82
hormones
    adrenocorticotropic, 255, 259, 266
    antidiuretic, 254–255, 259, 264
    endocrine, 252, 254, 259–260, 265
    estrogen, 257, 260, 262, 449
    fight-or-flight, 257
    FSH, 255, 259
    glucagon, 258, 377
    growth, 255, 259
    insulin, 258, 377
    luteinizing, 255, 259
    melatonin, 258
    oxytocin, 254–255, 259, 266, 474

parathormone, 257, 260
    parathyroid, 257
    pituitary, 255–256
    sex, 257, 260, 262, 449
    testosterone, 428
    thyroid, 256
    tropic, 254–255
    TSH, 255, 259
horny layer, 88
human chorionic gonadotropin
        (HCG), 469
human immunodeficiency virus
        (HIV), 327
human papillomaviruses (HPV), 466
humerus, 122
humoral immunity, 320
hydr/o, 191
hydrocele, 431, 432
hydrocephalus, 191, 192
hydrocortisone, 260
hydronephrosis, 417
hydrosalpinx, 462
hydrothorax, 355
hymen, 451
hyoid bone, 118
hyper-, 58, 67, 68
hyperbilirubunemia, 317
hypercalcemia, 262
hypercapnia, 352
hypercglycemia, 267
hypercholesterolemia, 317
hyperchromia, 314
hyperclycemia, 262
hyperemesis, 390
hyperemesis gravidarum, 473
hyperesthesia, 196
hypergonadism, 263
hyperhidrosis, 95
hyperkalemia, 263
hyperkeratosis, 95
hyperkinesia, 168
hyperkinesis, 197
hyperlipidemia, 317
hyperopia, 223
hyperparathyroidism, 264
hyperplasia, 58
hyperpnea, 354
hypertension, 284
hyperthyroidism, 264, 265
hypertrophy, 169
hypertropia, 225
hypo-, 58, 67, 68
hypocapnia, 352
hypochromia, 314
hypodermic, 95
hypoesthesia, 195
hypogastric, 58, 83
hypoglycemia, 263
hypoinsulinism, 263

hyponatremia, 263
hypospadias, 433
hypotension, 284
hypothalamus, 182, 183, 252, 254–255
hypotropia, 225
hypoxia, 348
hysterectomy, 457, 466
hyster/o, 29, 457
hysterosalpingectomy, 460
hysterosalpingogram, 460
hysterotomy, 457

I

-ia, 37
-iasis, 215
-ic, 84
-ician, 45, 46
idiopathic seizures, 199
ile/o, 385
ileocecal valve, 373
ileostomy, 385, 392
ileotomy, 385
ileum, 373
iliac, 83
ili/o, 83, 134
iliofemoral joint, 126, 135
iliosacral joint, 134
ilium, 122
immobilization, 145
-immune, 326
immune system, 319–320
    abbreviations, 328
    common diseases of, 327
    common roots, 24
    effects of aging on, 327
    term analysis and definition, 325–326
immun/o, 260
immunodeficiency, 325
immunoglobulins, 320
immunology, 325
immuno/o, 325
impotence, 432
in-, 58, 63, 422
incisions, 58, 59
incisors, 370–371
incontinence, 422
incus, 230
indigestible, 63
indurated prostate, 435
-ine, 455
infections, 104
inferior, 76, 78, 84
inferior love, 343
inferior vena cava (IVC), 286
infer/o, 82
infra-, 58, 67, 68
infraclavicular, 132
infracostal, 58
infrapatellar, 135

infundibulum, 255, 451
inguinal, 83
inguinal hernia, 385
inguinal nodes, 321, 324
inguin/o, 82
inhalation, 338
inner ear (labyrinth), 231
inner eye, 210–213
insertion, 160
inspiration, 338
insulin, 258, 260, 267, 377
insulin/o, 263
integrative function, 178
integumentary system, 87–114
    abbreviations, 105
    anatomy and physiology of skin,
        88–90
    common injuries and diseases, 104
    common roots, 18
    cosmetic surgery, 101–103
    effects of aging on, 103
    glands, 91–92
    hair, 90–91
    nails, 91, 92
    term analysis and definition, 93–101
inter-, 58
interarticular, 139
interatrial septum, 292
intercellular, 58
internal os, 451
internal sphincters, 375
internal urethral sphincter, 410
interphalangeal joints (IP joints),
        122–123, 133
interstitial cells, 428
interstitial cell-stimulating formone
        (ICSH), 255, 259
interstitial fluid, 321, 326
interstitial pneumonia, 357
interventricular septum, 297
intervertebral, 132
intervertebral discs, 121
intestin/o, 379
intra-, 58, 67
intra-articular fracture, 144–145
intracranial, 58
intraocular, 219
intraocular lens, 226
intraocular pressure (IOP), 213
intrauterine, 461
introitus, 451
involuntary muscles, 159
involution, 471
-ion, 45, 167
-ior, 84
iridectomy, 217
irid/o, 217
iridocyclitis, 217
iris, 210, 211, 212

iritis, 217
ir/o, 217
ischemia, 295
ischium, 122
isch/o, 295
-ism, 93
is/o, 215
-ist, 45
isthmus, 256
-itis, 37
-ium, 93

J

jejunal, 385
jejun/o, 385
jejunum, 373
joint capsule, 126
joint cavity, 126
joints, 126–128, 135–139

K

kal/o, 263
keratin, 88
keratinized cells, 88, 91
keratin/o, 95
keratinocytes, 88, 95, 103
kerat/o, 95, 218
keratoconjunctivitis, 218
keratoconus, 218
keratomycosis, 218
keratoplasty, 218
ketoacidosis, 267
ketones, 267
kidneys, 407–409
    effects of aging on, 422
    urine production in, 411–412
-kinesia, 168, 197
kinesimeter, 164
kinesi/o, 164
kinesiology, 164
-kinesis, 197
knee, 123
Kupffer's cells, 376
kyph/o, 128
kyphosis, 140, 141

L

labial, 386, 457
labia majora, 451–452
labia minora, 451–452
labi/o, 386, 457
labioglossopharyngeal, 386
labyrinthitis, 232
labyrinth/o, 232
lacrimal apparatus, 213–214
lacrimal bones, 118–119
lacrimal ducts, 213–214
lacrimal glands, 213–214
lacrim/o, 218

lactation, 471
lactiferous ducts, 452–453
lactiferous sinuses, 452–453
lact/o, 457
lactogenesis, 457
lapar/o, 386, 457
laparoscope, 56, 386
laparoscopy, 386, 457, 458
laparotomy, 386
large intestine, 369, 375
laryngeal, 346
laryng/o, 25, 346
laryngopharynx, 340
laryngospasm, 346
laryngotracheobronchitis, 352
larynx, 338, 341, 342
laser surgery, 101
laser therapy, 100
lateral, 76, 78
lateral malleoulus, 123
later/o, 53
left atrium, 287
left ventricle, 287
lei/o, 164
leiomyoma, 164
leiomyosarcoma, 164
lens, 211–212
lens accomodation, 212
leukemia, 317, 318–319
leuk/o, 92, 315
leukocytes, 310, 311, 312, 315
leukocytopenia, 317
leukocytosis, 316
leukoderma, 98
leukoplakia, 391
leukopoiesis, 312
levels of organization, 16, 17
Leydog cells, 428
ligaments, 127, 160
ligati/o, 457
lingual tonsils, 325, 340
lingu/o, 26, 386
lipd/o, 314
lip/o, 18, 95
lipoma, 38, 95
liposuction, 95, 102
-lith, 390
lith/o, 386, 414
litholytic agent, 386
lithotripsy, 386, 414
liver, 369, 376–377, 392
liver spots, 103
lobar, 346
lobar pneumonia, 357
lobectomy, 346
lobes, 343
lob/o, 346
-logist, 45
-logy, 45, 462

longitudunal fissure, 182, 184
lord/o, 128
lordosis, 141
lower esophageal sphincter, 372
lower extremity, 123–124, 134–135
lumbar puncture, 194
lumbar vertebrae, 119–120
lumb/o, 131
lumbodynia, 131
lumbosacral joint, 131
lumpectomy, 465
lung cancer, 357
lungs, 338, 342–344
    circulation through, 286–289
    effects of aging on, 356
lunula, 91
luteinizing hormone (LH), 255, 259
lymph, 320, 321
lymphadenitis, 325
lymphaden/o, 24, 325
lymphadenopathy, 321, 325
lymphangi/o, 24, 325
lymphangiogram, 40
lymphangiography, 325
lymphangitis, 326
lymphatic capillaries, 321
lymphatics, 321
lymphatic system, 320–325
    abbreviations, 328
    common diseases of, 327
    common roots, 24
    term analysis and definition, 325–326
lymph ducts, 321, 324
lymphedema, 326
lymph nodes, 321, 322
lymph/o, 24, 326
lymphoblast, 316
lymphocytes, 312, 319–320
lymphoid tissue, 320
lymphoma, 326
lymph vessels, 322, 323
-lysis, 37, 421
lysozyme, 213
-lytic, 379

M
macro-, 65, 68
macrocephalia, 65
macrophages, 89, 312
macula lutea, 210, 211
macular degeneration, 228
magnetic resonance imaging (MRI),
    191, 192
magnet/o, 191
major calyces, 408–409
mal-, 66, 67
-malacia, 37, 140
malaise, 66

male reproductive system, 427–435
    abbreviations, 435
    anatomy of, 427–429
    common diseases of, 434–435
    common roots, 28
    effects of aging on, 434
    term analysis and definition, 429–433
malleus, 230
mammary, 47, 457
mammary glands, 449, 452–453
mamm/o, 29, 457
mammography, 41, 42, 457
mammoplasty, 458
mandible, 118–119
mandibular, 130
mandibul/o, 130
mast cells, 89
mastectomy, 458, 465
masticate, 370
mast/o, 29, 457
mastodynia, 36
mastopexy, 458
maxilla, 118–119
maxillary, 130
maxill/o, 130
meat/o, 415
meatotomy, 415
meatus, 409, 429
medial, 76, 78, 84
medial malleolus, 123
mediastinal cavity, 343
mediastin/o, 347
mediastinoscopy, 347
medical terms
    analysis of, 6
    with no prefix, 6
    with no root, 7
    parts of, 5
    with two roots, 7
medi/o, 82
medulla oblongata, 182, 183
medullary, 415
medull/o, 415
-megaly, 38
melanemesis, 390
melanin, 88, 91, 103
melan/o, 95
melanocytes, 88, 95, 103
melanocyte-stimulating hormone
    (MSH), 255, 259
melanoma, 100, 104
melatonin, 258, 260
memory cells, 320
memory keys, 4
menarche, 453, 461
menibg/o, 192
meninges, 185, 187
meningiomas, 197, 199
meningitis, 192

meningocele, 195
meningoencephalitis, 192
men/o, 454, 459
menometrorrhagia, 459
menopause, 449, 454, 459, 465
menorrhagia, 459
menorrhea, 459
menses, 449, 453
menstrual cycle, 453–454
menstrual period, 453, 454
menstruation, 449, 453
-mesis, 36
meta-, 59
metacarpals, 122–123
metaplasia, 59
metastasis, 59
metatarsals, 123–124
-meter, 41
-metrist, 215
metr/o, 29, 459
metroptosis, 459
metrorrhagia, 459
-metry, 41, 473
micro-, 34, 66, 68
microencephaly, 40
microscope, 66
micturition, 409–410
midbrain, 182
middle ear, 230–231
middle lobe, 343
mineralocorticoids, 257, 260
minor calyx, 408–409
mi/o, 218
miosis, 218
miotic, 218
mitral valve, 279
Mniere's disease, 236
modified radical mastectomy, 465
Mohs' surgery, 100
molars, 370–371
mono-, 64, 67, 314
monocyte, 64
monocytes, 312
monoplegia, 197
mons pubis, 451–452
-mortem, 54
motor function, 178
motor neurons, 178
mtor impulses, 178
muc/o, 347
mucolytic, 347
multi-, 64, 67
multiform, 64
multigravida, 473
multipara, 473
multiple sclerosis (MS), 199
murmur, 284
muscles, 159–162
muscle spasms, 121

muscular, 164
muscular dystrophy (MD), 170
muscular system, 158–176
    abbreviations, 170
    common diseases of, 169–170
    common roots, 20
    effects of aging on, 169
    skeletal attachments, 160
    skeletal muscles, 161–162
    term analysis and definition, 163–169
muscul/o, 20, 164
musculoskeletal, 165
muyel/o, 19
myalgia, 165
myasthenia, 166
myc/o, 96
mydriasis, 218
mydriatic, 218
myein-, 215
myelinated axons, 180
myelin/o, 189
myelin sheath, 180, 198
myel/o, 21, 128–129, 193, 315
myelogenous, 315
myelogram, 193
myelography, 41, 196
myeloid, 315
myeloma, 128
myelomeningocele, 195
myeloradiculitis, 193
myeloschisis, 193
my/o, 20, 165
myocardial, 293
myocardial infarction (MI), 287, 299
myocardial ischemia, 295
myocardium, 280–281
myoclonus, 166
myoma, 38
myometrium, 459
myoneural, 193
myopathy, 165
myopia, 223
myositis, 165
myos/o, 165
myotome, 44
myotonia, 166
myring/o, 233
myringotomy, 233
myri/o, 218

N

nails, 91, 92
nasal bone, 118–119
nasal cavity, 338, 339
nasal conchae, 118–119
nasal septum, 339
nas/o, 25, 347
nasogastric tube, 384
nasolacrimal, 218, 347

nasopharyngeal, 347
nasopharynx, 340
nat/o, 53, 472
natr/o, 263
nearsightedness, 223
necr/o, 96
necrotic tissue, 96
negative prefixes, 63
nehropexy, 44
neo-, 66
neoplasm, 7, 66
nephr/o, 415
nephroblastoma, 418
nephrolithiasis, 415
nephrolithotomy, 415
nephrons, 411–412
nephropathy, 415
nephropexy, 417
nephroptosis, 38, 417
nephrosis, 38
nephrotomography, 417
nerve cells, 178, 180–181
nerves, 178, 179, 187, 188
nervous system, 177–208
    abbreviations, 200
    central nervous system (CNS),
        182–187
    common diseases of, 199
    common roots, 21
    divisions of, 178, 179
    effects of aging on, 198
    functions of, 178
    nerve cells, 180–181
    peripheral nervous system, 187–188
    synapses, 181–182
    term analysis and definition, 189–198
neuralgia, 193
neur/o, 21, 193
neuroglia, 180, 198
neurohormones, 254–255
neurohypophysis, 266
neurologist, 45, 193
neurology, 193
neurolysis, 193
neurons, 178, 180–181
neuropathy, 40
neurotransmitters, 181
neutrophils, 312
nipple, 452–453
noct/o, 413
nocturia, 422
non-small cell lung cancer, 357
noradrenaline, 257, 260
norepinephrine, 257, 260
norm/o, 314
normochromia, 314
nose, 338, 339
nuclear medicine scan, 41
nucleus pulposus, 121

nulli-, 455
nulligravida, 473
nullipara, 473
numbers, prefixes referring to, 64–65

O

oblique muscle, 213–214
O blood type, 313
obstetical conditions, 474–475
obstetrics, 468–475
   abbreviations, 475
   parturition, 469–471
   pregnancy, 468–469
   term analysis and definition, 471–474
occipital lobe, 182
occiptial bone, 118–119
ocul/o, 21, 219
odont/o, 387
-oid, 46
-ole, 46
olecranal, 133
olecran/o, 133
olecranon process, 122
olfactory neurons, 339
oligo-, 345
oligomenorrhea, 459
oligopnea, 354
oligospermia, 430
oliguria, 422
-oma, 38, 98, 197
onych/o, 18, 96
onychomycosis, 96
o/o, 460
oocyte, 460
oophor/o, 29, 460
oophororrhagia, 460
oophorectomy, 44
open fracture, 144–145
open reduction, 145
open reduction internal fixation
   (ORIF), 145
ophthalm/o, 21
ophthalmologist, 219
ophthalmoscopy, 219
-opia, 223
-opsia, 223
-opsy, 42, 462
opthalm/o, 219
optic, 220
optic disc, 211
optician, 220
opt/o, 220
optometrist, 220
-or, 46
oral cavity, 369, 370–371, 387
orbital cavity, 213–214
orchid/o, 28, 430
orchidopexy, 430
orchidoplasty, 44

orchi/o, 430
orchitis, 430
orex/i, 387
organ donor, 46
organism, 17
organization, levels of, 16, 17
organ of Corti, 231
organs, 16, 17
   See also specific organs
organ systems, 16–17
origin, 160
or/o, 26, 387
oropharyngeal, 348
oropharynx, 340
ortho-, 142
orthodontist, 387
orthopedics, 142
orthopnea, 354
-ory, 215
osetoclast, 140
-osis, 38, 140
osse/o, 129
ossicul/o, 233
ossiculoplasty, 233
ossification, 116
osteitis, 129
oste/o, 19, 129
osteoarthritis (OA), 7, 136, 144
osteoblasts, 116, 140
osteochondritis, 129
osteoclasis, 140
osteoclasts, 116
osteocytes, 116, 129
osteogenesis, 116, 140
osteoid, 46
osteoma, 129
osteomalacia, 140
osteomyelitis, 128
osteoporosis, 141, 144
osteosarcoma, 142
osteotome, 129
osteotomy, 129
ostomy, 392
otalgia, 35, 233
otitis media, 231, 233
ot/o, 21, 233
otorhinolaryngology, 350
otorrhea, 39, 233
otosclerosis, 233
otoscope, 234, 235
-ous, 46
outer eye, 213–214
oval window, 231
ovarian cyst, 460
ovaries, 449, 449–450
ovari/o, 29, 460
ov/o, 460
ovoid, 460
ovulation, 449, 454

ovulatory period, 453
ovum, 449
oximeter, 348
oxl/i, 347
ox/o, 347
oxy-, 266, 455
oxygentated blood, 278, 287
oxytocin, 254–255, 259, 266, 474

P

pacemaker, 283
pachy-, 198
pachymeningitis, 198
palate, 370
palatine tonsils, 325, 340
palpebral, 220
palpebr/o, 220
pan-, 66
pancarditis, 293
pancreas, 252, 253, 258, 260, 369, 377
pancreatic duct, 377
pancreatic juice, 377
pancreatitis, 388
pancreat/o, 264, 388
pancreatogenic, 264
pancytopenia, 317
panhypopituitarism, 264
panhysterectomy, 66
pansinusitis, 350
papilla, 90–91
papillae, 370
papilledema, 220
papill/o, 92
papilloma, 100
para-, 59, 189
para, 471
-para, 473
parametrium, 459
paranasal, 59
paranasal sinuses, 339
paraplegia, 198
parathormone (PTH), 257, 260
parathyroid hormone (PTH), 257, 260
parathyroid/o, 21, 264
parathyroids, 252, 253, 257, 260
paresthesia, 196
parietal bones, 118–119
parictal layer, 281
parietal lobe, 182
parietal peritoneum, 378
Parkinson's disease (PD), 199
paronychia, 96–97
parotoid gland, 376
paroxysmal dyspnea, 342
-partum, 474
parturition, 469–471
patella, 123
patell/a, 135
patellapexy, 135

patell/o, 135
path/o, 18
pathological fracture, 144–145
pathologic conditions, suffixes used to
    indicate, 35–40
-pathy, 38
-pause, 455
pectoral girdle, 118, 122, 132–133, 348
pector/o, 348
ped/o, 128
pelv/i, 134
pelvic, 84
pelvic cavity, 74–75
pelvic girdle, 118, 122, 134
pelvic inflammatory disease (PID), 451
pelvic ultrasonography, 474
pelvimetry, 41, 473
pelvi/o, 19
pelv/o, 19, 134
-penia, 38, 317
penis, 429
-pepsia, 391
peptic ulcers, 392–393
per-, 59
percutaneous, 59
percutaneous transluminal coronary
    angioplasty (PTCA), 290–291
peri-, 59, 67
pericardial fluid, 281
pericarditis, 293
pericardium, 278, 281, 293
perilymph, 231
perimetrium, 459
perinanal, 380
perine/o, 460
perineorrhaphy, 460
perineum, 451–452
perineuritis, 59
periodontist, 387, 453
periosteum, 129
peripheral, 76, 79
peripheral endocrine glands, 252–253,
    256–260
peripheral nervous system, 178, 179,
    187–188
peristaltic waves, 372
peritoneal cavity, 378
peritoneal dialysis, 423, 425
peritone/o, 388
peritoneum, 378–379
peritonitis, 388
periungual, 98
-pexy, 44
Peyer's patches, 320, 322
phac/o, 220
phacoemulsification, 226
phacomalacia, 220
-phagia, 390
phagocytes, 320

phagocytosis, 180, 312, 321
phak/o, 220
phalanges, 122–124
phalang/o, 133
phall/o, 28
pharmacist, 45
pharmac/o, 34
pharyngeal, 47, 388
pharyngeal tonsils, 325
pharyng/o, 25, 26, 348, 388
pharyngoesophageal sphincter, 372
pharyngoglossal, 348
pharynx, 338, 340, 369, 371
-phasia, 197
phleb/o, 23, 295
phlebostenosis, 40
phlebothrombosis, 295
-phobia, 38
-phonia, 353
-phoresis, 317
phosolipds, 311
phot/o, 221
photocoagulation, 221
photophobia, 221
phrenic, 84, 348
phren/o, 25, 82, 348
phrenotomy, 348
physician, 45
physi/o, 34
physiology, 16, 45
-physis, 141, 266
pia mater, 185, 187
pilmonary arteries, 286
pil/o, 18, 97
pilosebaceous, 97
pineal gland, 252, 253, 258, 260
pituitar/o, 21, 264
pituitary gland, 252, 254, 255–256
placental delivery, 469
placenta previa, 474
-plakia, 391
planes of the body, 81–82
plantar, 76, 77, 79
plantar flexion, 167–168
-plasia, 46
-plasm, 54
plasma, 310, 311
plasma cells, 89
-plastic, 314
plastic surgery, 101–103
-plasty, 44
platelets, 310, 311, 312
-plegia, 54, 197
pleur/a, 348
pleural cavity, 343
pleuralgia, 348
pleur/o, 348
plicae circulares, 373, 374
plurals, 10–13

-pnea, 354
pneumatic, 348
pneumat/o, 348
pneum/o, 25, 349
pneumoconiosis, 349
pneumonia, 37, 349, 357
pneumon/o, 25, 349
pneumopleuritis, 349
pneumothorax, 355
-poiesis, 46, 317
-poietin, 318
poikil/o, 314
poikilocytosis, 316
polio-, 189
poliomyelitis, 193
poly-, 64, 67, 422
polyadenoma, 64
polycystic kidneys, 422
polydipsia, 265
polymorphonuclear leukocytes, 312
polymyositis, 165
polyneuritis, 193
polyphagia, 390
polythelia, 461
polyuria, 422
pons, 182
-porosis, 128, 141
post-, 60, 67
posterior, 76, 78, 84
posterior lobes, 255
posterior pituitary, 255, 259
poster/o, 82
postmortem, 60
postnatal period, 472
postpartum, 474
postpartum period, 471
postprandial, 391
-potence, 432
practioner, 45
practiyion/o, 34
-prandial, 391
pre-, 60, 67
pre-eclampsia, 475
prefixes, 5, 6, 53
    miscellaneous, 65–66
    negative, 63
    with opposite meaning, 67–68
    referring to direction and position,
        54–62
    referring to numbers, 64–65
    with same meaning, 67
pregnancy, 468–469
prehypertension, 284
prenatal, 60, 472
prepuce, 429
presby-, 215
presbycusis, 235
presbyopia, 223
primary bronchi, 342

primary lung cancer, 357
primi-, 455
primigravida, 471, 473
primipara, 474
pro-, 60, 67
proct/o, 388
proctoclysis, 388
proctologist, 388
prodrome, 60
progesterone, 449
prognosis, 60
prolactin (PRL), 255, 259
pronati/o, 163
pronation, 167–168
prone, 76, 79
pronunciation guide, 4–5
prostate cancer, 435
prostatectomy, 430, 435
prostate gland, 428, 429, 434–435
prostatic-specific antigen (PSA), 435
prostatitis, 430
prostat/o, 28, 430
prosthetic device, 137–138
protein/o, 413
proteinuria, 422
prothrombin, 312, 376
proximal, 76, 78, 84
proxim/o, 82
pseudo-, 215
pseudocyesis, 473
pseudophakia, 220
-ptosis, 38
-ptysis, 38, 355
pubis, 122
pulmonary angiography, 353
pulmonary capillaries, 343
pulmonary edema, 349
pulmonary semilunar valve, 279,
     280, 286
pulmonary trunk, 286
pulmonary veins, 287
pulmon/o, 25
pulp, 370–371
pulse, 284
pulse points, 285
punctae, 213–214
pupil, 210, 211
pupillary, 221
pupill/o, 221
Purkinje fibers, 282, 283
purulent otitis media, 233
pyelogram, 418
pyelonephritis, 418
pyloric sphincter, 372–373
pyloric stenosis, 388
pylor/o, 388
pyloromyotomy, 388
pylorospasm, 388
py/o, 97

pyoderma, 98
pyogenic, 97
pyosalpinx, 462
pyothorax, 355
pyrexia, 199
pyuria, 422

Q
quadri-, 64
quadrilateral, 64

R
radiation therapy, 318, 465
radical hysterectomy, 466
radicul/o, 193
radi/o, 133, 260
radiocarpal joint, 126, 133
radioimmunoassay (RIA), 265
radiotherapy, 100
radius, 122
ras/o, 97
re-, 379
rect/o, 26, 389
rectocele, 36, 462
rectostenosis, 389
rectouterine, 461
rectouterine pouch, 451
rectum, 375, 450
rectus muscle, 213–214
red blood cells (RBCs), 310, 311, 318
reduction, 145
refraction, 211–212
refraction errors, 227
remodeling, 116
renal, 47
renal arteries, 287
renal capsule, 407
renal columns, 408–409
renal dialysis, 423
renal failure, 423
renal fascia, 407
renal hypoplasia, 418
renal medulla, 408–409
renal papilla, 408–409
renal pelvis, 408–409
renal pyramids, 408–409
renal tubules, 412
renal veins, 287
ren/o, 27, 418
reproductive system
     female, 29, 448–467
     male, 28, 427–435
reproductive tract, 427
respiration, 338
respiratory system, 337–367
     abbreviations, 358
     bronchi and lungs, 342–344
     common diseases of, 356–357
     common roots, 25

effects of aging on, 356
     nose, nasal cavities, and paranasal
          sinuses, 339
     pharynx larynx, and trachea, 340–343
     structures of, 338
     term analysis and definition, 345–355
reticul/o, 315
reticulocyte, 310–311, 315
reticulocyte count, 311
retina, 210, 211
retinal detachment, 221, 222
retin/o, 222
retinopathy, 222
retinopexy, 222
retinoschisis, 222
retro-, 60, 379, 464
retroflexion, 464
retrograde, 390
retrograde urogram, 419
retroperitoneal, 388, 407
retroperitoneal position, 378
retroversion, 60, 464
rhabd/o, 165
rhabdomyolysis, 165
rhabdomyoma, 165
rhabdomyosarcoma, 165
Rh antigen, 313
rheumatoid arthritis (RA), 136–137
rhinitis, 350
rhin/o, 25, 350
rhinoplasty, 350
rhinorrhea, 350
Rh negative, 313
Rh positive, 313
rhythm/o, 295
rhytidectomy, 97, 103
rhytid/o, 97
right atrium, 286
right ventricle, 286
RLQ, 85
rods, 210, 211
root canal, 370–371
roots, 5, 6
     anatomical, 18–29
     combining forms, 9
-rrhage/rrhagia, 39
-rrhaphy, 44
-rrhea, 39
-rrhexis, 39
rugae, 372–373
RUQ, 85

S
saccule, 231
sacr/o, 131
sacrococcygeal joint, 131
sacroiliac joint, 122
sacrum, 119–120
sacs, 231

sagittal plane, 81–82
salivary glands, 369, 376, 389
salping/o, 29, 234, 460
salpingo-oophorectomy, 460
salpingopexy, 460
salpingoscope, 234
-salpinx, 462
-sarcoma, 141
sarcomas, 104
sarcopenia, 169
scapulae, 122
scapul/o, 133
-schisis, 189
sclera, 210, 211, 212
sclerectomy, 222
scler/o, 92, 222, 295
scleroderma, 98
-sclerosis, 39
sclerotherapy, 295
scoli/o, 128
scoliosis, 141
-scope, 42
-scopy, 43
scrotum, 428, 429
sebaceous glands, 91, 92, 103
seb/o, 97
seborrhea, 97
sebum, 91
secondary bronchi, 342
secondary lung cancer, 357
second-degree burns, 104
second heart sound (S₂), 284
secretory period, 453, 454
section, 45
sect/o, 34
secundi-, 455
secundigravida, 473
secundipara, 474
seizure disorders, 190–191, 199
semen, 429
semi-, 64, 67
semicircular canals, 231
semicircular ducts, 231
semicomatose, 64
semilunar valves, 279
seminal vesicles, 428, 429
seminiferous tubules, 428
sensorineural deafness, 236
sensory function, 178
sensory impulses, 178
sensory neurons, 178
sept/o, 53
septum, 278–279
serum, 311
sex hormones, 257, 260, 262, 449
sexually transmitted diseases (STDs),
    466–467
shin, 123
shock, 104

sialadenitis, 389
sialaden/o, 389
sial/o, 389
sialolith, 390
sigmoid colon, 375
sigmoid/o, 389
sigmoidoscopy, 389
simple mastectomy, 465
sinoatrial node (SA node), 282, 283
sinus/o, 350
sinus, 350
sinusotomy, 350
-sis, 93
skeletal muscles, 159–162
skeletal system, 115–157
    abbreviations, 146
    anatomy and physiology of bone, 116
    appendicular skeleton, 118, 122–126,
        132–135
    axial skeleton, 117–121, 125, 129–132
    bursae, 127
    common diseases of, 144–145
    common roots, 19
    description of the skeleton, 117–126
    effects of aging on, 144
    joints, 126–128
    ligaments, 127
    term analysis and definition, 128–142
skin, 88–90
    See also integumentary system
skin biopsy, 93
skin cancer, 98–99, 100, 104
skull, 118, 118–119
skull bones, 129–130
slipped disc, 121
small cell lung cancer, 357
small intestine, 369, 373–374
somatotropic hormone, 266
somatotropin, 259
somatropin, 255
son/o, 53
-spadias, 433
-spasm, 40
sperm, 427
spermatic cord, 431
spermat/o, 413, 430
spermatocele, 431
spermatocidal, 431
spermatogenesis, 428
sperm/o, 430
sphenoid bone, 118–119
sphincter of Oddi, 377
sphygmomanometer, 284
-sphyxia, 355
spinal, 84
spinal canal, 74–75
spinal cavity, 74–75
spinal cord, 178, 179, 185, 186
spinal nerves, 187, 188
spinal tap, 194

spin/o, 19, 194
spir/o, 350
spirometer, 350
spirometry, 350, 351
spleen, 320, 322, 323
splen/o, 24, 326
splenomegaly, 326
splenorrhagia, 326
splenorrhaphy, 326
splenorrhexis, 39
spondylitis, 37, 132
spondyl/o, 19, 132
spondylopathy, 132
squamous cell carcinoma, 98–99, 104
stapedectomy, 235
staped/o, 235
stapes, 230–231
-stasis, 44, 318
steat/o, 18, 97, 389
steatoma, 97
steatorrhea, 389
stem cells, 312
stem cell transplantation, 319
-stenosis, 40
stent, 290
stern/o, 131
sternoclavicular joint, 132
sternotomy, 131
sternum, 121
steth/o, 350
stethoscope, 350
-stitial, 326
stomach, 369, 372–373
stomatitis, 37, 389
stomat/o, 26, 389
-stomy, 44
strain, 170
stratum corneum, 88
stress incontinence, 423
stroke, 299
sub-, 60, 67, 68
subarachnoid space, 185, 187
subcostal, 131
subcut, 105
subcutaneous, 60, 93
subcutaneous layer, 88, 89
subcutaneous tissue, 90
subdural, 190
subdural space, 185, 187
sublingual, 60, 386
sublingual gland, 376
submandibular gland, 376
submandibular nodes, 321, 324
subq, 105
subscapular, 133
sudoriferous glands, 91
suffixes, 5, 6, 34
    adjectival, 46–47
    general, 45–46

to indicate diagnostic procedures, 40–43
to indicate pathologic conditions, 35–40
to indicate surgical procedures, 43–44
sulci, 182, 184
superficial, 76, 79
superio, 76, 78
superior, 84
superior lobe, 343
superior vena cava (SVC), 286
super/o, 83
supinati/o, 163
supination, 167–168
supine, 76, 79
supra-, 61, 67, 68
suprapatellar, 135
suprarenal, 61
surgical procedures, suffixes used to indicate, 43–44
suspensory ligaments, 211–212
swallowing, 371
sweat glands, 91
sym-, 66
symblepharon, 216
symmetry, 66
symphysis pubis, 122
syn-, 66, 68
synapses, 181–182
synarthrotic, 66
synovial fluid, 126
synovial joint, 127
synovial membrane, 126
syphillis, 467
systole, 284
systolic pressure, 284

T

tachy-, 66, 68
-tachy, 298
tachycardia, 66, 298
tachypnea, 354
tarsals, 123–124
-taxia, 198
teeth, 370–371
temporal bones, 118–119
temporal lobe, 182
tempor/o, 128
temporomandibular joint (TMJ), 118–119, 130
tendinitis, 165
tendin/o, 20, 165
tendinous, 165
tend/o, 20
tendons, 160
ten/o, 165
tenodesis, 166
tenosynovi/o, 166
tenosynovitis, 166

tenotomy, 44, 166
tens/o, 163
term analysis, 4
tertiary bronchi, 342
testerone, 255, 260
testes, 427, 428
testicles, 427
testicular, 431
testicul/o, 28, 431
test/o, 28
testosterone, 428
tetra-, 66, 189
tetraplegia, 66, 198
thalam/o, 194
thalamocortical, 194
thalamus, 182, 183
thelitis, 461
thel/o, 461
-therapy, 100
-thermy, 169
thighbone, 123
third-degree burns, 104
thoracic, 84
thoracic cage, 118, 121, 130–131
thoracic cavity, 74–75, 343
thoracic vertebrae, 119–120
thorac/o, 25, 132, 351
thoracocentesis, 43, 351
thoracodynia, 351
thoracolumbar, 132
thoracoplasty, 351
thoracotomy, 351
-thorax, 355
thromb/o, 295, 315
thrombocytes, 310, 312, 315
thrombocytopenia, 317
thrombolysis, 315
thrombophlebitis, 295
thrombopoiesis, 312
thrombosis, 315
thrombus, 295
thym/o, 326
thymosin, 323
thymus gland, 320, 322, 323
thyr/o, 264
thyroid gland, 252, 253, 256–257, 259
thyroiditis, 264
thyroid/o, 21, 264
thyroid-stimulating hormone (TSH), 255, 259
thyrotomy, 264
thyrotropin, 255, 259
thyroxine, 255, 257, 259
tibia, 123
tibi/o, 135
tibiofibular joint, 135
tinnitus, 236
tissue, 16, 17
    connective, 89
    epithelium, 88

necrotic, 96
subcutaneous, 90
T lymphocytes (T cells), 319–320
-tocia, 474
-tocin, 474
-tome, 44
tom/o, 189
-tomy, 44
tongue, 370
tonic, 166
ton/o, 166, 222
tonometry, 222
tonsillar, 352
tonsillectomy, 44, 352
tonsillitis, 352
tonsill/o, 24, 352
tonsillotome, 352
tonsils, 320, 322, 325, 340
top/o, 472
total abdominal hysterectomy, 466
toxins, 104
trabecula, 213
trabecul/o, 222
trabeculoplasty, 222
trachea, 338, 341–342
trache/o, 25, 352
tracheoesophageal, 352
tracheostomy, 44, 352, 353
tracheotomy, 352, 353
trans-, 61, 413
transaortic, 291
transduction, 229
transection, 61
transurethral, 419
transurethral resection of the prostate (TURP), 434
transverse colon, 375
transverse plane, 81–82
-tresia, 379
tri-, 65
tricuspid, 65
tricuspid valve, 278–279, 280, 286
triglyceride, 311
trigone, 409
trigonitis, 418
trigon/o, 418
triiodothyronine, 255, 256, 259
-tripsy, 379
-trophy, 169
-tropia, 224
-tropic, 266
tropic hormones, 254–255
-tropion, 225
tubal ligation, 457, 458
tub/o, 454
tummy tucks, 102–103
turbinates, 118–119
tympanic membrane, 229, 234

tympan/o, 235
tympanoplasty, 235
Type 1 diabetes, 267
Type 2 diabetes, 267

U

ulcers, 392–393
-ule, 46
ulna, 122
ulnar, 133
uln/o, 133
ultra-, 61, 474
ultrasonography, 61–62
-um, 93
umbilical cord, 468
umbilical hernia, 385
umbilic/o, 379
undifferentiated cells, 312
ungu/o, 18, 98
uni-, 64, 67
unilateral, 64
upper esophageal, 372
upper extremity, 122–123, 133
urea, 407
uremia, 419
ure/o, 264
ureter, 408
ureterectasis, 418
ureter/o, 27, 418
ureteroileostomy, 418
ureterolith, 418
ureteropathy, 38
ureterostenosis, 418
ureters, 407, 409
uretha, 409–410
urethra, 407, 408, 450
urethral orifice, 450
urethr/o, 27, 419
urethroplasty, 419
urethrorrhagia, 419
uretral, 418
urge incontinence, 423
-uria, 421
uric acid, 407
urinalysis, 421
urinary, 419
urinary bladder, 407, 408, 409–410, 450
urinary incontinence, 422, 423
urinary retention, 424
urinary system, 407–426
    abbreviations, 425–426
    common diseases of, 423–425
    common roots, 27
    effects of aging on, 422

kidneys, 407–409
    term analysis and definition, 413–422
    ureters, urinary bladder, and urethra,
        409–410
    urine production, 411–412
urination, 409–410
urine, 407
urine production, 411–412
urin/o, 419, 421
ur/o, 419
urogram, 419
urologist, 420
-us, 189
uterine cancer, 465–466
uterine fibroid, 456
uterine inertia, 475
uterine tubes, 449
uter/o, 29, 461
uterovesical, 461
uterus, 449, 450, 451
utricle, 231
UV, 105
uvea, 210, 211, 212
uveitis, 223
uve/o, 223
uvula, 370

V

vagina, 449, 450, 451
vaginitis, 461
vagin/o, 29, 461
vaginomycosis, 461
valvul/o, 295
valvuloplasty, 295
varic/o, 296
varicocele, 432
varicose veins, 296
vascular system, 321
vascul/o, 23, 296
vas deferens, 428
vasectomy, 431
vas/o, 28, 297, 431
vasoconstriction, 297
vasodilation, 297
vasopressin, 255, 259
veins, 278, 284, 285, 286
ven/o, 23, 297
venous, 47, 297
ventral, 76, 78, 84
ventral cavity, 74–75
ventricles, 278–279
ventricul/o, 194, 297
ventriculoperitoneal shunt, 388

ventriculostomy, 194
ventr/o, 83
venules, 46, 284, 297
versi/o, 454
-version, 54
vertebrae, 119–121, 131–132
vertebral column, 118, 119–121
vertebr/o, 19, 132
vertigo, 232, 236
vesic/o, 420
vesicosigmoidostomy, 420
vesicoureteral reflux, 420
vestibule, 231
villi, 373, 374
visceral, 84
visceral layer, 281
visceral muscle, 159
visceral peritoneum, 378
viscer/o, 18, 389
visceromegaly, 38
visceroptosis, 389
vitrectomy, 223
vitre/o, 223
vitreous humor, 213, 223
vocal cords, 341
voiding disorders, 423–435
voluntary muscles, 159
vomer, 118–119
vowels, combining, 7–9
vulva, 451–452
vulvectomy, 461
vulv/o, 29, 461
vulvorectal, 461

W

white blood cells (WBCs), 310, 311,
    312, 318
windpipe, 341–342
wrinkles, 103

X

xiph/o, 131
xiphoid, 131

Y

-y, 40

Z

zer/o, 92
zeroderma, 98
zygomatic bone, 118–119
zygote, 451